The Nation's Doctor

The role of the Chief Medical Officer 1855–1998

Sally Sheard
Senior Lecturer in History of Medicine
Department of Public Health and School of History
University of Liverpool

and

Sir Liam Donaldson
Chief Medical Officer
Department of Health

Foreword by

Sir Denis Pereira Gray
Chairman
The Nuffield Trust

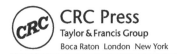

CRC Press
Taylor & Francis Group
Boca Raton London New York

CRC Press is an imprint of the
Taylor & Francis Group, an **informa** business

First published 2006 by Radcliffe Publishing

Published 2018 by CRC Press
Taylor & Francis Group
6000 Broken Sound Parkway NW, Suite 300
Boca Raton, FL 33487-2742

ISBN-13: 978-1-84619-001-8 (pbk)

Visit the Taylor & Francis Web site at
http://www.taylorandfrancis.com

and the CRC Press Web site at
http://www.crcpress.com

British Library Cataloguing in Publication Data

A catalogue record for this book is available from the British Library.

Typeset by Anne Joshua & Associates, Oxford

Contents

Foreword ix

Preface xi

    Structure of the book xii

    Healthy government and the governance of health xiv

    A note on sources xvii

About the authors xix

Acknowledgements xx

1 **A doctor at the heart of government** 1

    Staffing the new state medicine 7

    The insecure system 9

    A Ministry of Health? 10

    The formation of the Local Government Board 11

    Conclusion 14

2 **The line of succession** 17

    After John Simon: restructuring the post of Medical Officer 19

    A bigger pool: the appointment of 'external' CMOs 22

    1935: MacNalty vs. Jameson 28

    Jameson: 'the nation's doctor' 30

    Charles and Godber: succession crises 32

    Professionalisation of civil service appointments 34

    Conclusion 37

3 **Navigating the corridors of power** 39

    Newman and the status of the CMO 41

    Managing the tripartite relationship 43

    The smoking and lung cancer issue 44

    Size matters: re-establishing a strong CMO 56

    Whitehall in the post-Fulton period 59

    Selection of Permanent Secretaries 61

    Accountability 62

    Conclusion 63

4 **Making advice count** 67

    Valuing expertise in Whitehall 67

    The market value of the CMO 72

    Managing the National Health Service 74

    The Department of Health and Social Security 75

    The impact of Whitehall reviews 78

    A new Department of Health 79

    Reviews of senior medical civil servants 80

    The 1994 Banks Review 83

    The National Health Service 86

The importance of location 87
Conclusion 89

5 A doctor's doctor? 91
The emergence of 'state medicine' 92
Medical Royal Colleges 95
The British Medical Association and the National Health Service 96
Engaging with the doctors' trade union 99
Post-NHS relationships 103
One of Us? Castle, Yellowlees and the pay beds dispute 107
Conclusion 112

6 Engaging external expertise 117
The Ministry of Health and the Medical Research Council 118
External influences on policy 120
The Nuffield Trust and the King's Fund 121
AIDS: a plague for the twentieth century 123
The BSE crisis 134
Conclusion 145

7 The nation's doctor 147
John Simon and freedom of speech 148
The tradition of the Chief Medical Officer's Annual Reports 149
On the state of the public health 154
Guidance for the medical profession 155
Jameson: the fireside CMO 156
Don't die of ignorance 161
Conclusion 163

8 Reflections: a job is what you make it 165
The essential qualities 165
Seizing the day 166
Redefining the health agenda 167
A National Medical Service? 169
The wider arena 172
Crisis management 173
Life after CMO? 175

Appendix 1: CMO profiles 177

Appendix 2: Secretaries of State for Health and Ministers of Health
in the Ministry of Health, the Department of Health and Social
Security and the Department of Health 211

Appendix 3: Permanent Secretaries in the Ministry of Health, the
Department of Health and Social Security and the Department of
Health 213

Appendix 4: CMO chronology and allied historical events 215

Index 229

List of figures

Figure A   CMO lifespan and time in office.

Figure 1.1   The arrival of cholera in America in the nineteenth century.

Figure 1.2   'A court for King Cholera.'

Figure 3.1   'Couldn't we tell 'em that we've discovered *clean* tobacco . . .?'

Figure 3.2   Ministry of Health poster warning which linked the cost of smoking with lung cancer.

Figure 3.3   The Medical Research Council's 50th anniversary in 1963.

Figure 3.4   Godber's attempt to introduce fluoridation to Britain's water supplies.

Figure 3.5   Sir Kingsley Wood, Minister of Health, receives artificial sun-ray treatment in 1936.

Figure 4.1   The Ministry of Health, c. 1930.

Figure 4.2   Alexander Fleming House, designed by the Hungarian-born architect Ernö Goldfinger for the Department of Health and Social Security in 1968.

Figure 5.1   Members of the British Medical Association, represented as gladiators, conceding the introduction of the National Health Service to Aneurin Bevan, represented as Nero.

Figure 5.2   'The Express Panel Doctor.' The National Insurance Act of 1911 introduced limited free medical services, but there were concerns about their quality.

Figure 5.3   'Chief Mourner.' Barbara Castle's role in the 1974 NHS crisis.

Figure 5.4   Henry Yellowlees with the Secretaries of State for Health he served.

Figure 6.1   Department of Health and Social Security AIDS leaflet, 1987.

Figure 6.2   An AIDS press conference.

Figure 6.3   'Patience my son, I'm still trying to remember when I last had casual sex!'.

Figure 6.4   'The Classic Civil Servant': Kenneth Calman poking fun at himself.

Figure 7.1   Jameson giving a speech at the opening of new kitchens at the London Hospital in Whitechapel, London, after they were damaged during the Blitz. 8th August 1945.

Figure 8.1   World Health Assembly in New Delhi, 1961.

Figure A1   John Simon.

Figure A2   Edward Cator Seaton.

Figure A3   George Buchanan.

Figure A4   Richard Thorne Thorne.

Figure A5   William Henry Power.

Figure A6   Arthur Newsholme.

Figure A7   George Newman.

Figure A8   Arthur MacNalty.

Figure A9   Wilson Jameson.

Figure A10   John Charles.

Figure A11   George Godber.
Figure A12   Henry Yellowlees.
Figure A13   Donald Acheson.
Figure A14   Kenneth Calman.

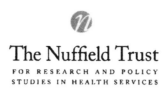

The Nuffield Trust

FOR RESEARCH AND POLICY
STUDIES IN HEALTH SERVICES

The Nuffield Trust is one of the leading independent health policy charitable trusts in the UK. It was established as the Nuffield Provincial Hospitals Trust in 1940 by Viscount Nuffield (William Morris), the founder of Morris Motors. In 1998 the Trustees agreed that the official name of the trust should more fully reflect the Trust's purposes and, in consultation with the Charity Commission, adopted the name The Nuffield Trust for Research and Policy Studies in Health Services, retaining 'The Nuffield Trust' as its working name.

The Nuffield Trust's mission is to promote independent analysis and informed debate on UK healthcare policy. The Nuffield Trust's purpose is to communicate evidence and encourage an exchange around developed or developing knowledge in order to illuminate recognised and emerging issues.

It achieves this through its principal activities:

- bringing together a wide national and international network of people involved in UK healthcare through a series of meetings, workshops and seminars
- commissioning research through its publications and grants programme to inform policy debate
- encouraging inter-disciplinary exchange between clinicians, legislators, academics, healthcare professionals and management, policy makers, industrialists and consumer groups
- supporting evidence-based health policy and practice
- sharing its knowledge in the home countries and internationally through partnerships and alliances.

To find out more, please refer to our website or contact:

The Nuffield Trust
59 New Cavendish St
London
W1G 7LP
Website: www.nuffieldtrust.org.uk
Email: mail@nuffieldtrust.org.uk
Tel: +44 (0)20 7631 8458
Fax: +44 (0)20 7631 8451

Charity number: 209201

List of Trustees

Foreword

The story of the office of the Chief Medical Officer (CMO) has never been told before.

Covering a period of about 150 years, this book traces the work of consecutive CMOs in England, illuminating both the development of the office and the interpretation of the role by 14 different doctors.

The complexities of the role are described in relation to the progressive rise of state medicine in the UK. In addition to the interplay of politics, Sheard and Donaldson describe two triangles. The first is the institutional relationships between the Government, the public and the medical profession, where they see the CMO as a focal point. Simultaneously, the CMO is constantly involved in an inter-personal triangle of relationships with the leading Health Minister of the day and the Permanent Secretary of the Health Department. They see the relative successes and failures of each office holder in terms of how far they mastered the Whitehall machine and expressed their personality within these two triangles.

An advantage of this scholarly, historical, perspective is the way the continuity of key aspects of the CMO's role have been emphasised. Professional independence, the right of access to ministers, and the right to report in public were hard won and were not always sustained. Some CMOs achieved landmarks during their term of office including John Simon and Sir William Jameson who made the first, wartime, broadcast on health and who bravely tackled sexually transmitted diseases. Jameson played a key role facilitating the introduction of the NHS. Sir George Godber was 'a giant', who achieved unique personal and professional authority in the office.

The office of CMO emerged in the nineteenth century, largely through the need to tackle infectious diseases like cholera. Despite an expectation in the mid-twentieth century that infectious diseases were surmountable, the work of Sir Donald Acheson was particularly focused on AIDS and his successor, Sir Kenneth Calman, was also confronted by another new infectious disease in the BSE crisis. Infectious conditions continue to be a concern for CMOs, right up to the MRSA issue of today.

The authors are frank about setbacks in the development of authority, such as when one CMO was excluded from the Health Department's negotiating team with the medical profession.

Of all the countries in the OECD group, the position of health and healthcare within British government is unique. Health and economic policy are the two aspects of government most characterised by analysis and discussion and by formal government 'policies'. No western government pays for a higher proportion of health costs through central taxation. Hence the British government's CMO can be exceptionally influential.

The UK is alone in the scale of its comprehensive, free-at-the-time-of-use and politically directed Health Service. Yet, paradoxically, the British health system, perhaps best set up to foster health promotion and general enhancement of the health of the people, has sometimes been distracted by the pressing day-to-day issues of the NHS.

Most of the CMOs had a common 'restlessness of spirit' and a 'hunger to tackle current issues' and the authors lighten their well-referenced text with a series of anecdotes, both witty and thought provoking. Several books have been written about individual CMOs. However, this is the first to study the role of the office over 150 years, illuminated by highlights of the work of 14 successive post holders.

The Trustees of The Nuffield Trust thank Dr Sally Sheard and Sir Liam Donaldson for their innovative work and are pleased to support this important book.

Sir Denis Pereira Gray OBE, HonDSc, FRCGP, FMedSci
Chairman, The Nuffield Trust
September 2005

Preface

The office of Chief Medical Officer (CMO) is one of the most critical roles within the British government and medical system. It has developed into the focal point for advice to government and to the public on a wide range of medical and public health issues. The holder is now the recognisable, non-political face of state medicine – the 'Nation's Doctor'.

From an initially short-term disease surveillance function in 1855, the post has been actively restructured by each of the fourteen CMOs (all men) in response to advances in scientific and medical knowledge, changes in government and the professionalisation of medicine. By the beginning of the twentieth century, it had matured into a permanent, vital element of the Whitehall machine – particularly as a focal point for contact between the government and the medical profession and the legitimisation of medical advice.

This study suggests that the CMO has had a far larger part to play in the development and delivery of health policy in Britain than has hitherto been acknowledged. Part of the explanation for this relative obscurity is that previous frames of analysis have been administrative or disease based. Away from the heroic exploits of the nineteenth-century sanitarians like Chadwick, Duncan, Snow and Simon there is an anonymous bureaucracy, through which only a very few will shine.[1] A trawl through the indices of the authoritative histories of British public health and health services by Fox, Honigsbaum, Klein, Rivett, Webster and others yields remarkably few references to CMOs.[2] These narratives have constrained the history of the individual in the administrative development of healthcare.

[1] Edwin Chadwick (1800–1890) was the architect of the new Poor Law of 1834 and of the subsequent period of sanitary reform: see RA Lewis, *Edwin Chadwick and the Public Health Movement* (London, Longman, 1952); SE Finer, *The Life and Times of Edwin Chadwick* (London, Methuen, 1952); C Hamlin, *Public Health and Social Justice in the Age of Chadwick* (Cambridge, Cambridge University Press, 1998). Dr William Henry Duncan (1805–1863) was England's first local Medical Officer of Health in Liverpool in 1847: see WF Frazer, *Duncan of Liverpool* (London, Hamish Hamilton, 1947; new edition Preston, Carnegie Publishing, 1997). Dr John Snow (1813–1858) pioneered anaesthesia in Britain and was also a gifted epidemiologist. He was the first person to correctly identify cholera as a water-borne disease: see P Vinten-Johansen, H Brody, N Paneth, S Rachman and M Rip, *Cholera, Chloroform and the Science of Medicine. A Life of John Snow* (New York, Oxford University Press, 2003).

[2] D Fox, *Health Policies, Health Politics; the British and American Experience, 1911–1965* (Princeton, New Jersey, Princeton University Press, 1986); F Honigsbaum, *The Division in British Medicine: a history of the separation of general practice from hospital care* (London, Kogan Page, 1979); R Klein, *The New Politics of the NHS* (London, Longman, 1995); G Rivett, *From Cradle to Grave: fifty years of the NHS* (London, King's Fund, 1998); C Webster, *The Health Services Since the War, I. Problems of Health Care. The National Health Service before 1957* (London, HMSO, 1988); C Webster, *The Health Services Since the War, II. Government and Health Care – The British National Health Service, 1958–1979* (London, HMSO, 1996); C Webster, *The NHS: a political history* (Oxford, Oxford University Press, 1998).

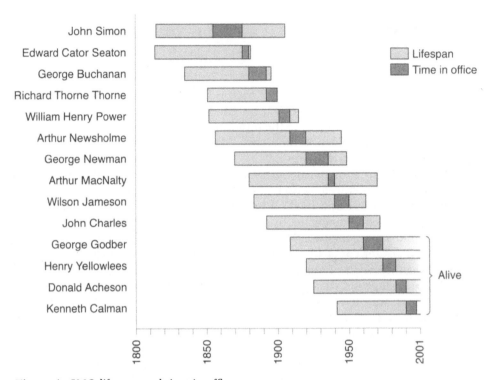

Figure A CMO lifespan and time in office.

A revised model of the development of the British system of state medicine is required. An explicit examination of the role and authority of the CMO reveals a fuller, more satisfactory picture of the changing experiences of health in Britain. Personality and personal ability then emerge as critical issues. The metaphor of the 'CMO as gatekeeper' is incisive in analysing the relationship between the government and the medical profession and the translation of expert advice into policy. Health in Britain has probably been subjected to more conscious 'policy formation' than almost any other area of government activity. It demands attention both for its own sake as well as for the broader picture of the process of government. This analysis enables a repositioning of this significant group of professionals at the centre of the Whitehall system and a move towards a useful analysis of the development of medical authority in Britain.

Structure of the book

We have stepped back from a simple chronological approach to the careers of the fourteen CMOs who have held this post between its formation in 1855 and 1998. This study is constructed around a number of key themes with an integral element of chronology which eases the general reader into an appreciation of the long-term development of the role of CMO. The early chapters deal with why the post was initially established and how each of the fourteen CMOs has been selected. Subsequent chapters develop wider themes. These sections – on the tripartite relationship with the Permanent Secretary and Minister, on the policy-making function, on building a medical civil service and on reporting health – highlight the activities of particular CMOs, those activities which present relevant case studies for the theme in question.

This considered, thematic approach has been adopted to ensure that at least one substantial feature of each CMO's tenure is discussed in detail. Some are more prominent than others. Sir John Simon as the founding father of state medicine looms large throughout the nineteenth century; Sir George Newman's persistence in ensuring the CMO's status within the new Ministry of Health dominates the inter-war period; Sir Wilson Jameson's mediating role in the formation of the National Health Service (NHS); Sir John Charles, Sir George Godber and Sir Henry Yellowlees illustrate the benefits and pitfalls of working with Permanent Secretaries and Ministers. Sir Donald Acheson and Sir Kenneth Calman provide a perspective on obtaining expert advice and the formulation of health policy. The disadvantage of this approach is that the casual reader may depart from a single chapter with an unrepresentative impression of an individual's period in office. To balance this thematic approach, a short biography for each CMO has been provided in an appendix at the end of the book. Here, the reader may peruse all the CMOs chronologically, with the benefit of a timeline of key dates in history.

The 14 leading actors in this story cover a 143-year period, but there is often considerable overlap between them – professionally and, occasionally, socially. Simon's long life meant that he witnessed the activities of the next five CMOs; Newman was instrumental in the appointment of Jameson; Jameson recalled his outstanding student Godber when he was looking for an assistant in planning for the NHS; Yellowlees and Acheson had both worked at the Middlesex Hospital early in their careers. Rarely have they been from outside a small, London-based medical circle.

There is also a wider group of supporting actors (but only a few actresses) in this complex plot. They are the Ministers and civil servants who, together with the CMO, form the senior management team for health in central government. The Permanent Secretaries (and the CMOs are intermittently included in this Whitehall group) are non-political, and as their title suggests, *permanent* appointments. Consequently most have had a relatively long spell in office (see Appendix 2).

On the political side, as with the CMOs, there are those who stand out. The average length of a Ministerial appointment is amazingly short – estimated at two and a half years since the First World War.[3] To put this into context, between the formation of the Ministry of Health in 1919 and 1997 there were 33 Ministers or Secretaries of State for Health, but only eight CMOs (see Appendix 3). For this reason the focus of Ministers is often on short-term, quick fixes to problems which Departments see as requiring long-term solutions. The relative influence of Ministers of Health within Westminster has also waxed and waned. There have been long periods when health has not had direct representation within the Cabinet (before 1919, 1952–62, 1964–68). At these times, the influence of the CMO as a prime advocate for the public's health was even more critical.

---

[3] R Rose, 'The political economy of cabinet change', in F Vibert (ed.), *Britain's Constitutional Future* (London, Institute of Economic Affairs, 1991), pp. 45–72.

Healthy government and the governance of health

The story unfolds mainly in Whitehall, the geographically and culturally defined epicentre of British government. This is a close, even claustrophobic environment, in which personality and face-to-face contact have become increasingly significant. Yet there are also other dimensions. As state medicine developed in the late nineteenth century, the CMO became responsible for increasingly vigorous national health surveillance and intervention. The international dimension to the CMO post also grew alongside the rapid and massive expansion in overseas trade in the nineteenth century. Some CMOs had to negotiate international agreements on, for example, infectious disease and the health of migrant workers.

Yet the intrinsic framework remains state medicine: the principle of public medical services, delivered through government agencies and financed through systems of public taxation. State medicine provided the initial motivation for the CMO post and its subsequent security. Using this organising principle, it is possible to identify a sequence of significant periods following John Simon's appointment in 1855. They fall into a broad synthesis within Whitehall periods. First, from the mid-nineteenth century there was a steady expansion in state responsibility for basic healthcare services – smallpox vaccination, Poor Law medical services, notification and treatment of infectious diseases. This coincided with, and in part stimulated, the expansion of the professional civil service through the appointment of technical (medical) experts and career mandarins, as well as the development of a clear selection and promotion strategy within Whitehall. This was also a time of the genesis of Ministerial responsibility and civil servant anonymity.

It would be wrong, however, to present this as a simple account of the rise of Victorian Whitehall. Many of these health services were conceptualised and delivered locally with little central government involvement. This period was the heyday of local government, in which the town hall exerted considerable financial authority and provided its Medical Officer of Health with increasing resources to develop preventive medicine, once the immediate crises of the insanitary urban environments had been brought under (local government) control. In 1871, the Local Government Board was formed to consolidate this new concern with systematic surveillance and improvement to extra-metropolitan areas. It required increasing numbers of technical staff and a complex administration. As one of the largest state employers of the nineteenth century, it helped to engender an essentially legalistic, information-collecting view of the purpose of a permanent bureaucracy – into which the CMO easily fitted.

By the end of the nineteenth century, Whitehall had progressively developed a system of Boards for specific governmental purposes. These were staffed by permanent civil servants and reported to Ministers who, in turn, represented their interests in government and Parliament. Out of a proliferation of specialist Boards emerged the Ministries of the early twentieth century. The creation of a Ministry of Health was finally achieved, after several years of planning, in 1919. It was the result of one CMO's ambitious collaboration – not that of Newsholme, the CMO 'proper' at the Local Government Board, where the majority of health business was located, but of Newman, CMO to the Board of Education, who recognised the enormous potential which a dedicated Ministry offered to him personally and to the wider cause of improved national health.

Yet despite this stronger Whitehall base, with direct Cabinet representation for health for the first time, the CMO did not have complete control over health services in Britain. The majority of public health functions remained with the Medical Officers of Health in local government. The chain of command to the Ministry, although present, was not a robust one and the CMO could not always dominate. Medical Officers of Health were, after all, the employees of their local authority, not civil servants. This inter-war period of strong local autonomy and relatively weak central government control is perhaps a good one in which to test a hypothesis that the integrity and personal authority of the CMO has been crucial to the development of Whitehall and health services.

The importance of 'public health' relative to health services is one issue which has dogged all CMOs. To what extent is health the result of health services, lifestyle choices, life circumstances, family history? Public health as a discipline has mirrored the rise of the CMO – from a formative 'sanitary reform' era following the first national Public Health Act, through periods which have focused in more detail on the role of the individual in securing their health and that of their community, to a renewed emphasis on health inequalities and the economic and social determinants of poor health in the late twentieth century. The role of public health practitioners, too, has mirrored some of the experiences of the CMOs as they have developed 'preventive medicine', later to be rearticulated as 'health education' or 'health promotion'. The political and financial support for public health has ebbed and flowed along with the image and career prospects of the public health practitioner – especially the local Medical Officer of Health. From their heyday in the late nineteenth century, when armed with the new science of bacteriology, the Medical Officers of Health appeared unassailable; their territory has since been encroached upon by general practitioners, social workers and environmental health experts. Attempts to reinvigorate the discipline through social medicine in the 1940s and community medicine in the 1970s and 1980s were not entirely successful. The CMO, as a figurehead, whether willingly or not, has been intimately associated with the fortunes of the discipline of what today is again called 'public health'.

How does this account fit into the bigger picture of the development of government in Britain? Certainly, by the mid-twentieth century, a relatively stable Whitehall system is recognisable, albeit one which continued to rely for its senior civil servants largely on an upper-class, Oxbridge-educated élite. The post-war period has been recognised as one of 'consensus politics, the zenith of the welfare state and the managed economy'.[4] From the 1960s, the CMO's position in Whitehall has also had to accommodate the advent of the 'special adviser'. Increasing use has been made of these political appointments, such as that of Brian Abel-Smith at the Department of Health and Social Security in the 1960s and 1970s. They have usually enjoyed direct access to Ministers. More recently, there has been wider acceptance of advice from 'policy networks' and 'think-tanks', which by the 1990s tended to reflect a broader intellectual climate.

Whitehall has also come under increasing pressure to reform itself, most notably in the aftermath of the Fulton Committee report of 1966, and through

---

[4] D Kavanagh and P Morris, *Consensus Politics from Atlee to Thatcher* (Oxford, Blackwell, 1989).

the rise of Raynerism which promised efficient management in the 1980s.[5] A formative step was taken with the issue, in 1993, of the Civil Service Management Code, which clarified for the first time the long-standing tradition that a civil servant's duty is 'first and foremost to the Minister of the Crown who is in charge of the Department in which he or she is serving'.[6]

The more rigorous budgetary controls of the 1960s heralded a phase of planning which was more within the control of the mandarins than the Ministers. However, the eventual outcome of pressure on departmental budgets through to the 1980s and 1990s reduced long-term planning, with relatively fewer strategic interdepartmental committees. CMOs have had duties not only in the Department of Health, but also in other government departments including the Home Office and the Ministry for Agriculture, Fisheries and Foods to name the most significant. They therefore have had the capacity to forge links which may be beyond the capabilities of other senior civil servants, although as the bovine spongiform encephalopathy (BSE) crisis illustrates, this requires co-operation on both sides of Whitehall doors. There is ample evidence here to substantiate a view of Whitehall in the later period covered by this history as a 'beautifully designed and effective braking mechanism'.[7]

The CMO has fitted into the civil service framework not only as a senior civil servant, with the rank and status of a Permanent Secretary, but also as a technical expert. He had not only to have considerable professional skills, but also to be aware when they were insufficient and where to go, within Britain and at times internationally, to get the necessary expertise. This function of soliciting expert advice has increased considerably, as medical and scientific knowledge has grown, and as new problems, such as AIDS (acquired immune deficiency syndrome) and BSE, have emerged. Many of the issues examined here thus illustrate the result of years of CMO 'networking' – knowing who is the leading expert in a particular field, or approaching people with the talent to help develop innovative health services. Some of this expertise can be provided from within the medical civil service, but more recently there has been a heavier reliance on external experts, prepared to give their time and advice precisely because of the prestige of working with the CMO inside the Whitehall policy-making machine.

The CMO's required qualification as a medical practitioner has located him within another significant narrative, that of the rise of the medical profession through the nineteenth and twentieth centuries. It is impossible to separate completely the professionalisation of medicine from the growth of the British welfare state. The two are intertwined and mutually dependent. Beginning with the provision of Poor Law medical services in the early nineteenth century, the state progressively adopted responsibility for a wide range of healthcare services.

[5] Derek Rayner (later Lord Rayner) was brought in by Margaret Thatcher in 1979 to conduct a number of Whitehall reviews. He had also previously worked for the Heath government. 'Raynerism' became synonymous in the 1980s with the drive for efficiency and the removal of 'paper – the tyranny of the past'. See P Hennessy, *Whitehall* (London, Pimlico, 2001) for a detailed analysis of Rayner's position in the British bureaucracy and his activities.

[6] HM Treasury, *Civil Service Management Code* (HM Treasury/Cabinet Office, 1993), section 4.1, annex A, paras 3–4.

[7] S Williams, 'The decision makers', in Royal Institute of Public Administration (ed.), *Policy and Practice: experience of government* (London, RIPA, 1980), p. 81.

There have been two subsequent periods of notable services expansion. First, the Liberal Government's welfare legislation of 1905–1914, which *inter alia* initiated national health insurance, school medical inspections, as well as mother and infant welfare services. The second sea change came through the National Health Service Act in 1946. This established the principle of a comprehensive medical service, free at the point of delivery for the entire population. It was achieved through the nationalisation and consolidation of three separate types of hospital (voluntary, Poor Law and municipal) and the contracting of doctors. Thus, as the medical profession formed increasingly tighter partnerships with the government, the CMO's role as mediator has developed.

What emerges from this study is a multifaceted portrait of a senior government official, operating as an adviser, manager, co-ordinator, arbitrator, communicator and medical practitioner. A good CMO has also been required to be a politician, to use that word in its purest sense. He had to have an aptitude for knowing the flow of the political tide within Whitehall and Westminster: to be able to evaluate alternative ideas, trade policies and steer a course which was not always the best possible, but which represented the best achievable. This study offers a framework within which the functions of the CMO can be interpreted. It identifies the varying spheres of influence within which the CMO worked, and, most crucially, the importance of authority and credibility, both within Whitehall and the medical profession, in addition to the inherent authority which this senior Whitehall post accrued over the 143-year period.

To return to our initial tentative hypothesis, the various case studies presented here suggest that through such analysis, or at the bare minimum, awareness, it is possible to influence the effectiveness of government. There is also a wider concept of government as a living organism, whose 'health' requires careful management to ensure effective mechanisms for the selection and development of staff, and for the promotion of appropriate policies. 'Healthy government' is a significant concept which has rarely been directly addressed. The CMOs can provide a fascinating insight into this elusive issue.

A note on sources

The phrase 'there is no history, only histories' is one which is more commonly used in self-defence than in a truly positive way. What we mean by this is that one rarely writes without a purpose. Several of the CMOs have already produced their 'histories' of the post, or of their experience, notably Simon's *English Sanitary Institutions*, Newsholme's *Fifty Years in Public Health*, Newman's *The Building of a Nation's Health* and MacNalty's *The History of State Medicine in England*.[8] Some of these are what might now be disparagingly termed 'whiggish' accounts – suggesting (sometimes consciously) a relentless improvement in health due to the activities of their predecessors in the post. Most of them are uncritical celebrations of state medicine, measured through declining mortality rates and improving life expectancy. Yet they are useful documents, providing a contemporary perspective on health issues at different points in time.

[8] J Simon, *English Sanitary Institutions* (London, Cassell & Co, 1st edn, 1890); A Newsholme, *Fifty Years in Public Health* (London, George Allen and Unwin, 1935); G Newman, *The Building of a Nation's Health* (London, Macmillan, 1939); AS MacNalty, *The History of State Medicine in England* (London, The Royal Institute of Public Health and Hygiene, 1948).

As this study seeks to place the role of the CMO within the broader perspective of the development of Whitehall, the medical profession and a state medical service, it therefore draws on documents which are kept in that temple to bureaucracy, the National Archives at Kew in London.[9] Many fruitful (and frustrating) hours have been spent reading through the minutiae of Whitehall life in the various files for the Local Government Board, Ministry of Health, Department of Health and Social Security, Cabinet Office and other government departments. It is easy to slip into a happy familiarity with the handwriting of prominent civil servants. A long day's work on the archive may equate to several years of one person's work on a particular issue.

Yet this is no easy journey. There is a paucity of information for both the beginning and end of our period. The archives from the mid-nineteenth century are incomplete, with tantalising cross-references to documents which no longer exist within the National Archives files. For the late twentieth century, the cut-off point is much more abrupt: Whitehall's '30 years rule' means that fat files, ripe for history, are locked away, only to be opened on a rolling basis. Even then, there are potential further delays – sensitive issues and personal files usually have a much longer closure period.

To gain some insight into the period since 1974, it was necessary to exploit other sources. Newspapers and the medical press are useful indicators of events, particularly crises. Diaries, too, can play a part, although civil servants and privy councillors are also supposed to abide by the '30 years rule' (Richard Crossman's publication in 1975 of the first volume of his diaries was a flagrant violation of this principle). But the best source is undoubtedly oral testimony from the people involved. Those individuals who kindly gave their time and knowledge are listed in the acknowledgements.

Sally Sheard
Sir Liam Donaldson
September 2005

---

[9] All of the documents referred to in the text and footnotes are located at the National Archives, Kew, London (formerly known as the Public Records Office) unless otherwise indicated.

About the authors

Sally Sheard is Senior Lecturer in History of Medicine at the University of Liverpool. Her research interests include British nineteenth- and twentieth-century health, especially the political economy of health services and the development of medical authority.

She co-edited *Body and City: histories of urban public health* (Ashgate, 2000) and *Financing British Medicine since 1750* (Routledge, forthcoming 2005), and has published articles in medical and history journals. She has developed an innovative history of medicine course for undergraduate medical students at the University of Liverpool and a range of academic outreach activities, including radio and television broadcasts and guest museum curatorships.

Sir Liam Donaldson was appointed as the 15th Chief Medical Officer for England and the United Kingdom's Chief Medical Adviser in 1998. During his tenure, he has introduced a wide range of innovations and reforms impacting on both public health and healthcare quality. These have included: the country's first comprehensive health protection strategy (*Getting Ahead of the Curve*); a ground-breaking report on patient safety (*An Organisation with a Memory*); the creation of the concept of clinical governance; a programme to empower patients with chronic disease to manage their own conditions (*The Expert Patient Programme*); reports leading to legislative change in relation to organ and tissue retention and use, to permit regulated use of stem cells for research (*Stem Cell Research: Medical Progress with Responsibility*) and a new approach to medical litigation (*Making Amends*); and a new system of training for doctors in the early years after qualifying (*Unfinished Business – proposals for reform of the Senior House Officer grade*).

Sir Liam's Annual Reports *On the State of Public Health* have strongly championed the need for action on key areas of the nation's health. For example, his calls for action on obesity and on the need for smoke-free public places and workplaces triggered an extensive public debate on the growing concern about these issues and the need for action to address them.

He has also made important contributions on the international front both in relation to public health but also quality and safety of healthcare. He has become a leading international voice on patient safety and Chairs the World Alliance for Patient Safety (an umbrella organisation created by the World Health Organization).

Sir Liam has made numerous key note addresses at conferences in the United Kingdom and around the world. He is an experienced broadcaster and author of a standard text book of public health (*Essential Public Health*) and numerous papers in peer review journals. He holds an honour Chair in Applied Epidemiology at the University of Newcastle upon Tyne, England and has been a recipient of ten honorary doctorates from Universities in the United Kingdom.

Acknowledgements

The idea for this book originated in September 1998. The Nuffield Trust agreed to fund a short period of research to locate related archives and undertake oral history. Thanks are due to the Nuffield Trust, and in particular its Secretary, John Wyn Owen, for their willingness to fund an essentially historical study, which it is hoped will provide critical context for the current and future structure of this central medical function.

All the retired CMOs for England have been willing to be involved with this project, through interviews and the loan of related material. Sir George Godber, Sir Henry Yellowlees, Sir Donald Acheson and Sir Kenneth Calman collectively have 38 years' experience as CMO. Their excellent memories have corrected some of our false assumptions and provided wonderful insights into their time in office.

Much of this book highlights the position of the CMO as a senior civil servant within Whitehall, specifically how they have worked with the Permanent Secretaries and Ministers of State, and constructed effective teams to work with them. Amazingly, with only a couple of exceptions, all of those approached were happy to be interviewed for this research: Dr Michael Abrams, Dr Sheila Adam, Professor John Ashton, The Right Honourable Kenneth Clarke, Dr John Evans, Dr Gillian Ford, Sir Norman Fowler, Sir Christopher France, Sir Graham Hart, Dame Deirdre Hine, Dr Alistair Mason, Dr Jeremy Metters, Dame Yvonne Moores, Sir Patrick Nairne, The Right Honourable the Lord Owen, Dr Geoffrey Rivett, Dr Elizabeth Shore, Sir Kenneth Stowe, Lord Waldegrave of North Hill, Lord Warner of Brockley, Professor Graham Winyard.

To balance the Whitehall accounts, a number of health professionals, academics and commentators gave their views on the role of the CMO: Dr Roy Acheson, Dr Ian Bogle, Niall Dickson, Dr Paddy Donaldson, Professor Walter Holland, Sir Donald Irvine, Dr John Horder, Professor Rudolf Klein, Gordon McLachlan, Robert Maxwell, Professor Jerry Morris, Professor Andrew Semple, Nick Timmins and John Wyn Owen. They have all been patient with the questions and generous with their time.

A number of different archives and libraries have been used for this research and we are grateful to them for their assistance in locating relevant material: the National Archives, the Wellcome Trust Contemporary Medical Archives Centre, the British Medical Association, the libraries of the Royal College of Physicians, the Royal College of Surgeons, the House of Lords, the University of Liverpool and the Liverpool Medical Institution. Dr Eileen Smith, the CMO's Intelligence Officer at the Department of Health, and Ms Lee Morris, the CMO's Senior Personal Secretary, both deserve special thanks for their willingness to go in search of obscure bits of Whitehall information and for making numerous drafting amendments.

As this research progressed, tentative hypotheses were aired through seminars at the University of Lancaster, the Wellcome Unit for the History of Medicine at the University of Manchester and at the London School of Hygiene and Tropical Medicine.

This research was also discussed at the CMO's Residential Event in December 2001, and at a symposium held at the Nuffield Trust in October 2002. Our thanks go to all those who engaged in these discussions and also to colleagues who have commented on various drafts, especially Professor Virginia Berridge, Alan Doran, Dr Dan Fox, Dr Muir Gray, Dr Anne Hardy, Dr Jeremy Metters, John Wyn Owen, Dr Geoffrey Rivett and Hugh Taylor.

Finally, many thanks to the family and friends who have supported the research and writing at home and away.

Sally Sheard
Sir Liam Donaldson
September 2005

In memory of
Raymond 'Paddy' Donaldson (1920–2005) and John Edwardson (1910–2005)
Two exemplary public servants.

Chapter 1

A doctor at the heart of government

With hindsight it is too easy to see the appointment of John Simon in 1855 as Medical Officer to the General Board of Health as part of a natural progression towards a system of state medicine in Britain. Yet on the eve of his resignation in 1876, the position he had nurtured as the top medical civil servant was no more secure than on his appointment 21 years earlier. Nonetheless, the status and duties which Simon had carved out for himself still underpin the position of the Chief Medical Officer today. They deserve closer examination.[1]

The creation of the post of Medical Officer was a response to the great nineteenth-century cholera and fever epidemics. The rapid unplanned urbanisation in the early nineteenth century produced in Britain an insanitary, overcrowded environment in which infectious diseases thrived. The arrival of three epidemics of cholera in Europe in 1832, 1848 and 1854 each provoked an atmosphere of fear and short-lived reformist compulsions. Likewise, successive outbreaks of typhus fever put pressure on local authorities.[2] Although the relatively low cholera mortality rates belied the reputation of 'King Cholera', the fear it engendered was useful to Edwin Chadwick in his mission to introduce a programme of state-funded sanitary reform. Through the 1848 Public Health Act, the first public health systems were established, nationally and, to a limited extent, locally.[3] They were fundamentally environmentalist programmes, in which medicine, personified by the local Medical Officer of Health, played a subordinate role to that of the Sanitary Engineer. Chadwick's vision of a sanitary environment required minimal input from the nascent medical profession. Yet the threat of diseases such as cholera meant that medicine could not be completely divorced from the government's schemes. Epidemics shifted the focus of attention swiftly from the environment to the individual and legitimated the intrusion of the doctor into the formation of public health policy.

John Simon received his medical education at King's College, London and initially worked as a lecturer and surgeon at St Thomas's Hospital. In 1848 the City of London established a public health department and Simon moved to the new Medical Officership. It was a part-time appointment so he maintained his lectureship and a private practice. Simon used his new office to collect and interpret mortality and morbidity data and to advise on sanitary reforms. He established through his reports a reputation as a national expert in this field. Simon's stature in public health circles was in direct contrast to the opinions held

---

[1] The definitive biography of John Simon is that by Royston Lambert, *Sir John Simon and English Social Administration* (London, MacGibbon & Kee, 1963).

[2] M Pelling, *Cholera, Fever and English Medicine, 1825–1865* (Oxford, Oxford University Press, 1978) provides a good analysis of the early nineteenth-century epidemics.

[3] 1848 Public Health Act. 11 & 12 Vict. c.63.

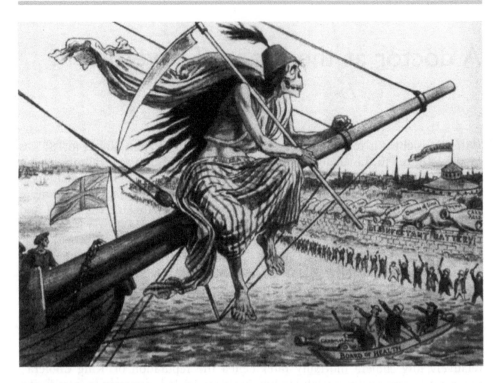

Figure 1.1 The arrival of cholera in America in the nineteenth century.

of Chadwick, who was a domineering and unpopular administrator at the General Board of Health. The Board initially had no medical representation at all and Chadwick's dogmatic adherence to a strictly environmentalist approach to sanitary reform was continually criticised by the medical profession, members of Parliament and the press. When the Board's renewal came up for consideration in 1854 (under the terms of the 1848 Act), the position of Chadwick and its *modus operandi* were no longer tenable.[4] A new Board of Health was constituted comprised of a group of *ex officio* Ministers, a permanent salaried President and a permanent inspectorship. This meant that for the first time England had an established central health administration with Ministerial representation.

The new President of the General Board of Health, Sir Benjamin Hall (1802–1867), gave medical advice a far more prominent place than it had achieved under Chadwick during the tenure of the first Board. He was responding to pressure from the public and the medical profession, and by aligning himself closely with doctors he could distance himself from the anti-medical Chadwick. Hall 'leant heavily' on Simon for advice from the outset of his Presidency.[5] His immediate concern was the cholera epidemic of 1855 and he appointed twelve

---

[4] Chadwick resigned, and although he held no further government office, he continued to be a vociferous critic of the medicalisation of public health until his death aged 90 in 1890. RA Lewis, *Edwin Chadwick and the Public Health Movement* (London, Longman, 1952); SE Finer, *The Life and Times of Edwin Chadwick* (London, Methuen, 1952); C Hamlin, *Public Health and Social Justice in the Age of Chadwick* (Cambridge, Cambridge University Press, 1998).

[5] Lambert, *Sir John Simon*, p. 229.

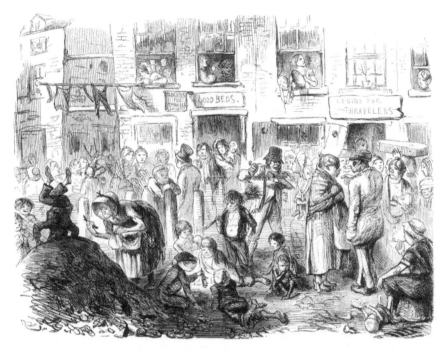

A COURT FOR KING CHOLERA.

Figure 1.2 *Punch* cartoon from 1852 illustrating the insanitary conditions in Britain which made the transmission of the disease so easy. © Punch Cartoon Library and Archive.

doctors as cholera inspectors and a Medical Council to investigate the scientific basis of the epidemic. Simon used his position as Medical Officer of Health for London to gain constant access to Hall and to push for more permanent sanitary measures. Hall won a further Act in 1855 and with it the power to appoint a Medical Officer to the Board of Health.[6] He had no hesitation in asking Simon to fill the new post. It was a significant year for public health. New legislation enabled the appointment of local medical officers of health throughout London.

Simon had all the attributes desirable for this innovative government post. He was practical rather than doctrinaire. He had proved the value of his 'scientific' approach during the cholera epidemic of 1854 in London. He was the personification of preventive medicine in the eyes of both the public and the medical profession. In August 1855, the Treasury finally sanctioned the appointment of 'a gentleman eminent in his profession, who enjoys the confidence of that profession as well as that of the public' at a salary of £1500 per annum.[7] Simon was offered the post on condition that he resigned from his post as Medical Officer of Health for the City of London and gave up his private practice. He accepted, and was allowed to keep his position as Lecturer at St Thomas's Hospital which he saw as a useful connection with practical medicine.

[6] 1855 Nuisances Removal and Diseases Prevention Act. 18 & 19 Vict. c.121.
[7] MH 13/259. 04.09.1855, G Arbuthnot to W Cowper. Cowper had replaced Hall as President of the Health Department earlier in 1855.

Simon began his new position as Medical Officer to the General Board of Health with a clear personal vision of what he should be able to achieve. He interpreted his role to include the development as well as the implementation of policy. This was not a new idea – Simon had expressed this ambition in the Preface to his collected *Reports of the Medical Officer of Health for the City of London* in 1854. The fundamental principle which he campaigned for was that the sanitary problem 'should be submitted in its entirety to some single department of the executive, as a sole charge . . . there should be some tangible head, responsible not only for the enforcement of existing laws, such as they are or may become, but likewise for their progress from time to time to the level of contemporary science, for their completion where fragmentary, for their harmonisation where discordant'.[8]

His aims from a central office were now wider than he had been permitted in his City of London post. The techniques of delivery, though, were much the same – systematic co-operation between authorities, preventive action linked to regular notification of morbidity and mortality data, systematic inspection cycles, investigations on special topics, publication of annual reports specifically designed to inform the public and the press as well as fulfilling his obligation to Parliament. Simon recognised that to achieve these aims he needed to adopt a gradual approach. Swift change would provide ammunition to those in Britain who feared 'centralisation', whereas a slower pace of change would be more likely to succeed without raising too much attention. The paradox of Simon's appointment was that although his own position was statutory (under the 1855 Public Health Act), the future of the General Board of Health to which he was attached was fragile. The stability of central health machinery had not fully recovered from its poor image under Chadwick's leadership. Between 1855 and 1858 there were sustained calls from within Parliament for the new administration to be dismantled.[9] The government's only recourse was to push through continuance Acts to save the Board from extinction.

Simon was fortunate that the Permanent Secretary to the Board was Tom Taylor (1817–1880), who fully supported his vision for an extension of the health policies of central government.[10] From the Board's small offices at 8 Richmond Terrace, Whitehall, Simon was able to arrange the routine inspection work and to extend his advice to other government departments.[11] He also used his new national position to issue Instructional Minutes on qualifications for the posts of Sanitary Engineers and Medical Officers of Health. Through these official circulars he elaborated his preferred model of sanitary reform, which favoured scientific medicine rather than sanitary engineering. He was also able to call upon professional organisations, including the Association of Metropolitan Medical

---

[8] J Simon, *Reports of the Medical Officer of Health for the City of London*, 1854, p. xxvii.

[9] See C Hamlin, *Public Health and Social Justice in the Age of Chadwick* (Cambridge, Cambridge University Press, 1998) for a detailed analysis of Chadwick's impact on the politics of sanitary reform.

[10] See R Lambert, 'Central and local relations in Mid-Victorian England: the Local Government Act Office, 1858–1871', *Victorian Studies*, 1962, pp. 121–50 for more detail on this early period of state medicine.

[11] Simon advised the Colonial Office on a system of sanitary organisation for Hong Kong based on that which he had developed for London. He also provided help with the reorganisation of health legislation in the Bahamas and other colonies and issued international sanitary circulars.

Officers of Health (formed in 1856), the Social Science Association (formed in 1857) and the Epidemiological Society of London (formed in 1850), to lobby Parliament in support of his proposed legislation. He became close to these pressure groups during his years as Medical Officer of Health for London.[12] To some extent then, Simon can be seen to have played the role of Trojan horse – moving the energy of these outside associations into Whitehall administration, and creating the impetus for sanitary reform.

In 1858 the position of medicine in central government was reviewed again. Simon had used the publication of his *Sanitary Papers* to launch a risky attack on the system in which he was employed. He criticised the shortage of staff for investigations and the lack of planning for sanitary legislation. Parliament and the newspapers saw him as a centralist, who favoured imposing a national model of health administration on a reluctant country. Although he was jeopardising his own job security, Simon's justification was his concern for the long-term development of state medicine. The gamble paid off. The 1858 Public Health Act enabled Simon and his department to be transferred intact under the protective wing of the Privy Council.[13] However, the 1858 Act did not make the central health administration permanent, and the Whig Government was not in favour of extending its initial temporary arrangement.

All this changed with the fall of the Whig Government in June 1859 and the return to power of Palmerston and the Conservatives. The new President of the Privy Council, Robert Lowe (1811–1892), was quickly persuaded by Simon of the indispensable nature of the medical work of the Council. He successfully obtained the 1859 Public Health Act through which Simon's position was made more secure. It was a short parliamentary Act, with only eight sections, four of which were the direct result of Simon's intervention. Section two transferred responsibility for inspection of smallpox vaccination to Simon at the Privy Council and was worded in such a way as to remove related duties from the Poor Law Board on the grounds of medical competency. Section three allowed the Privy Council to make 'such enquiries as they see fit in relation to any matter concerning the public health in any place or places, and to the observance of the regulations and directions issued by them under this Act'.[14] This section legitimated Simon's right to initiate his own inquiries and once again extended the boundaries of state interference in local health affairs.[15] Section four transferred Simon to the Privy Council as Medical Officer at a salary of £1500 per annum and allowed the Council 'from time to time [to] employ such other persons as they deem necessary for the purpose of this Act'. Significantly, Simon had persuaded the Bill's proponents to drop the word 'temporarily' from this clause, enabling him to appoint medical advisers on a more permanent basis than originally envisaged.

Section five was also vital to the success of Simon's plans, in providing that 'the Medical Officer, shall from time to time report to the Privy Council in relation to any matters concerning the public health, or such matters as be referred to him

[12] Simon was the first President of the Association of Metropolitan Medical Officers of Health, and he hosted its meetings in his Whitehall offices until 1863. Lambert, *Sir John Simon*, p. 246.

[13] 1858 Public Health Act. 21 & 22 Vict. c.97.

[14] 1859 Public Health Act. 22 & 23 Vict. c.3. Section 3.

[15] Although it did not sanction direct intervention, it allowed the CMO's department to pursue policies of investigation and recommendation.

for that purpose'. The precise wording of the section was crucial. It gave Simon independent authority from the Privy Council to issue reports. He was completely free from control by his political chiefs, and responsible solely to Parliament. The Medical Officer had gained through the 1859 Act a position of 'privileged immunity'.[16]

The 1859 Public Health Act thus established the Medical Officership as a unique component of the British government system. Its loose legislative language conferred the privilege on the holder of the post of Medical Officer to interpret it as widely as he wished. Unlike other civil servants, Simon had secured the right to initiate investigations, criticise the legislature and propose his own reforms. He had a freedom of speech and independence unique within Whitehall. It was the envy of other senior civil servants who worked through advice to Ministers and commissions and who could not put their names to policy initiatives.

The success of the post of Chief Medical Officer ever since, and the very public recognition of the holder, owes much to the forms of words that John Simon secured in section five of the 1859 Public Health Act. Through the statutory *Annual Reports*, he could now expound his views on sanitary reform and state medicine with complete immunity from political censure. Enemies such as Chadwick outside the Whitehall system were at bay. The success of public health policy now rested almost entirely with John Simon through his interpretation of his role in the light of the 1859 Act. He needed to consolidate his position as medical expert and secure the endorsement of the public, the medical profession and Whitehall. One way in which he achieved this was through maintaining his position at St Thomas's. He had contact with other doctors, access to the latest medical and scientific ideas, and continued his research into tuberculosis from this academic base. He published papers and participated in medical societies. Most importantly, he continued to find time to maintain his reputation as a 'practical sanitarian'.[17] His medical qualifications were prized at a time when the employment of experts in government was still a novelty and his professional opinions were beyond the criticism of his superiors. Above all, his communication skills, particularly his ability to influence the right people, were critical.

Simon's relationship with the medical profession was exemplary, partly because there were as yet few issues on which they could disagree with the government. Having a medical man of Simon's stature inside Whitehall was a sufficient achievement to placate most of the medical sceptics. The *British Medical Journal* and the *Lancet* were unwavering in their support for him as the 'profession personified'. His reputation was founded on his connections with international luminaries such as Justus von Liebig and Max von Pettenkofer, and his own personal achievements in practical medicine.[18] Simon realised the support that the medical profession could give and used bodies such as the British Medical

[16] Lambert, *Sir John Simon*, p. 283.
[17] Simon found time in 1870–71 to organise a model field hospital during the Franco-Prussian War. *British Medical Journal*, 1870, (II), 422. *The Times*, 17.08.1870; 23.08.1870; 06.09.1870; 14.09.1870; 23.09.1870.
[18] Justus von Liebig (1803–1873) was a German chemist who made major contributions to organic analysis and laboratory techniques. Max von Pettenkofer (1818–1901) was a German chemist and hygienist, recognised as one of the founders of epidemiology.

Association and the Medical Officers of Health Association to lobby the government for his proposals. There was a marked similarity, both in personnel and policy, in the 1850s and 1860s between Simon's Privy Council office and such professional pressure groups. The role which Edward Cator Seaton (later to become a CMO himself) played in the development of government smallpox vaccination policy exemplifies this approach. He was informed by his activities in the London Epidemiological Association, an organisation which petitioned Simon formally with its recommendations.

New powers under the 1859 Act allowed Simon to bring into his Richmond Terrace department some of his closest medical colleagues. He constructed a team around him of both medical and non-medical staff. They were completely devoted to his work and inspired by his own personal enthusiasm and commitment. He used the location of his office in Whitehall to establish frequent and informal contact with politicians, both within the Privy Council and other government departments. He called on these carefully nurtured friendships in later years when the security of his position was once again in doubt.

Staffing the new state medicine

In 1856 Simon had persuaded St Thomas's Hospital to create the first Lectureship in Public Health. It was an important initiative, which demonstrated Simon's philosophy on state medicine. He insisted that progress could only be achieved through scientific inquiry and education – both of the public and the medical profession. In addition to pushing for the creation of the lectureship, Simon was also influential in the choice of appointment. He successfully campaigned for it to be awarded to his close associate Dr Edward Headlam Greenhow (1814–1888). Simon was adept at exploiting the skills of his friends for the wider cause of public health. For example, he asked Greenhow to analyse unpublished mortality data collected by the Registrar General. Greenhow demonstrated the value of these district-level data in a report to the Social Science Congress in 1857. He also published, in 1858, *On the Study of Epidemic Disease, as Illustrated by the Pestilences of London*.[19] Simon reworked this research and published it as a parliamentary 'blue book'.

Simon employed a number of eminent medical men to conduct investigations and produce reports for him. As Lambert noted, he had 'a genuine belief in the dynamic power of mere information, in the inevitability with which accumulated knowledge would induce progress'.[20] Yet Simon insisted that information must be of the correct type, employing state-of-the-art science rather than the 'crude generalisations' previously used by Chadwickian reformers. The Registrar General's office also played a key role in providing statistical analyses in support of various conflicting sanitary theories, and was not always the ally that Simon needed.[21]

[19] EH Greenhow, *On the Study of Epidemic Disease, as Illustrated by the Pestilences of London* (London, T Richards, 1858).
[20] Lambert, *Sir John Simon*, p. 264.
[21] For a good study of the role of the Registrar General's Office, see S Szreter, 'The GRO and the Public Health Movement in Britain, 1837–1914', *Social History of Medicine*, 1991, 4, 434–6.

Once Simon had gained security of tenure for himself and for his department at the Privy Council, he began to identify deficiencies in existing public health policies. The most fundamental weakness was the way responsibilities were scattered between four of the main offices of state: the Privy Council (quarantine, and since 1858 a Medical Department), the Home Office (Factory, Burial Registration and Local Government offices), the Poor Law Board (workhouse infirmaries, medical officers, smallpox vaccination and nuisance controls) and the Board of Trade (supervision of water companies from 1852 and Alkali manufacture from 1863). There were other smaller authorities, too, which all combined to give England and Wales a much inferior system of health administration than Scotland and Ireland.[22] Linked to these different establishments were a variety of medical officers, with diverse backgrounds, duties and training. Simon wanted all of them under his direct control.

This fragmentation of responsibility was the main motivation for the formation of the Royal Sanitary Commission in 1868, but it was also set up to consider the position of the health function within the Privy Council. A 'hot house' for a variety of government initiatives (including education, and the spawning of the Board of Trade), the Privy Council's consultative function had been transformed during the 1860s to encompass a wide range of administrative and legislative duties. Parliament was no longer content to sanction its *ad hoc* growth. Simon, however, had found the fluidity of the Privy Council particularly useful. He was able to secure some of his most important initiatives through Orders in Council rather than by the tortuous parliamentary Bill route. His work was also assisted by the appointment of one of his close associates, Arthur Helps (1813–1875), as Clerk of the Privy Council in 1860.

In 1858 Simon had cemented his dominant role within the Privy Council when he was given control of the medical staff. In stressing to his political chiefs the technical nature of the work of his department, he thereby established the principle that no medical staff should be employed or allocated work without his consent. Through this significant administrative arrangement, Simon effectively emasculated the other senior civil service positions within the Privy Council such as the Permanent Secretaryship.[23] With this precedent established, and with section four of the 1859 Act allowing him to employ medical inspectors, Simon set about constructing a highly skilled and dedicated team to carry out routine and special investigations. He had met most of them through the Epidemiological Society, the Sanitary Science Association or the London hospitals. Many were already well-established public health authorities, such as Greenhow and Edward Cator Seaton (1815–1880).

Simon also recruited younger doctors at the beginning of their careers. Through this route he brought into his department, among others, George Buchanan (1831–1895), Medical Officer of Health for St Giles; John Burdon Sanderson (1828–1905), Medical Officer of Health for Paddington and John Bristowe (1827–1895), Medical Officer of Health for Camberwell and physician at St Thomas's Hospital. They provided him with a wide variety of medical and scientific skills and all were content to work for the relatively low fees offered (most were

---

[22] Lambert, *Sir John Simon*, p. 305.
[23] PC 8/139, 25.03.1868; 01.04.1868. J Simon to Duke of Marlborough re: control of medical staff.

contracted on a daily rate) for the prestige of being part of Simon's chosen band of men.[24] Simon ignored his earlier promise to the Treasury not to employ permanent Medical Inspectors. Greenhow was employed on a rolling basis full-time, as was Seaton from 1860 when he gave up his private practice in Sloane Street to begin a detailed investigation for Simon into smallpox vaccination.

By 1861 Simon was pushing so much health-related business through the Privy Council office that he was given the authority personally to sign Orders, Regulations and Directions resulting from Health and Medical Acts. He had in effect been given the status of a Permanent Secretary within the Privy Council, in charge of his own department and equal to the senior lay administrative staff. From his new position as permanent head of the Medical Department of the Privy Council, he also secured the right of constant and direct access to Ministers of State. This was a formal ratification of the informal relationship he had cultivated so carefully with his political superiors. However, Simon was astute enough to recognise that a change in government or Minister might bring into office those less inclined to allow a Medical Officer such a high degree of autonomy and he needed to insure for this eventuality.[25] This fundamental principle, of independent access to Ministers, has continued to be a cornerstone of the authority of the post of CMO.

The insecure system

Simon subsequently devoted much of his attention to the 1866 Sanitary Act, and then to the deliberations and direction of the 1868 Royal Sanitary Commission. Although this had failed to achieve its purpose of producing an integrated, comprehensive, compulsory public health system, it went some way towards furthering Simon's goals. However, despite the clear progress being made within the Department at the Privy Council, the political climate of Britain at the time was not supportive of state medicine. In July 1866, the Conservative Lords of the Privy Council suggested demoting Simon from his position as independent Secretary.[26] Although he was protected by the Lord President of the Council (the Duke of Buckingham), Simon spent an uncertain few months waiting to see if sufficient pressure could be applied by the medical profession and his other allies outside government. In 1868, the threat to his independence and authority was renewed. This time, the new Lord President, the Duke of Marlborough, did nothing to protect his Medical Officer. The earlier political acceptance of the concept of 'state medicine' seemed less substantive.

On 18 February 1868 Simon was deprived of his secretarial status and his powers of authenticating Orders were transferred to the Clerk of the Council.[27] Marlborough went further in March of that year, personally selecting a vaccination inspector without Simon's involvement. Simon complained that his technical authority was being compromised, but Marlborough retorted that Simon's proper position in the Department was not sufficiently senior to have responsi-

---

[24] C Fraser Brockington, *Public Health in the Nineteenth Century* (Edinburgh, E&S Livingstone Ltd., 1965).
[25] Second Report of the Royal Sanitary Commission, PP.1871, xxxv, Q.9767.
[26] Lambert, *Sir John Simon*, p. 409.
[27] PC 4/21. 18.02.1868.

bility for appointing staff. Although Marlborough did not venture any further involvement with the medical staffing of the Department, he deliberately frustrated Simon's plans for large-scale sanitary inquiries. In December 1868 Disraeli's Conservative Government was replaced by a Liberal administration under Gladstone and Simon once again anticipated a renewal of activity in his department, with support from this long-standing ally.

A Ministry of Health?

During his years as Medical Officer at the Privy Council Simon had been sensitive to the information and advice supplied by his team of Medical Inspectors. He changed his views on compulsory health initiatives, having witnessed the advances which had been made through the introduction of compulsory smallpox vaccination. He slowly adopted a view that rigorous and systematic local inspections, followed by compulsory remedial activity, were essential in the formulation of proper policies for sanitary reform and the development of state medicine. Simon increasingly favoured central government supremacy in areas of health policy, and concluded that the autonomy of local government could not be left unchallenged. He advocated the formation of a Ministry of Health, with a medical person (himself) as a Superintendent-General of Health. Thus, from 1868, he used his extensive networks of contacts within Whitehall (including his former colleague Robert Lowe, now Chancellor of the Exchequer) to lobby for a proper solution to the incomplete measures achieved through the 1866 Sanitary Act.[28] The fundamental weakness of this Act was the permissive nature of many of the key clauses, for example the requirement to employ local public health staff.

Simon began by demanding a thorough reorganisation of his Medical Department at the Privy Council. He wanted to secure better and more stable working conditions for his team of Medical Inspectors who were becoming increasingly frustrated with the financial and other constraints on their local investigations. Greenhow had left the team in 1862 and others were threatening to find permanent and more financially rewarding employment elsewhere. Simon successfully petitioned the Treasury to fund two permanent medical inspectorships to which he appointed George Buchanan and John Netten Radcliffe (1830–1884). In this way, he retained his two most distinguished colleagues. He also secured, in 1869, a regular grant for laboratory-based research – essential for his vision of health policies with sound scientific pedigrees.

A positive sign of the reintegration of state medicine into the British political culture came in July 1869, when the Liberal Ministers in the Privy Council passed a formal minute reinstating Simon as a Secretary in the Department, with authority to sign his own Orders.[29] He was once again in charge of medical administration and on a par with the other senior civil servants. He now began to target other governmental functions which affected his plans, including the quality of the data generated by the Registrar General's office and the work of medical officers of the Poor Law Board. The Royal Sanitary Commission of 1868 also broadly supported Simon's chosen course of action.

[28] 1866 Sanitary Act. 29 & 30 Vict. c.90.
[29] PC 4/21. 02.07.1869; T.1/1869/21,400. 07.07.1869.

From 1870 Simon embarked upon a campaign to unite all public health functions within an administration under his control. He suggested that he should have responsibility for the medical work of the Local Government Act Office, a small department also located under the administrative umbrella of the Privy Council. Simon wrote to the Home Secretary, requesting that all medically-related inquiries should be put through the Medical Department before they were delegated to the engineering and legal offices of the Local Government Act Office. He further suggested that the Home Office should consult the Medical Officer about any planned Bills and regulations which had a health component. The rationalisation of the Medical Department and the Local Government Act Office was achieved through an agreement in 1870. Simon gained much more than was at first apparent to the Whitehall administrators. He had effectively placed the medical expert above the engineering expert in the battle for control of sanitary reform and he had produced the blueprint for the anticipated revolution in local government.

The formation of the Local Government Board

Although Simon had himself benefited from some of the vague drafting of mid-nineteenth-century legislation (particularly the 1859 Public Health Act), he was unhappy with the 1871 Local Government Board Act.[30] He found himself once again subordinate to lay administrators. This Act, which had the potential to provide the skeleton 'Ministry of Health' which Simon had demanded, subsumed public health within the wider – and longer established – ideology of the Poor Law Board. The Act came out of the investigations of the 1869 Royal Sanitary Commission, which had been convened largely to placate the Sanitary Science Association and the British Medical Association. Simon later likened the mess of piecemeal sanitary legislation at the end of the 1860s as 'parquetry . . . unsafe to walk upon'.[31]

The Sanitary Commission was short-sighted in its inquiries. It took minimal evidence from those government departments which had health functions. Simon, in giving his evidence to the Commission, appeared to be hedging his bets. He favoured the association of his department with the Poor Law Board, and it is likely that he was gambling on achieving domination of the medical components of this Board (as he had done with the Local Government Act Office). He proposed keeping the Medical Department as a separate unit, under his control. He also argued that he should maintain his position as Secretary with direct and unrestricted access to Ministers. When the Royal Commission reported in 1871, it seemed to Simon that he had achieved the best of both worlds – continuation of both the powers of the 1859 Public Health Act and of his recently enlarged independent department.

In practice, however, the Royal Commission had no administrative solution for the merger of the Medical Department and the Poor Law Board which would ensure Simon's autonomy. Medical inspections were routinely carried out by the Poor Law inspectors. This made a case for the Board also to adopt the inspection work done by Simon's team. An amalgamation of medical and engineering inspection teams was inevitable. Simon by then lacked the political support

---

[30] 1871 Local Government Board Act. 34 & 35 Vict. c.70.
[31] J Simon, *English Sanitary Institutions* (London, Smith, Elder, 2nd edn, 1897), p. 323.

needed to make his mark on the new arrangements. When the Local Government Act was passed in July 1871, Simon negotiated the partial transfer of his duties to the new Board, but left at the Privy Council responsibility for regulation of the medical profession and scientific research. Simon also insisted that his post remained as Medical Officer to the Privy Council – a calculated investment to provide security if things did not go well at the new Board.[32]

The Act left the details of the new Local Government Board to the discretion of the President. James Stansfeld (1820–1898), who was appointed to this role, was sympathetic to Simon's pleas for continued authority in appointing staff and managing the work of the Medical Department. They worked together to create the 1872 Public Health Act which introduced some new public health initiatives (including the formation of Port Sanitary Authorities), and also provided for the appointment of Medical Officers of Health in all local administrative districts.[33] But the sections were vague and lacked the rigorous control which Simon was intent on securing over the local Medical Officers of Health.

With the malleable Stansfeld in post as the President of the new Local Government Board, the Prime Minister, William Gladstone (1809–1898), offered the post of Permanent Secretary as a consolation prize to his close colleague John Lambert (1815–1892, former Chief at the Poor Law Board). Lambert had been passed over for appointment as Permanent Secretary at the Treasury. Gladstone also rewarded another associate, Henry Fleming, by making him Joint Secretary with Lambert. There was little room for John Simon at this level in the new administration. *The Times* commented that the Board 'was practically the old Poor Law Board under another name'.[34] Simon's influence was radically curtailed and he lost the intimate contact with Stansfeld which would have allowed him to influence the direction of policy at the new Board. His position as adviser to Stansfeld was usurped by Edwin Chadwick and Florence Nightingale. Between them they orchestrated a campaign to move the focus of sanitary reform away from medicine and back towards the environmental strategies of the 1840s.[35]

John Lambert was a strong and influential administrator, who would not tolerate Simon's demands to retain his Medical Department intact within the new Board. Lambert's political connections and civil service status were sufficient to stifle Simon's plans and cut off his access to Ministers. In fact, the wording of the 1871 Bill had been changed. The original allowed the Acts and Instruments of the Board to be executed by the Secretary or by 'any other authorised officer'. The eventual Act permitted only Secretaries or Assistant Secretaries to perform these functions. Simon's proposals for policy and all his correspondence now passed across Lambert's desk and many of his suggestions were quietly ignored. Even worse, Stansfeld (briefed by Lambert) now argued that the 1859 Act was never intended to give Simon such wide discretionary powers, and that he had no independent authority to issue annual reports 'on his own mere notion'.[36] Simon

---

[32] Simon stipulated that £500 of his £2000 salary should be paid to him from the Privy Council budget, thus securing his continued employment with that government department. T 1/1872/6,151. 15.02.1872.
[33] 1872 Public Health Act. 35 & 36 Vict. c.79.
[34] *The Times*, 04.04.1874.
[35] Lambert, *Sir John Simon*, p. 521–3.
[36] MH 19/211. 06.04.1876, J Lambert to Treasury.

had been demoted to a subordinate position within the reformed 'Poor Law Board'. All his achievements in establishing a major role for medical expertise at the heart of government seemed to have been lost.

Simon's decision in 1869 to retain the post of Medical Officer at the Privy Council was now central to the salvation of state medicine and vindicated his tactical astuteness in creating this safe haven. His was still a statutory post-holder under the Public Health Acts of 1855 and 1859. This allowed him to report independently of superior authorities. Lambert could not touch Simon's position at the Privy Council. It gave him equality through the civil service rank of Permanent Secretary, direct access to Ministers, and, incidentally, a higher total salary than Lambert's. Simon turned his attention to regaining access to Stansfeld, by using his status as a Secretary at the Privy Council. Stansfeld began to see that he needed to have direct advice from his Medical Officer, and that Lambert's involvement was seriously hindering the work of the Local Government Board. Delays were occurring in the investigation of outbreaks of disease and in the approval of schemes for sanitary reform (such as waterworks and sewerage systems). Stansfeld stopped short of granting Simon's request for a fixed weekly meeting, and, indeed, there were numerous instances of Lambert advising on medical matters without any reference to Simon. As the *Lancet* noted: 'Mr Simon . . . has been relegated to some departmental limbo.'[37]

Despite the return of Disraeli's Conservative administration in 1874, the anti-medical stance of the Local Government Board was well-entrenched. Simon's lack of authority was regularly bemoaned by the medical and national press and the various sanitary reform pressure groups. The new President of the Local Government Board was George Sclater Booth (1826–1894) – well-intentioned towards sanitary reform but no match for Lambert's continuing dominance as Permanent Secretary. Although Simon was not allowed to resume his privilege of unrestricted Ministerial access, he at least had some influence on Sclater Booth. Once again, he was allowed to make independent reports under section five of the 1859 Public Health Act. Simon used his three annual reports between 1874 and 1876 to return to his former passionate advocacy role, in which he openly criticised the policy initiatives of his superiors at the Local Government Board.

According to his contemporaries, Simon did not cope well with being marginalised from sanitary administration at the Local Government Board. His outspoken reports were a way to vent his anger and frustration but they did not provoke the parliamentary reaction he had hoped for. He was further distanced from Lambert within the Board. It is testimony to Simon's stature within the medical profession that he continued to receive its support during a period when he had little influence with either Sclater Booth or Lambert. There was little alternative: Simon was the only potential contact for the nascent British Medical Association and other organisations. Yet it must also reflect his character and, in particular, his tenacity. He had reversed the fortunes of state medicine over a 20-year period and his continued devotion to scientific research and publication was as strong as ever. Despite the administrative frustrations, Simon was intimately involved with the production of the most important piece of health legislation of the late nineteenth century – the 1875 Public Health Act, which finally produced

---

[37] *Lancet*, 24.04.1875, (I), 582.

an acceptable degree of coherence from the existing pieces of legislation.[38] Simon preferred the big picture, rather than the routine administration which he publicly complained was 'tedious'. With the 1875 Act, Simon had delivered his vision for comprehensive sustained public health activity to address the big health problems of the time. The requirement to appoint public health officers in all local administrative districts was a particularly important measure which stood the test of time: it was not reviewed again on such a systematic scale until 1936.[39]

Simon's frustration with government attitudes to his work peaked in 1876, when the Conservative administration requested that the research undertaken at the Privy Council be transferred to the Local Government Board, and to Lambert rather than Simon's control. Simon sent Sclater Booth an ultimatum, demanding that he support all of his demands for control over staff, research and sanitary administration at the Board. He had no bargaining power, and his resignation, which Lambert had long hoped for, was willingly accepted by Sclater Booth.

Simon left office on 25 May 1876, aged 59 years, after 21 years' service in central health administration. He was awarded a civil service pension and the Companion of the Bath – perhaps a fairly paltry honour relative to his achievements.[40] His departure aroused substantial comment. *The Times* observed in a special feature article written later that summer:

> There is obviously no place for Mr Simon in a Department, or under a Government, by which science is held to be superfluous except when it is practically useless, or by which it is at best regarded as a reserve force for the rectification of blunders, or as a means of securing, in a dignified and imposing manner, the door of a stable from which the steed has already been stolen.[41]

Conclusion

Although Simon's resignation in 1876 was seen by some as an admission of defeat, he clearly no longer had the stamina to continue to battle against the system. He lacked the enthusiasm to exploit the potential offered by the Local Government Board and the new sanitary legislation for further development of public health. Unlike Chadwick, Simon did not have the patience for the 'minutiae of implementation'.[42] He lived another 28 years and continued to exert a considerable influence on the professionalisation of medicine in Britain through his position as Crown Member of the General Medical Council (1876–1895) and his election as President of the Royal College of Surgeons (1878–79). Most crucially, however, he maintained an involvement with the development of state medicine through his continued close association with three of his successors at the Local Government Board: Seaton, Buchanan and Thorne Thorne.

[38] 1875 Public Health Act. 38 & 39 Vict. c.55.
[39] 1936 Public Health Act: 'An Act to consolidate with amendments certain enactments relating to public health', 26 Geo. 5 & Edw. 8. c.49.
[40] Lambert, *Sir John Simon*, p. 571.
[41] *The Times*, 07.09.1876.
[42] C Hamlin, 'State medicine in Britain', in D Porter (ed.), *The History of Health and the Modern State* (Amsterdam, Rodopi, 1994), p. 133.

Simon's legacy was the transformation of central health administration between 1855 and 1876, making it more interventionist, exploratory and consistent. He had the vision to operate through administrative developments rather than the potentially contentious legislative procedure. He achieved a considerable degree of integration between national and local health administration: for example the introduction of accepted systems of disease surveillance and strategies for sanitary reform. This was underpinned by the main principles of public health enquiry and reporting within a predominant culture of *laissez-faire*. These principles remained unique to the Medical Department at the Local Government Board during the second half of the nineteenth century.

Simon was responsible for initiating the process of systematic verification of facts as a basis for intervention, a fundamental principle which has since become firmly established within the culture of government. Simon constructed a system in which the expert was indispensable, and this technical authority proved a dynamic force in the extension of the state's activities in the late nineteenth century. He was astute in maintaining some autonomy for his scientific research by locating it at the Privy Council.[43] Yet as Hamlin has noted, however well-intentioned Simon's vision for scientific authority in government, many of the investigations he directed were less than satisfactory. Burdon Sanderson's work on microbes in disease lacked the means to culture, isolate and identify microbes, whilst Thudichum worked without reference to new European techniques and concepts of structural organic chemistry.[44]

Yet Simon's heritage of systematic surveillance and the principle of evidence-based public health reform was substantial enough to endure the subsequent political and administrative attacks. Later CMOs were able to retain a central role in the formulation of health policy. By the early twentieth century the principle of consulting expert advisers outside Whitehall had become established practice. As will be seen in the chapters that follow, this gave the medical profession an additional relationship with the state, in which the CMO has played a pivotal role.

[43] This tradition was maintained through the formation of the Medical Research Committee in 1913, becoming in 1920 the Medical Research Council. In this way it did not become too closely associated with a political/executive department and thus remained beyond the manipulation of Ministers.

[44] Hamlin, 'State medicine in Britain', p. 150.

Chapter 2

The line of succession

By the time John Simon resigned in 1876, the post of Principal (Chief) Medical Officer had acquired a reputation as the most significant medical position in Britain, with its own integral authority. Despite the continuing lack of security and internal Whitehall confusion over its status and future, the post now carried a degree of respect which made it an attractive career goal for aspiring medical men. There was a clear sense of career progression and succession planning within the Medical Department at the Local Government Board. Although the financial incentives were weak – Simon's successors had diminished salaries – there were other rewards.

The requirement for a highly respected and competent medical professional has been perhaps the one enduring criterion for choosing a CMO. Yet as the Whitehall system became more sophisticated there was intermittent recognition that CMOs ought to have civil service experience to be effective. Likewise, as the functions of the post have incorporated increasing responsibility for health *service* policy and delivery, there has, at times, been only a loose adherence to its traditional public health heritage. This chapter explores the background to the selection of each of the fourteen CMOs, how their skills have been valued by Whitehall and Westminster, and illustrate the enduring power of personal connections and personality.

Simon's long public service was finally recognised on his retirement in 1876 with the award of the Companion of the Bath (CB). His admirers thought this insufficient but it established the precedent of conferring an award on holders of this senior civil service position. Simon was finally knighted, but ten years after his retirement. This acknowledged the CMO position as one of the most prestigious in government, equal in status to the Permanent Secretaries, who customarily received the highest levels of award in the honours system. All subsequent CMOs, with the exception of Edward Seaton (who died a few months after ill-health forced his early retirement), received a knighthood in recognition of their service. The type and timing of the honour has varied (see Table 2.1).

When Simon resigned in 1876, he left behind a small, loyal group of medical officers within the Medical Department of the Local Government Board. From this group, four of his successors were subsequently drawn. Many were his contemporaries and they had accumulated the same epidemiological knowledge and experience that Simon had acquired through his previous posts.[1]

---

[1] See J Brand, *Doctors and the State. The British Medical Profession and Government Action in Public Health, 1870–1912* (Baltimore, Johns Hopkins University Press, 1965) for a detailed study of these Local Government Board Medical Officers.

Table 2.1 Awards to CMOs

	Date of appointment	Date of departure	Date of honour	Type of honour
Simon	1855	1876	1876	CB
			1887	KCB
Seaton	1876	1879		
Buchanan	1880	1892	1892	KT
Thorne Thorne	1892	1899 (died in post)	1897	KCB
Power	1900	1908	1908	KCB
Newsholme	1908	1919	1917	KCB
Newman	1919	1935	1911	KT
			1918	KCB
			1935	GBE
MacNalty	1935	1940	1936	KCB
Jameson	1940	1950	1939	KT
			1943	KCB
			1949	GBE
Charles	1950	1960	1950	KT
			1955	KCB
Godber	1960	1973	1962	KCB
			1971	GCB
Yellowlees	1973	1984	1975	KCB
Acheson	1984	1991	1986	KBE
Calman	1991	1998	1996	KCB

CB, Companion of the Bath
KT, Knight Bachelor
KCB, Knight Commander of the Bath
KBE, Knight Commander of the British Empire
GCB, Knight Grand Cross of the Bath
GBE, Knight Grand Cross of the British Empire

Edward Cator Seaton (1815–1880), George Buchanan (1831–1895), Richard Thorne Thorne (1841–1899), and William Henry Power (1842–1916) were all recruited into the Local Government Board's Medical Department by Simon to staff his nationwide medical inspections. Simon fostered a strong *esprit de corps*. Despite his nominal superiority, he considered his colleagues equal to himself in technical ability. Perhaps this was easier because of their closeness in age – Simon was born in 1816 and outlived the next three CMOs.

By the 1870s a distinct career progression for ambitious public health doctors was emerging. This involved a period as a local Medical Officer of Health (perhaps preceded by a hospital attachment) and then progression into a medical inspectorship at the Local Government Board. The value of this experience was acknowledged by the medical community and used to sanction the philosophy of detailed local inspection which Simon championed.

After John Simon: restructuring the post of Medical Officer

When Simon resigned, the Local Government Board – and Lambert in particular – was forced to consider the statutory obligations surrounding the post of Medical Officer. The post was initially left unfilled, in breach of the 1858 Public Health Act, while Lambert considered how best to reconstruct the role so that it could not be exploited as Simon had done so successfully. The new post was in effect downgraded to a level equivalent to that of an engineering inspector in the Local Government Board. The statutory rights to initiate investigations, form policy, manage staff and issue reports were removed. The salary of the post of Medical Officer was reduced to £1,200 a year (although Simon had been receiving £2,000 by 1876). Simon's carefully protected 'department within a department' was also dismantled. The clerical and administrative staff were relocated to other departments within the Board, finally fulfilling Lambert's plans.[2]

The reconfigured post was filled by Edward Cator Seaton later in 1876. He had been one of Simon's protégés (although he was actually a year older than Simon) and had been an integral part of his team. Seaton had worked with Simon initially in the Epidemiological Society of London, where he served as Secretary and later as President. He made his epidemiological reputation through his research into smallpox, publishing *A Handbook of Vaccination* in 1868.[3] Simon had appointed him as the first vaccination inspector for London under the compulsory 1853 Vaccination Act.[4] From 1858, Seaton undertook, at Simon's request, many investigations for the Medical Department of the Privy Council. His inspectorship was made permanent in 1865 with specific responsibility for the National Vaccine Establishment.[5] He moved with Simon to the new Local Government Board in 1871 as Senior Assistant Medical Officer. When Simon resigned in 1876, Seaton's delayed succession was undisputed, albeit to a much restructured and emasculated role. The hierarchy of medical inspectorships was broken when no one was appointed to fill the vacancy he left as Senior Assistant Medical Officer.

It is likely (but impossible to prove from the remaining archives) that Seaton was deliberately chosen as Simon's successor because he lacked the professional stature and political skills necessary to secure his authority within Whitehall. His term of office as Medical Officer was short. Although Lambert was keen to quash the power of the Medical Officer, he could not deny that the Department's work was steadily increasing following the implementation of the legislation of the 1860s and 1870s. Seaton commented in early 1877: 'Eleven months' experience in the present duties of my office enable me to state that these have taxed me more than I had anticipated . . . partly because the business of the Department has been greatly increasing.'[6] In 1879, after only three years in office, he took six

[2] MH 113/7. Lambert to Smith, 29.03.1876.
[3] EC Seaton, *Handbook of Vaccination* (London, Macmillan, 1868).
[4] 1853 Vaccination Act. 16 & 17 Vict. c.100.
[5] This had been established by Parliament in 1808 to supply free vaccine and vaccination against smallpox. This was the first time the state had provided a vaccination service. The initial annual grant of £3,000 paid for the production of sufficient vaccine lymph to supply practitioners throughout the country, but in practice it struggled to keep pace with demand.
[6] MH 19/212. Seaton minute, 31.01.1877.

months' sick leave and went abroad to recuperate from 'hemiplegia' (stroke). He died in 1880, aged 65 years.[7]

Seaton was replaced by George Buchanan, who had also been brought into the Medical Department of the Privy Council as a temporary inspector in 1861 at the relatively young age of 30 years. Simon had recognised his aptitude for epidemiological investigations. He also had useful experience as Medical Officer of Health for the London district of St Giles in the 1850s and at the London Fever Hospital. Buchanan had been one of the founding members of the Association for Metropolitan Medical Officers of Health, formed in 1856 with Simon as President. Despite his initial unhappiness with the casual, temporary nature of his employment at the Privy Council (EH Greenhow had resigned over this in 1862), which was beyond Simon's control, Buchanan was persuaded to stay. He was appointed to one of the two new general health inspectorships in 1869 and moved with Simon to the Local Government Board, where he was employed on local investigations.

The intimacy of Whitehall's medical community at this time is clear from the close connections forged both professionally and socially. Buchanan married his predecessor Seaton's daughter in 1865 and they set up home in Harley Street, where he developed a private practice to supplement his income from his Privy Council inspections. When Seaton died, Buchanan had the appropriate experience and connections in London to be the natural successor. He had consciously developed his relationships with the Royal Colleges and maintained an involvement with such organisations as the Epidemiological Society.

Buchanan served as CMO for twelve years from 1880 to 1892. Over this time, the work of the Medical Department at the Local Government Board slowly regained some of the independence from the lay Secretariat that had been lost. Buchanan worked hard to redress the serious understaffing of the Medical Department. The lack of staff meant that he and his Assistant Medical Officer, John Netten Radcliffe, routinely worked six-day weeks.[8] Surprisingly, Buchanan was actively supported by Lambert in his demands to the Treasury for more funding and staff. The Treasury consistently stifled the efforts of the medical staff to conduct investigations and disseminate their findings. They refused to sanction expenditure on lithographs and illustrations for reports, and insisted on reducing the number of copies printed of each report, so that circulation was mainly within Whitehall rather than to all sanitary districts. These were essentially cost-cutting measures, but they highlight the low priority given to health at the broader governmental level.[9]

The preparation of the annual reports was always delayed and provoked criticism from the medical press which complained that Buchanan had no time to 'discuss at length any one subject of public health in the broad catholic spirit that illuminated Mr Simon's blue books'.[10] Buchanan was also unable to provide

[7] Obituaries: *Lancet*, 31.01.1880, (I), 188–9; *British Medical Journal*, 31.01.1880, (I), 188.
[8] MH 113/8. Buchanan to LGB President, 22.06.1882; representations made by the Medical Department of the Local Government Board, 01.10.1883.
[9] For a more detailed analysis of this issue, see RM McLeod, 'The frustration of state medicine, 1880–1899', *Medical History*, 1967, XI, 15–40, and RM MacLeod, *Treasury Control and Social Administration* (London, Bell and Sons, 1968).
[10] *British Medical Journal*, 28.01.1882, (I), 124.

the swift feedback that his inspectors and local authorities required. Lambert retired as Permanent Secretary in 1882 and was replaced by Hugh Owen (1835–1916), a former Poor Law clerk.[11] Sir Charles Dilke came in as the new Liberal President, and they were both generally more supportive of Buchanan and his staff, but were equally ineffective in getting additional inspectors or higher salaries from the Treasury.

When Netten Radcliffe retired in 1883, Buchanan promoted Richard Thorne Thorne to be his Assistant Medical Officer.[12] He was now so short-staffed that there was a two-year backlog of inspections. The smallpox vaccination inspection service was suffering because he had to redeploy its team to study outbreaks of other infectious diseases. Research into diphtheria was halted completely by the lack of staff. In 1885, however, the Treasury was provoked into providing additional resources by the threat of cholera. Finally, in 1887, a review into the medical staffing within the Local Government Board led to more staff, but no increase in the salaries for Medical Officers which remained out of line with those of Poor Law Officers, or medical posts outside Whitehall.

Buchanan retired at the age of 60 years in 1892, unwilling to extend his time in such an unrewarding post. He had been consistently denied any opportunity of expanding the administration he had inherited from Seaton. All his activities were hampered by Treasury control. The dislocation of the inquiry and report functions undoubtedly handicapped the understanding of infectious diseases during this period – Dr Parsons' report on the influenza epidemic of 1889–90 was not published until 1892. The *British Medical Journal* commented on the publication of the annual reports: 'Why this portentous delay should recur year after year is quite inexplicable to the public mind. Under the present dilatory method of publication, the value of the reports is sensibly diminished.'[13]

When Buchanan retired, he recommended to the Permanent Secretary that Richard Thorne Thorne should succeed him. Thorne Thorne had been employed full-time in the medical civil service since his appointment as an inspector in 1871. Like his CMO predecessors, he had previously worked for Simon on an intermittent basis during his time as a physician at the London Fever Hospital (where he was a colleague of George Buchanan). He had not been a local Medical Officer of Health, unlike his predecessors. This posed a challenge to his credibility with this important group of front-line staff. The climate was slightly more favourable at the Local Government Board by the early 1890s, partly because the 'old guard' of the former Poor Law Board had retired. A younger generation welcomed the involvement of experts in administration.[14] However, there were still crises which exposed the chronic under-resourcing of the department. The most acute was the impending cholera epidemic. Thorne Thorne used this to secure extra staff and funding for inspections, but not enough to enable him to delegate the backlog in personal workload that had accumulated. He also requested substantial increases in salaries for himself and his senior staff – an

[11] See McLeod, 'The frustration of state medicine', p. 20, and MacLeod, *Treasury Control and Social Administration*, for further details on Owen and his achievements at the Local Government Board.
[12] *Lancet*, 30.06.1883, (I), 1139.
[13] *British Medical Journal*, 14.03.1891, (I), 594.
[14] McLeod, *Treasury Control*.

issue which had rumbled on intermittently since the reductions imposed in 1876.[15]

Thorne Thorne died unexpectedly in 1899. He was 58 years old. He was widely regarded as an outstanding CMO, who had developed the nascent role inherited from Buchanan.[16] Thorne Thorne had been fully aware of the potential authority and influence of his office. Internationally, he forged sanitary agreements, representing the United Kingdom at the Sanitary Conventions in Rome in 1885, Venice (Paris sitting) in 1892, Dresden in 1893, Paris in 1894 and Venice in 1897. At home he steered the General Medical Council in drafting regulations for the training and conduct of doctors. A clear example of the prestige and authority of his CMO-ship was the wide reporting of his activities and his death in newspapers such as *The Times*. His name often appeared in the Court Circular column as well as in more routine reports of government business.

The issue of eligibility for the post of CMO remained unproblematic throughout the era of the Local Government Board. Simon had stamped such a strong impression on the office, and the attributes required to fulfil it, that there was never any serious discussion of appointing someone from outside the medical civil service. Even after the death of Thorne Thorne in 1899, his successor, William Henry Power, came from the ranks of Medical Inspectors. Power had been another of Simon's protégés. He had joined the inspectoral team in 1871 and his position was made permanent in 1875. In 1887 he was promoted to Assistant Medical Inspector with responsibility for training junior medical staff. A gifted epidemiologist, he appears to have had a fairly minor role in the management of the department until his succession as CMO in 1899.[17] Power's career undoubtedly benefited from his close friendship with Buchanan. Buchanan's daughter recalled his frequent visits to the family home in London at 24 Nottingham Place. He would often call in the morning from his home on the north side of Regent's Park to accompany Buchanan on his walk to the office in Parliament Street and return with him in the evening.[18]

A bigger pool: the appointment of 'external' CMOs

When Power retired in 1908 there was a marked change in recruitment policy. Power was regarded as a competent CMO, but some suggest that his reticence in building relationships outside the Local Government Board was unhelpful to the medical profession and the progression of public health policies.[19] When Power's retirement was imminent, the President of the Local Government Board, the progressive John Burns (1858–1943), head-hunted the pioneering Medical Officer of Health for Brighton, Arthur Newsholme (1857–1943). Burns thought

[15] MH 113/8. Thorne Thorne to Buchanan, 16.01.1888.
[16] Obituaries: *British Medical Journal*, 23.12.1899, (II), 1771–3; *Lancet*, 23.12.1899, (II), 1748–9, 1762–6; *Transactions of the Epidemiological Society of London* n.s. vol. 19, 1899–1900, 210–13; *Dictionary of National Biography Supplement III*, (London, 1901), p. 382.
[17] Obituaries: *Lancet*, 05.08.1916, (II), 244–6; *British Medical Journal*, 05.08.1916 (II), 203–7.
[18] A Smith, *A Memoir of the Buchanan Family and in particular of George Buchanan KT 1831 to 1895*. (Private printing at Aberdeen University Press, 1941, manuscript in the British Library.)
[19] MacLeod, *Treasury Control*, pp. 38–54. Power obituaries: *Lancet*, 05.08.1916, (II), 244–6.; *British Medical Journal*, 05.08.1916, (II), 203–7.

that Newsholme would bring a fresh, innovative approach to the role of CMO and would be supportive of the new Liberal 'welfare system' which was currently being developed.[20] Although Beatrice Webb sought to claim the credit that she had pushed Newsholme into Burns' gaze, Burns had previously offered him a position as a Medical Inspector.[21] On that occasion, Newsholme had declined. The offer of the top post, which would give him unprecedented involvement in the formulation of health policy of national importance, could not so easily be refused. Burns was deliberately rejecting the senior internal 'candidates' Franklin Parsons and Bruce Low, a position that upset senior civil servants and the Medical Department. In contrast, the medical and popular press welcomed the prospect of a genuine outsider becoming CMO.[22]

Administrative inertia pervaded the cumbersome Local Government Board at the beginning of the twentieth century, but the transition from 'sanitarianism' to a new focus on personal medical services was gathering momentum. In 1905, the Liberal Government of Lloyd George started to introduce a range of welfare policies, including school medical inspections and clinics for infant and child welfare, tuberculosis as well as sexually transmitted diseases. The *Lancet* noted the challenge for the new CMO, Newsholme, in 1908. The post, it commented, was 'the highest and the most onerous' in public service, and adding 'it would be interesting to know how many schemes of constructive sanitary policy in matters both large and small, which have entailed endless inquiry and work by Simon's successors, could be unearthed from the Board's pigeonholes'.[23] Newsholme's memoirs, published in 1936, record the unremitting distractions of reading reports (some 13,000 papers in 1908–09), daily communications with Medical Officers of Health and receiving official delegations on health issues. With an ever-increasing workload, he found limited time for strategic planning.[24] There were also demands for the CMO to be involved in the growing field of inter-national public health policy.

Newsholme's tenure as the last CMO under this old regime helped to forge a closer relationship between state and medical profession, in part driven by the increasing state provision of medical services. The most significant innovation was the Panel Doctors Scheme. This enabled medical services and sickness benefit to be distributed under the 1911 National Insurance Act.[25] The CMO had helped to plan all these developments in state medicine. This cemented a new role of intermediary between Whitehall and the medical profession.[26]

The extension in state medicine challenged not only the vested interests of the medical profession (provision of services such as infant and child healthcare had

[20] An additional impetus to go 'outside' the LGB for a replacement was because the two most senior staff under Power (Franklin Parsons and Bruce Low) were also nearing retirement age.
[21] JM Eyler, *Sir Arthur Newsholme and State Medicine* (Cambridge, Cambridge University Press, 1997), p. 219.
[22] Ibid., p. 221. Eyler cites an article in the *London Daily News* 'Dr Newsholme's Appoint-ment and What it Means', 20.01.1908, p. 6.
[23] *Lancet*, 25.01.1908, (I), 242.
[24] A Newsholme, *The Last Thirty Years in Public Health* (London, George Allen & Unwin Ltd, 1936), p. 50.
[25] 1911 National Insurance Act. 1 & 2 Geo V. c.55.
[26] Eyler, *Newsholme*, pp. 227–38.

formed part of their income), but also increased antagonism between several government departments over control of these new public services. The Local Government Board had the responsibility for most medical aspects of central government, its legitimacy reinforced by being home to Simon and his successors.[27] Yet by the First World War, the Board of Education (created in 1902), prompted by its Medical Officer George Newman, demanded control over infant welfare work, as a natural adjunct to its provision of school medical inspections. A prolonged, bitter dispute between these two Whitehall departments ensued. At its heart was the personal rivalry of their respective Chief Medical Officers. Arthur Newsholme had been appointed to the established post at the Local Government Board in 1908. George Newman (1870–1948), only a year earlier, had become CMO at the Board of Education, a new post.

Newman, his counterpart's junior by thirteen years, was a formidable rival. Well-versed in manipulating influential people to secure promotion, he was at home and politically well-connected within the Board of Education. His record of research on infant mortality, and his experience as Medical Officer of Health for the London Borough of Finsbury, were strengths. Yet he had little experience of school medical inspection. His appointment was seen by some as the result of lobbying by his supporters (the Webbs and Morant again). James Kerr, the School Medical Officer for the London County Council, claimed that he himself had already been promised the post.[28] Ironically, Newman had called on Newsholme to rally support for him from the public health community, through the journal *Public Health* (which Newsholme edited from Brighton).

As CMO to the Board of Education, Newman initially had fruitful working relationships with the CMOs at the Local Government Board, first Power and then Newsholme. For example, he welcomed Newsholme's advice on the development of the new school medical inspectorate, putting his long-standing interest in school hygiene into practice.[29] They agreed that school medical inspection should be integrated as a public health function with the work of local Medical Officers of Health, rather than being a 'stand alone' activity. Newman reinforced this message through an official Circular Letter.[30]

Newsholme should have had greater authority in state medicine than the fledgling Newman, given the range of services under his jurisdiction as CMO. However, the expansion of the Local Government Board had resulted in a stultifying administration. In contrast, politicians and senior civil servants saw the Board of Education as young and flexible; a good environment to nurture policies.[31] The harmony did not last long: 'With each passing year Newman needed Newsholme and the Local Government Board less, and his own political sense alerted him to much greater opportunity through an independent

---

[27] Some duties stayed with other departments, for example medical research with the Privy Council.

[28] *British Medical Journal*, 21.09.1907, (II), 760–1. 'The attitude of the Board of Education to school hygiene'.

[29] Newsholme had published a textbook on school hygiene in 1887, and an influential editorial in the *British Medical Journal*, 14.11.1903, (II), 1288, which he claimed authorship for in *Fifty Years*, p. 391.

[30] Board of Education circular 576, 22.11.1907. Quoted in *Lancet*, 30.11.1907, (II), 1557.

[31] C Bellamy, *Administering Central–Local Relations, 1871–1919: the Local Government Board in its fiscal and cultural context* (Manchester, Manchester University Press, 1988).

course.'[32] Newman cultivated the political world much more assiduously than Newsholme, aware that his career ambitions depended upon it. His diaries detail the minutiae of his contact with politicians and his interpretation of Whitehall gossip.[33] Even in 1908, his first year as CMO to the Board of Education, he was actively seeking opportunities for contact with Lloyd George (then Chancellor of the Exchequer). His reward was entry to an inner circle which discussed plans for national health insurance:

> A wonderful day w. Lloyd George . . . Ll.Geo. & the Tuberc. Children. He offered me the Vice Chairmanship of the Insurance Commission. We discussed the [National Insurance] Bill – Sanatoria, Health Committees, Children. He wished me to start the Insurance Scheme & afterwards to go to LGB. as Chf. M.O. I declined provisionally. He pressed me a great deal & so I said I wd. think abt. It. But it filled me w. anxiety and trouble. I said I wd. only go to LGB if I cd. take the chn. w. me.

On the same page of his diary he also pencilled a note:

> Lloyd George's ideas! for me!! L.G.B. & Ho. of Lords![34]

Newman's close contact with government Ministers led to offers of various promotions. In 1913, he declined the Chairmanship of the Board of Control for Lunacy and Mental Deficiency. Later the same year, his refusal to become Secretary of the Medical Research Council secured him a higher salary and more research funds for the Board of Education. By 1914 the dispute with Newsholme over the control for infant and children's health services had reached an impasse. Adjudication by Lord Haldane did not improve relations between the Boards and their respective CMOs.[35]

By this time, however, there was tentative exploration of the possibility of forming a 'Ministry of Health'. This was a piece of government machinery which Simon had tried for 60 years earlier. The Local Government Board and the Board of Education continued to wrangle over infant welfare through the First World War, but preparations continued and were put to the Cabinet in April 1917 by the President of the Local Government Board. Christopher Addison (1869–1951), one of Lloyd George's closest advisers on health, was the driving force behind the planning, but he was actually Minister of Munitions (and from July 1918, Minister of Reconstruction). Addison drafted the Ministry of Health Bill and was understood to be lined up as the first Minister of Health.

Newman was already well-acquainted with Addison through their work together at the Board of Education (where Addison had been Parliamentary Secretary) and also through his keen observation of Liberal party politics. Chief

[32] Eyler, *Newsholme*, p. 320.
[33] Newman's diaries are held at the National Archives (MH 139/1–6). They provide a very detailed account of his professional and social life. The historian Bentley Gilbert used them extensively for his study of the development of the British welfare state because there were so few other detailed accounts: BB Gilbert, *British Social Policy, 1914–1939* (London, Cornell University Press, 1970).
[34] MH 139/1. Newman diary, 05.11.1911.
[35] Eyler, *Newsholme*, p. 327.

Medical Officer at the planned Ministry of Health was Newman's next career target.[36] It was obvious that the separate health functions at the Board of Education and the Local Government Board would be merged. After all, the chronic in-fighting had been one of the stimuli for the creation of a dedicated Ministry. Newman's diaries reveal a frenetic period, late in 1916, of lobbying both of Ministers and senior civil servants. His candidacy was strengthened with Lloyd George's succession as Prime Minister (replacing Asquith) in January 1917. The challenge was how to move Newman into the new Ministry as CMO, with Addison as Minister and Robert Morant (1863–1920) as Permanent Secretary. The sticking point was what to do with Newsholme. Newman brusquely dismissed the idea that he could stay: his diary recorded that Newsholme was 'weak, vacillating, incompetent, untrustworthy and vain'.[37] He could only have conveyed similar sentiments to his government colleagues.

On 11 January 1919 Addison became President of the Local Government Board. From that position he must have made clear to Newsholme that Newman would be coming into the new Ministry. Newsholme would not serve under Newman and Addison therefore asked for him to retire. Newsholme at 62 years could have stayed until the then mandatory civil service retirement age of 65 years. When he eventually retired at the end of March 1919, he maintained a dignified silence on his removal and on his successor.[38] John Eyler's excellent biography of Newsholme rebalances inaccurate contemporary and historical assessments of his career, some of which were the deliberate result of Newman's own campaign for promotion.[39] These views, such as the accusation that Newsholme mismanaged the 1918 influenza epidemic, were perpetuated by historians like Frank Honigsbaum.[40] Other historians have painted a much more positive, dynamic picture of Newsholme. Gerry Kearns, for example, examines his innovative approach to tuberculosis as part of a 'family' of social diseases.[41]

Newman once again argued for the status and remuneration of the new post. He secured a higher salary and the rank of Secretary, which he had held at the Board of Education. He also took with him to the new Ministry the title of Chief Medical Officer. Newsholme's title (and that of his predecessors) had officially been Principal Medical Officer to the Local Government Board. Newman was eminently qualified to succeed Newsholme as the government's senior medical adviser. Since his appointment to the Board of Education in 1907, he had in effect been a second senior medical adviser, and had outranked Newsholme in civil service status. He even received his knighthood before Newsholme, in the 1911 New Year's Honours List. Addison and Lloyd George had been waiting for

[36] M Hammer, *The Building of a Nation's Health: the life and work of George Newman to 1921* (Unpublished D Phil. Thesis, University of Cambridge, 1995).

[37] MH 139/1. Newman diary, 29.10.1918.

[38] MH 78/92. Monro to Meiklejohn (Assistant Secretary, Treasury), 8.3.1919. See Eyler's *Newsholme* for a detailed account of Newman's scheming to replace Newsholme, and for Newsholme's subsequent 'third career' as an international public health statesman.

[39] JM Eyler, *Newsholme*.

[40] F Honigsbaum, *The Struggle for the Ministry of Health, 1914–1919*, Occasional Papers on Social Administration No.37 (London, G Bell, 1970).

[41] G Kearns, 'Tuberculosis and the medicalisation of British Society, 1880–1920', in J Woodward and R Jutte (eds), *Coping with Sickness: historical aspects of health care in a European perspective* (Sheffield, EAHMH Publications, 1995), pp. 145–70.

Newsholme's retirement since 1916, and his KCB in January 1917 was intended by the Prime Minister to be seen as a 'parting gift'.[42]

Newman's promotion to CMO at the Local Government Board on 1 April 1919 was the career pinnacle that he had relentlessly pursued. The potential authority which the post held within the Ministry of Health, which was constituted three months later, was reflected in the strong political interest shown by Cabinet members and influential pressure groups in the appointment.[43] Despite the extraordinary manoeuvring to create a 'dream team' for the new Ministry, it held together for only a year. Morant, the Permanent Secretary, died from influenza in March 1920 and Addison was forced to resign as Minister in 1921. Newman appeared to burn out, and his sixteen years as CMO did not produce the widely anticipated innovations in policy.[44] Perhaps the personality clashes with subsequent Permanent Secretaries (as discussed in Chapter 3) hampered him. Certainly, his self-confidence within the Whitehall machine was not evident to all. The *British Medical Journal*'s obituary for him in 1948 noted that:

> Entering the civil service at as late an age as 37, Sir George Newman never quite accommodated himself to its practice and traditions, which, with all their virtues and limitations have meant so much to the country. He was always the medical man rather than the civil servant . . .[45]

There was great irony in this statement. Newman had persistently eschewed the idea that government health policy should be made on medical criteria alone. He argued that it needed to reflect the impact of economic and social determinants of health.[46] Although he championed medicine and especially the triumph of scientific medicine, he was surprisingly blinkered to the politically unwelcome reports that linked high infant and maternal mortality in the 1930s to low family incomes. He also ignored the weight of evidence for diphtheria immunisation, which was delayed in Britain until 1942. This was 20 years after the success of the Canadian programme, although the delay mainly had to do with the financial constraints of inter-war governments.[47] Newman's later annual reports exude an

[42] MH 139/1. Newman diary, 20.02.1917. Eyler makes no mention of the circumstances or significance of Newsholme's KCB award. Newsholme in his memoirs simply notes the honours that he had received during his latter years as CMO, specifically mentioning his election to the Athenaeum Club in the same year that he was awarded the KCB, under rule II, which 'authorises the Committee of the Club to elect not more than nine new persons each year of distinguished eminence in science . . . for public services'. A Newsholme, *The Last Thirty Years in Public Health* (London, Allen and Unwin Ltd, 1936), p. 30.

[43] House of Lords Records Office, Lloyd George papers D/20/1/6 letter from Newman 30.05.1915; C/4/12/5 letter from Joseph Peace 24.04.1914.

[44] S Stacey, *The Ministry of Health 1919–1929: ideas and practice in a government department* (Unpublished D Phil., University of Oxford, 1984).

[45] *British Medical Journal*, 1948, (I), 1112.

[46] S Sturdy, 'Hippocrates and state medicine: George Newman outlines the founding policy of the Ministry of Health', in C Lawrence and G Weisz (eds), *Greater than the Parts: holism in biomedicine* (Oxford, Oxford University Press, 1998), pp. 112–34.

[47] J Lewis, 'The prevention of diphtheria in Canada and Britain, 1914–1945', *Journal of Social History*, 1986, 20, 163–76; C Webster, 'Healthy or hungry thirties?', *History Workshop Journal*, 1982, 5, 110–29; J Lewis, *The Politics of Motherhood: child and maternal welfare in England, 1900–1939* (London, Croom Helm, 1980).

air of complacency, of the 'inevitability of progress'. Perhaps this reflected the stultifying culture of the Ministry, or his own lack of vision. A golden opportunity for the development of health policy was slowly smothered by Newman's determination to cling on to authority (and status) for as long as he could.

1935: MacNalty vs. Jameson

Newman retired aged 65 years in 1935. The Ministry of Health was by then the acknowledged (if slightly emasculated) epicentre of health policy, co-ordinating related activities at the Board of Education and other government departments. A steady growth in local authority health services incorporated Poor Law hospitals from 1929. Newman's successor, Arthur MacNalty (1880–1969), stepped into a greatly expanded administration. He was an established medical civil servant of sixteen years' standing. Although the Ministry had expanded its staff, it was still low status and vulnerable to control by the powerful Treasury (dominated by its Permanent Secretary Sir Warren Fisher from 1919 to 1939). The Ministry of Health was not an attractive option for high-flying civil servants. One historian called it 'a monolithic and pyramidal administrative class with authority vested exclusively in its apex'.[48] This was in part Newman's legacy. The Ministry was 'a career backwater staffed by second-rate minds suitable to act only as instruments of regulation'.[49]

Like his predecessors, MacNalty had been a local Medical Officer of Health (at Essex County Council) before being hand-picked by Newsholme to join his team at the Local Government Board in 1913. At the inception of the Ministry of Health in 1919 he was Deputy Senior Medical Officer and in 1932, he became the first Deputy CMO. The post carried special responsibility for the co-ordination of the work of the medical staff.[50] This new post of Deputy CMO suggests the planning of a 'line of succession' within the medical civil service. Certainly previous appointments had generally been easy to predict from within the ranks of junior staff, notwithstanding the tussle between Newsholme and Newman. Now, by the early 1930s, there was a deputy role with a clear opportunity for someone to gain experience and make their mark as a potential future CMO. Yet even while MacNalty was being promoted internally, senior civil servants and politicians were looking elsewhere for Newman's successor. MacNalty, at 55 years, was comparatively old to fill this senior post. There were doubts, too, about his energy, drive and vision.

Whilst still in post, Newman had suggested a different successor: Wilson Jameson, Dean at the London School of Hygiene and Tropical Medicine (LSHTM). Newman was close to Jameson, seeing himself as mentor and friend to the younger public health academic. He was on the Board of Management at the LSHTM and well-acquainted with Jameson's talent. Newman's diaries record a number of social events between the pair and their wives. It is not clear whether

[48] Stacey, *The Ministry of Health*, pp. 141–4.
[49] C Webster, 'Conflict and consensus: explaining the British Health Service', *Twentieth Century British History*, 1990, 1, 115–51.
[50] MH 107/27. Establishment file for A MacNalty. 11.01.1933. Minute from Minister requesting the appointment of a deputy to the CMO, proposing that one of the current Senior Medical Officers be appointed with an additional allowance of £200 p.a.

Newman may have fallen out with MacNalty, or whether he seriously thought that his deputy was unsuited to the job. Although Jameson was short-listed in 1935, he was considered to lack the breadth of experience (and, crucially, in the civil service) to be appointable. It cannot have helped Jameson's candidacy that he was known to be negative about the Ministry's culture: 'The whole atmosphere is like a poorly run girl's school.'[51] This was a thinly-disguised reference to the chronic bickering between the medical and administrative staff, which had persisted since John Simon's era.[52]

MacNalty served for only five years, retiring as the eighth CMO, aged 60 years, in 1940. His early retirement, never fully explained, presented difficulties for the Ministry of Health. He asked to be given office space for his role as editor of the official medical history of the Second World War. He remained in the Ministry building, working on such projects for many years after his retirement as CMO. MacNalty was more caretaker than active policy maker, although he did help plan the wartime Emergency Medical Services.[53] However, on the crucial issues during these five years – the regionalisation of hospital services and the extension of state responsibility for healthcare – MacNalty was ominously silent. George Godber, a later CMO, recalls that MacNalty was 'an able physician but ineffective in the department. I suspect that he had been selected for the leadership to weaken the independence of the medical establishment'.[54] His name does not appear in discussion papers produced by the various think-tanks such as the Nuffield Provincial Hospitals Trust or the King's Fund, and the CMO is an almost invisible character in the histories of this formative period in the development of the NHS.[55] Newman's diary gives some insight into how he viewed MacNalty's appointment. He recounts his final pre-retirement meeting with the Prime Minister, Ramsay MacDonald:

> I thanked him for the GBE which Hilton had told me of. P.M. said he had not heard of it! . . . asked about my successor, assumed he had been nominated by me! I cleared his mind on that point, at wh. he expressed great surprise.[56]

MacNalty seems to have worried little about the falling reputation of the medical staff within the Department at that time. The historian Frank Honigsbaum, for example, scathingly assessed the contribution of Sir Weldon Dalrymple Champneys, then a Senior Medical Officer, and by implication the calibre of the Ministry's medical staff, more generally:

> He was a dilettante, known as a 'playboy' within the department, who had no experience of clinical practice or panel negotiations. The son of Sir Francis Champneys, the venerable obstetrician . . . his progress

[51] NM Goodman, *Wilson Jameson, Architect of National Health* (London, George Allen and Unwin, 1970), p. 81.

[52] For more discussion on this, see Chapter 3.

[53] CL Dunn, *The Emergency Medical Services*, vol. 1 (London, HMSO, 1952).

[54] Godber interview, 25.08.04.

[55] D Fox, *Health Policies, Health Politics: the British and American Experience, 1911–1965* (Princeton NJ, Princeton University Press, 1985); C Webster, *The Health Services Since the War*, vol. 1 (London, HMSO, 1988).

[56] MH 139/6. Newman diary, 28.03.1935.

within the Ministry probably owed more to his father's reputation than to his own. He was more interested in animal than human disease and was passed over twice for CMO . . . According to Godber, who shared an office with him, he never received an assignment that stretched his abilities.[57]

Jameson: 'the nation's doctor'

In 1940, Wilson Jameson was once again invited to apply for the post of CMO. He had by then acquired Whitehall experience (part-time medical adviser to the Colonial Office, chairmanship of the Medical Research Council Committees on Industrial Health and Preventive Medicine, and the Medical Advisory Committees to the armed services); also, there were no suitable internal candidates. This time the approach was made by the Minister of Health, Malcolm MacDonald, who had already consulted senior members of the medical profession including Lord Dawson, Sir Farquhar Buzzard, Sir Edward Mellanby and Sir George Newman.[58]

Jameson had accumulated, quite deliberately, an enormous range of experience in all types of medical posts and was ideally equipped for the post of CMO. An Aberdeen graduate, he came south to the Prince of Wales Hospital in Tottenham in 1909, then worked at the City of London Hospital for Diseases of the Chest in 1910. These were 'voluntary' hospitals, maintained through charitable donations and friendly society subscriptions. Jameson returned to Aberdeen in 1912 to obtain his MD (a thesis on hospital treatment of tuberculosis) and then expanded his medical training with a year's general practice in Eastbourne. He served as Junior Assistant Medical Officer to a Poor Law Union hospital in Hackney whilst simultaneously reading for his membership of the Royal College of Physicians, which he duly obtained in July 1913. A year later he was on the move again, to an Assistant Medical Officership to the Metropolitan Asylums Board at a Chelsea outpost of the Western Hospital for Infectious Diseases.

Jameson also continued part-time study: during 1914 he had attended the Diploma in Public Health Course at University College under Professor HR Kenwood. After obtaining his Diploma he began to lecture part-time for Kenwood, combining this with the post of Deputy Medical Officer of Health in Stoke Newington. The shortage of medical staff during the First World War enabled Jameson to run a new Hygiene Laboratory at the Army School of Sanitation at Aldershot, where he also researched. He was posted to France (and later Italy) in 1917.

Within the short space of seven years – and during unique wartime conditions – Jameson had gained the qualifications he needed to pursue a career in public health, and had accrued excellent experience in a range of hospital, local authority and academic posts. He further consolidated his professional reputation through appointments to various part-time teaching and examining posts, and wrote a textbook of hygiene for medical students.[59] His most significant appointment by then (the autumn of 1919) was as Medical Officer of Health and School

[57] F Honigsbaum, *Health, Happiness and Security* (London, Routledge, 1989), p. 214.
[58] Goodman, *Jameson*, p. 81; MH 139/6. Newman diary, 08.08.1940.
[59] W Jameson, *Synopsis of Hygiene* (London, Messrs Churchill, 1920).

Medical Officer in Finchley, London. From 1920 he also served as Deputy Medical Officer of Health for St Marylebone. Here, his chief, Dr Charles Porter, was well-known for his progressive views on health education and stimulating annual reports.

Jameson's broad interests extended to medical politics: a year after his appointment as a Medical Officer of Health, he formed a branch of the British Medical Association in Finchley and became its first Secretary.[60] Two years later, in 1922, he was called to the Bar, having joined Middle Temple and gained a third-class qualification. In later years, Jameson was sceptical on the merits of a Medical Officer of Health having a legal training, claiming that it was an unnecessary duplication of talent, which might not be looked on favourably by the Town Clerk. He had also described, though, his legal training as 'the most valuable education he ever had'.[61] His progression in the world of public health was achieved piecemeal, following a path which many CMOs have taken. In 1925, he moved as Medical Officer of Health to Hornsey, a bigger London Borough with a bigger salary, where he continued to produce innovative schemes. A health education campaign for clean food, the first of its kind in Britain, was launched on his behalf by the Minister of Health, Neville Chamberlain.

Four years later, he abandoned this practical public health career to move to the London School of Hygiene and Tropical Medicine as Professor of Public Health. He was made Dean in 1931, and during the next nine years worked to construct effective links between the LSHTM and the Ministry of Health. After useful experience as an adviser in Whitehall to the Colonial Office, he was almost over-endowed in the qualities and experience appropriate to the CMO post.

Jameson, 'at very short notice', became CMO on 12 November 1940.[62] He was still very reluctant to move to the Ministry of Health, and eventually agreed only after MacDonald personally stressed that he could not develop the plans for the post-war medical service without his help. Godber also succinctly noted in Jameson's obituary that he went to the Ministry 'as a duty rather than from inclination'.[63] His time was taken up almost immediately with emergency wartime arrangements for the City of London. In February 1941, for example, he set up an Epidemic Committee to study the spread of disease in air-raid shelters, which he visited most evenings as part of an inspection along with the Minister of Health, Malcolm MacDonald.

Jameson served for ten years until he reached the then official civil service retirement age of 65 years in 1950. He had successfully managed the wartime medical services, mediated the medical profession's participation in the National Health Service, and rejuvenated the reputation of the Ministry through his reorganisation of the Medical Department and employment of first-class staff. Through his innovative approach to communication, especially the use of radio broadcasts, he can without doubt be heralded as the first 'nation's doctor'. These achievements are discussed in more detail in Chapters 5 and 7.

---

[60] Goodman, *Jameson,* p. 49.

[61] Ibid., p. 50.

[62] Ibid., p. 82. Although I have found no reference in Ministry papers which substantiates that the appointment was made in a rush.

[63] *British Medical Journal,* 27.10.1962, (II), 1132.

Charles and Godber: succession crises

John Charles, who succeeded Jameson in 1950, had, like most other CMOs, been brought into the Ministry by his predecessor. His academic and practical work as Medical Officer of Health for Newcastle-upon-Tyne brought him an invitation from Jameson and he moved to Whitehall in 1944 as Deputy CMO, assisting in the detailed planning for the NHS. Charles' letter to Jameson, written after an informal discussion at the Athenaeum Club in March 1944, typifies his unassuming and hesitant demeanour:

> It has not been easy to decide, but I feel I should be guilty of a lack of proper spirit and courage if I declined to allow my name to go forward for consideration . . . I can only hope that your confidence in me will be justified. Personally I know that there is no one under whom I would more gladly do my share of the work of the days to come.[64]

No one thought that the other Deputy CMO, Sir Weldon Dalrymple-Champneys, the subject of Honigsbaum's deconstruction, would succeed Jameson. In contrast to his predecessors, Charles was a quiet CMO. His devotion to international health affairs and the ineffective civil service support he received (see Chapter 3) meant that he appeared to lack enthusiasm for internal matters at the Ministry. The government, however, found him a congenial CMO, particularly in his reluctance to antagonise the tobacco industry and the Treasury over the new research on links between smoking and health. His weakness on smoking is the most likely explanation for his remaining in post until the age of 67 years – two years after the mandatory civil service retirement limit.[65]

Charles' deputy, George Godber, had meanwhile been cultivating the sort of wide-ranging relationships which were crucial to a successful CMO. He came into contact with Jameson when he studied for the Diploma in Public Health at the London School of Hygiene and Tropical Medicine. He then worked in regional administration in the Ministry of Health, before being called to London to act as Jameson's personal assistant. His succession to Charles was a natural, if delayed, progression: he finally took over in 1960, serving as CMO for thirteen years until his retirement aged 65 years in 1973. There was, however, some dissonance: John Pater, the influential senior civil servant, tried to block Godber's appointment, whereas the eminent physician Henry Cohen (later Lord Cohen of Birkenhead) actively campaigned for Godber and claimed the credit when he became CMO. According to one close colleague of Godber's, it caused a long-term rift between the two, which was not healed before Cohen's death in 1977.[66]

Godber is considered by many to be the greatest of the CMOs. Godber himself gives that accolade to Wilson Jameson. It has been suggested that Godber's very success in the role of CMO, and especially the authority he wielded with the medical profession, made the choice of his successor a difficult one. He had become one of the most influential figures in British medicine, pushing perhaps

---

[64] MH 107/66. Charles Establishment file. Letter from Charles to Jameson, 09.04.1944.
[65] Senior medical civil servant interview, 13.07.1999. See also MH 107/66; Ministry of Health memo 25.06.1958: 'The Secretary has told me that the CMO would like to stay on for two years or so anyway, and we are content that he should.'
[66] Senior civil servant interview, 17.05.2000.

the conventional boundaries expected of the senior medical civil servant.[67] Certainly, when the short-list was drawn up for his replacement, the candidates seemed less substantial figures in comparison. Godber himself was actively involved in the succession planning. He had clearly been grooming Henry Yellowlees to take over upon his retirement. He had brought Yellowlees into the Department in 1963 as a Principal Medical Officer, and promoted him to Deputy CMO in 1967. Yet, as he neared retirement, Godber seems to have had second thoughts. Junior staff in the Department have commented that this was probably no more than a symptom of his desire for total control and not specific to Yellowlees: 'The nearer people got to having positions of responsibility the more George felt they weren't quite up to it.'[68]

Godber's style of management had already caused some difficulties within the bureaucracy and illustrates the problem of planning his replacement. He insisted on opening all his own post and dictating replies without involving the usual administrative machinery. Thus, members of the Department would subsequently find that there had been significant developments in areas which they nominally had responsibility for, which they had not been briefed about. One of Godber's senior staff recalled that she used to try and limit the 'fallout' by staying late in the office and going through the carbon copies of his correspondence so that she could give concerned parties some advance warning on what he had been planning.[69]

However, at the end of 1971 Godber used his weekly meetings with the Deputy CMOs to begin to discuss the burden of the workload which he carried as CMO. He put forward a scheme to create an additional CMO post – CMO2. Yellowlees was unhappy with several aspects of this plan, in particular the failure to define the roles of the Deputy CMOs and existing heads of divisions (Senior Permanent Medical Officers), and because he thought that it would create difficulties in lines of communication. He voiced these objections, but the plans continued to be developed along Godber's preferred lines.

Godber's doubts about his successor were perhaps also exacerbated by Yellowlees' recent period of ill-health, specifically a period of six weeks recovering from a serious coronary thrombosis in August 1972, and he clearly began to consider the potential of the other Deputy CMO, John Reid. Reid and Yellowlees each had different aptitudes. Yellowlees was well-known in the medical community and was strong on administration. Reid, in contrast, had the traditional public health pedigree, including the Diploma in Public Health and previous employment as a county Medical Officer of Health, which Yellowlees lacked. Reid was a highly respected public health academic, a qualification which Godber thought essential to the post of CMO.

Thus, when Yellowlees was discharged from hospital in September 1972 he learned that Godber had persuaded the Civil Service Department to create a new post of second Chief Medical Officer (shortened to CMO2), and that he was to be appointed to it. Although he had reservations about this strategy, Yellowlees accepted the revised post. According to senior staff who worked with Godber and

---

[67] Godber developed a reputation for inviting opinions from junior medical staff, and for his refusal to delegate work as his predecessors had done.

[68] Senior medical civil servant interview, 17.03.2000.

[69] Senior medical civil servant interview, 26.11.1999.

Yellowlees at the time, this was a traumatic period. Yellowlees felt deeply hurt that his 'inheritance' had been subdivided with Reid. In the event, this turned out to be a short, if uncomfortable, period for the Department. In March 1973 10 Downing Street announced that Godber would be retiring on 30 November and that he would be succeeded as CMO by Henry Yellowlees.

During the summer of 1973 when both Godber and Reid were away from the Department, Yellowlees set to work on his preferred staffing structure. He circulated a working paper on 6 July to Sir Phillip Rogers (Department Permanent Secretary), Mr Osmond (the Establishment Officer), with a copy Godber on his return. This paper made it clear that on Yellowlees' accession on 1 December 1973, his own vacated post of CMO2 would not be filled. Godber tried to get the paper rejected but failed.[70] Reid was thus left at the rank of Deputy CMO, which, it should be said, he had been in for less than a year. He finally got his CMO appointment in Scotland in 1977, with the encouragement and support of Yellowlees, who also arranged for him to take over the role as UK representative at the World Health Organization in Geneva – a responsibility previously held by the English CMO.

As one former senior civil servant succinctly put it, when Yellowlees became CMO 'he was still working in the shadow of the oak tree'.[71] If his appointment had been pushed through by the civil service to give them a more malleable CMO, then the plan had probably succeeded. Yellowlees' authority suffered because he was seen by the medical profession as essentially the government's doctor, rather than their representative – a dual role which Godber had played with ease. The government's view of Yellowlees was, however, perhaps the reverse: he was side-lined from some negotiations because they felt he was too close to the profession (see Chapter 5).

There had also been some internal dissatisfaction with the way in which Godber had brought Yellowlees into the Department to boost knowledge of hospital administration, and promoted him at the expense of insiders who had a traditional public health background. According to one senior medical civil servant, Yellowlees also came across as insecure because 'he hadn't got the ticket [the Diploma in Public Health]. To a more secure man this wouldn't have mattered but Henry never got over it, despite the fact that other senior staff like Gill Ford and Liz Shore didn't have it either'.[72] Yet he proved to be a competent CMO, handling a number of difficult issues during his ten years in office, initiating some important health-related policies, including the removal of lead from petrol, and campaigning successfully for the smallpox eradication programme at the World Health Organization.

Professionalisation of civil service appointments

Whereas Godber had masterminded his own replacement, Yellowlees was more removed from the process when he retired in 1983. There were by then four Deputy CMOs in the Department. They were all interviewed with the exception of Dr Gillian Ford who declared at an early stage that she did not wish to be

---

[70] Private information.
[71] Senior civil servant interview, 10.11.1999.
[72] Senior medical civil servant interview, 22.07.2002.

considered. Dr Ed Harris had expertise in toxicology and medicine, but was not a serious contender. Dr John Evans had better odds: he had been groomed as a potential CMO by the Permanent Secretary Ken Stowe by being moved into a Deputy Secretary post, succeeding James Collier, the toughest Deputy Secretary in the Department. Stowe's rationale for his nurturing of Evans was to produce a real figure of substance – 'a medical heavyweight' – to consolidate the Department's improved relations with the medical profession and the wider healthcare system. This fitted with Stowe's personal civil service ethos, which insisted that the Department of Health and Social Security required greater professionalism (which he masterminded through the appointment of Roy Griffiths to report on NHS management), and in particular a CMO who was an authoritative public health professional. But Evans suffered from ill-health. He used to joke with colleagues that he was more of 'a satsuma than a mandarin'.[73] He did not view himself as a potential CMO.

Dr Elizabeth Shore was perhaps the strongest internal candidate, with a solid background in the medical civil service. She had been trained up under Godber and Yellowlees, both of whom were proud to have nurtured a female doctor who had the potential to succeed them. However, Shore was married to the Labour politician Peter Shore, and although her name went forward to Downing Street for consideration, she was considered a politically sensitive risk.[74] Yellowlees was disappointed to see her miss out for this reason, but had already begun to search for a viable alternative outside the Department.

Yellowlees and Ken Stowe's preferred short-list was thus essentially narrowed down to two 'outsiders': Malcolm Godfrey, Dean at the Royal Postgraduate Medical School, and Donald Acheson, Dean of Medicine at Southampton University Medical School. Godfrey withdrew his application after initial discussions and subsequently moved to be Second Secretary at the Medical Research Council, a post with less direct political pressure and the opportunity to be, as one senior civil servant put it, 'a bigger fish in a smaller pond'.[75]

The post went to Donald Acheson, the academic outsider whom Yellowlees had known since working at the Middlesex Hospital, and whom he suggested should be included in the short-list because of his strong epidemiological and public health background. Acheson seemed initially an unusual choice, and has admitted his surprise in being 'headhunted' for this post, given his lack of experience of the civil service or of National Health Service administration.[76] Possibly this was part of his appeal to the civil service selection board, who were looking for a CMO who could foster relations with the medical profession without being seen to be 'in the pockets' of Whitehall.[77] Acheson came into Whitehall for three months at the end of 1983 to shadow Yellowlees in the routine departmental business. The CMO post was also restructured at this point, and Acheson was given a five-year contract, rather than the permanent tenure which his predecessors had enjoyed.

---

[73] Private information.

[74] Patrick Jenkin, the Conservative Secretary of State for Health, had even gone so far as to state that Shore's position was incompatible and that she should leave the civil service. There were, however, precedents for husband and wife both to work in Whitehall.

[75] Senior health professional interview, 16.02.2000.

[76] Acheson interview, 22.05.2002.

[77] Senior civil servant interview, 10.07.2000.

Acheson's handling of the acquired immune deficiency syndrome (AIDS) crisis in the 1980s marked him as a talented CMO, and in the event he held the post for eight years until his retirement at the age of 65 years in 1991. However, AIDS has tended to overshadow Acheson's other achievements, and perhaps also some of the issues which his 'outsider' status highlighted. Former colleagues have noted that he was 'rank conscious' – and that such an attitude within the civil service meant that he was reluctant to collaborate with juniors or to delegate to them. He therefore missed out on some potential high flyers within his staff.[78]

Yet senior members of the public health profession have remarked that Acheson's appointment in 1983 was a 'bold and brilliant move' by Whitehall, and having broken a line of internal appointments, it was easier still on his retirement to actively look outside the Department for his successor. Additionally, the civil service at this stage further modernised by contracting out the initial selection/head-hunting stage to a professional recruitment agency, Saxton Bampfylde. The agency's appointment analysis, prepared in March 1991, listed the principal duties of the CMO, the line management responsibilities, and stressed the significance of maintaining and developing relationships with the medical profession and international contacts. This latter area in particular had increased in significance since the development of European health legislation. The specific requirements for the post stated that: 'The CMO's fields of experience will include preferably epidemiology and public health medicine and substantial experience in the National Health Service. It will be essential for the CMO rapidly to become knowledgeable and influential in all these areas.'

The strong candidate for Acheson's replacement had no direct experience in either epidemiology or public health medicine, but clearly met one of the Permanent Secretary's (Sir Christopher France) criteria for the post. France wanted a candidate who would bring 'that extra dimension, a new window on the world'.[79] Kenneth Calman had been CMO for Scotland since 1989, previously having been at the University of Glasgow since 1974 as Professor of Oncology and later Dean of Postgraduate Medicine. Sir Graham Hart, the Scottish Health Department's Permanent Secretary, recommended him to France, although when Saxton Bampfylde made the initial telephone call to Calman he refused to speak to them, believing that they were a pharmaceutical company. He was eventually persuaded to attend for interview in Whitehall, despite a strong desire to remain in Scotland for personal reasons. However, when Sir Robin Butler rang to offer him the post he realised that it was an opportunity too good to pass over.

In 1991 there were other serious contenders to fill Acheson's shoes and the more open selection process brought forward some interesting candidates. However, the system was still ultimately controlled by Whitehall, with the Department's Permanent Secretary in the driving seat. France's first move was to compile a 'long list' by inviting nominations from the senior medical profession. His decision to solicit opinions first from the Royal College of Physicians, rather than from the Faculty of Public Health Medicine, drew immediate criticism from senior public health academics, dismayed that they were not one of the first ports of call in a discussion about an essentially public health post. In the event, several of the nominees when contacted declined to be considered for the short-list, apparently unhappy with the package offered.

[78] Senior medical civil servant interview, 09.05.2000.
[79] Interview, 04.04.2000.

It was hard to reconcile Saxton Bampfylde's person specification – 'a qualified medical practitioner of substantial professional distinction . . . high level of representational skills and professional standing' – with the civil service standard salary for a Second Permanent Secretary of £77,500 (December 1991). Some of the potential candidates from the mainstream health service would have already been earning substantially more than that with top-end consultant salaries and A+ distinction awards. The salary would only appear relatively attractive to internal candidates from the Department of Health, and these were scarce compared to the Godber and Yellowlees eras. Two strong candidates for the post were the Deputy CMO Dr Diana Walford (later Director of the Public Health Laboratory Service, then Principal of Mansfield College, Oxford) and Dr Michael O'Brien, who was a regional Director of Public Health. O'Brien withdrew for personal reasons, but Walford was a serious rival to Calman, considered by senior public health professionals to have all the right attributes to have been a very successful first female Chief Medical Officer for England.

Conclusion

Several themes run through the selection of all fourteen CMOs. There was a persistent concern with appointing a person whom the medical profession would respect, both for clinical ability but also for willingness to act as a channel of communication between the profession and the government. The civil service selectors also looked for intellectual ability coupled with physical stamina. The post acquired a reputation at a very early stage for long hours and punishing schedules. Most of the CMOs knowingly and willingly sacrificed any personal or social life to devote all their energies to this post. Some, like John Simon, were left after retirement feeling bitter about their devotion and the inadequate recompense. For others, like Seaton and Thorne Thorne, the stresses of the post undoubtedly shortened their lives – Thorne Thorne was even forced to give evidence to a Royal Commission from his deathbed.

There was an acceptance that to be an effective CMO complete devotion was essential to the post. George Godber even slept on a camp bed in his office for several nights each week (to save time travelling home to Bedford). He once surprised the Australian CMO who rang the Department to leave a message on the answerphone ready for the next morning, by answering the telephone himself in the middle of the night, a story that has passed into the Department of Health's folklore.[80]

As the demands have increased through to the end of the twentieth century, the position is now seen as one which is difficult to hold long-term, until retirement, in the style of Newman or Godber. Even Calman, having publicly declared in 1994 that he 'expected to be CMO until he retired', left the post in 1998 at the age of 57 years to become Warden and Vice Chancellor at Durham University.[81] It was not latterly always undertaken perhaps as a final career move, but while the incumbent still has the energy and enthusiasm for the long hours and the extensive travel required by international work. The selection of CMOs

---

[80] Senior health professional interview, 16.02.2000.
[81] R Smith, 'Health Profile: challenging doctors: an interview with England's Chief Medical Officer', *British Medical Journal*, 1994, 308, 1221–4.

was always a two-way process. Not all of those who were long-listed by the Permanent Secretaries were prepared to accept the personal sacrifices, or at times a relatively low salary. Part of the unofficial compensation was undoubtedly the personal satisfaction of being at the centre of Whitehall. When both Newman and Godber retired there were suggestions in the press that they should be made life peers, so being able to continue to provide their considerable wisdom on health issues through the House of Lords.[82] No CMO to date has yet received that honour.

---

[82] MH 139/3. Newman notes in his diary on 20.02.1935 ten 'fallings out' which he had had with Robinson which he thought lost him a peerage.

Chapter 3

Navigating the corridors of power

From the middle of the nineteenth century, the state accepted responsibility for an increasingly wide range of public services. This expansion of government activity required the development of a competent administrative system, which has come to be known simply as 'Whitehall'. What underpins most of the success (and failure) of the work of all the CMOs is their reliance upon the senior civil servant – the Principal Clerk, later known as the Permanent Secretary. At the heart of this relationship lies the sensitive and complex issue of right of access to Ministers. As one Permanent Secretary characterised his relationship with the CMO: 'We walk along the corridor arm in arm, but when we come to a door, I go through first.' This chapter examines the impact of both positive and negative partnerships on the development of specific health policies, especially the link between smoking and lung cancer, and the effect of Whitehall reforms in the late twentieth century on the role and image of senior civil servants.

The Permanent Secretary is the civil servant at the head of each Whitehall department. In the early days of the civil service, this post was often gifted to upper-class well-educated gentlemen, such as the Earl of Bathurst, who served as Principal Clerk to the Privy Council between 1827 and 1860. His replacement (and Simon's useful ally) Arthur Helps was of a different breed, reflecting the introduction of the career civil servant, although there was still a blurring between civil and political office holders. The principle of the civil servant remaining in post through changes in government was relatively new. By the 1870s, the Permanent Secretary 'had, in most departments, outstripped in importance his parliamentary counterpart'.[1] The television series *Yes, Minister* in the 1980s did much to personify the Whitehall mandarin. In the character of Sir Humphrey Appleby we encountered, as Peter Barberis so eloquently puts it:

> An essential glimpse of a persona that lives vividly in the memory: upper middle class, public school and 'Oxbridge' educated; cultured, clubbable, articulate and full of subtlety; a font of knowledge and wisdom; incorruptible yet capable of deception, manipulation and disingenuity when the mores of Whitehall are challenged by wayward ministerial initiative. And all within the cloak of anonymity, the skein of constitutional propriety.[2]

Barberis's book, *The Elite of the Elite* (1996), provided a much-needed analysis of this key governmental post. It uncovered the real Sir Humphreys and

---

[1] K Theakston, *Junior Ministers in British Government* (Oxford, Blackwell, 1987), pp. 19–29.
[2] P Barberis, *The Elite of the Elite: permanent secretaries in the British higher civil service* (Aldershot, Ashgate Press, 1996), p. xvi.

demonstrated that there is more than a grain of truth in the fictional represen-tation.[3]

The abolition of recruitment by patronage after 1870 did much to increase the anonymity of the civil servant. It effectively broke the personal allegiance between the Minister and the servant.[4] There had previously been an unspoken agreement within Whitehall that civil servants would not court attention or make their personal views public, but not all were prepared to work under these conditions. Edwin Chadwick flagrantly flouted them through his manipulation of Royal Commissions and publication of articles in national newspapers. However, there was some justification for the style of his personal crusade, coming at a time when government lacked a coherent system of Departments and accountable Ministers.[5] Chadwick's name was so openly linked to reform of the Poor Law and the introduction of public health systems that he could not be part of the civil service code of anonymity. His apparent excesses 'were a major factor in his removal and, ultimately, the General Board of Health's demise'.[6] He wanted it both ways – to be able to subvert ministerial policy, but at the same time not to be directly open to attack from his opponents, which he said was equivalent to 'hitting a woman'.[7]

As the lines of accountability were drawn in Whitehall with the formalisation of government departments with Ministers at their helms, the anonymity of the civil servant became an increasingly useful tool. It provided Departments with skilled, permanent staff who could advise Ministers. However, when the advice offered was refused, the civil servants found other ways to push forward their preferred agendas – supplying information indirectly to the press, instructing useful Members of Parliament, and, in extreme cases, motivating pressure groups outside Whitehall. Thus by the time the CMO post was firmly established in the late nineteenth century, there was already a cadre of 'statesmen in disguise' into which he was placed and had to work. As Denis Healey succinctly put it in a radio interview:

> I think that a Minister who complains that his civil servants are too powerful is either a weak Minister or an incompetent one.[8]

The CMO, while never being an ordinary civil servant, still had to fit into the conventions of Whitehall. His dual role as civil servant and technical adviser meant that he trod a delicate line between the Minister and the Permanent

---

[3] Although it should be noted that three of the Permanent Secretaries at the Department of Health and Social Security and the subsequent Department of Health – Sir Kenneth Stowe, Sir Christopher France and Sir Graham Hart – were not products of the private education system.

[4] SE Finer, 'The individual responsibility of Ministers', *Journal of Public Administration*, 1956, XXXIV, 380.

[5] The New Poor Law of 1834 operated until 1848 without parliamentary representation. Even after the creation of the Board of Health in 1848, the Minister could be overruled by its official. This was not corrected until 1854.

[6] RA Lewis, *Edwin Chadwick and the Public Health Movement, 1832–1854* (London, Longman, 1952), p. 358.

[7] Quoted in G Kitson Clark, '"Statesmen in Disguise": reflexions on the history of the neutrality of the civil service', *Historical Journal*, 1959, II, 32.

[8] Quoted in P Nairne, 'Mandarins and Ministers: a former official's view', in P Barberis (ed.), *The Whitehall Reader* (Buckingham, Open University Press, 1996), p. 81.

Secretary. His unique freedom of speech will be discussed in more detail in Chapter 7. The purpose of this chapter is to examine how the relationship between the CMO and the Permanent Secretary responded to pressures within Whitehall and to changes within the world of medicine.

Newman and the status of the CMO

By the early twentieth century government activity and the civil service had increased substantially. Still essentially controlled by a select élite, coterminous perhaps with London's 'club land', friendship and social networks were as important for advancement in Whitehall as ability. George Newman, who came into Whitehall initially as Chief Medical Officer to the Board of Education in 1907, knew only too well that his future career depended upon carefully cultivated connections. His selection as CMO for the Local Government Board, in preparation for its transformation into a new Ministry of Health, reflected this (see Chapter 2), but his work to secure his status and relationship with the Ministry's first Minister and Permanent Secretary deserves closer attention. It is these two issues which have been resurrected on several occasions by subsequent CMOs to secure their own positions in Whitehall.

Newman had a unique vision of how the state should expand its role in medicine which went well beyond the scope of John Simon's nineteenth century ambitions.[9] After the shock of the 1904 Parliamentary Report on Physical Deterioration, which had been stimulated by the poor physical condition of the army recruits for the Boer War, there was public and political acceptance that the state had a duty to ensure some basic living conditions and access to healthcare. Newman's experience as a Medical Officer of Health, and then as Medical Adviser to the Board of Education, convinced him that preventive medicine should be central to every government's agenda. This determination, combined with a strong Quaker philosophy of public duty, made him singularly ambitious, aware that he could only advance his cherished causes from a position of authority.[10]

Newman's diaries chronicled the minutiae of contacts both personal and professional. They provide a unique perspective on this driven man from the time of his appointment to the Board of Education, until his retirement in 1935. They expose the Whitehall network to the extent that Newman as CMO fitted into it. The spontaneity and informality of Whitehall business in the early twentieth century is perhaps surprising. Newman moved relentlessly between critical coteries meeting in government buildings and Pall Mall clubs.[11] He was

[9] S Sturdy, 'Hippocrates and State Medicine: George Newman outlines the founding policy of the Ministry of Health', in C Lawrence and G Weisz (eds), *Greater than the Parts: holism in biomedicine* (Oxford, Oxford University Press, 1998), pp. 112–34.

[10] M Hammer, *The Building of a Nation's Health: the life and work of George Newman to 1921* (Unpublished D Phil. Thesis, University of Cambridge, 1995).

[11] He was elected to the Athenaeum Club on 01.03.1919 – two weeks after his appointment by Addison as CMO had been announced in *The Times* (15.02.1919). The Athenaeum is perhaps the most prestigious of the London clubs, and was used by several of the CMOs to conduct unofficial business and to entertain guests. Godber, however, declined his invitation to join, stating that he was already a member of the Oxford and Cambridge Club, which he had chosen because it was the nearest one to the Bakerloo line underground station and thus convenient for getting to and from the office (interview 13.07.1999).

already Lloyd George's favoured political health adviser when he involved himself in the planning for the new Ministry with Christopher Addison, its Minister-elect, and Morant, who was promised the Permanent Secretaryship.

The team of Addison, Morant and Newman which headed the new Ministry in 1919 thought it held all the important cards. It was a golden opportunity to ditch the cumbersome baggage of the Local Government Board and recast the relationship between the administrative and medical staff. Addison even addressed a meeting of the medical staff on 7 July 1919 to confirm their position and line management and, most significantly, the status of the CMO.[12] Morant was equally supportive, agreeing that Newman should have direct access to Addison. Addison had also agreed that Newman was to retain the rank of Permanent Secretary *ad hominem* to reflect his parity in the Ministry with Morant. Addison's personal papers reveal an even more astonishing degree of support for Newman. Morant had written to Addison in 1919 offering to leave the Ministry if it helped to secure Newman's position: 'As you remember, I always said I was willing if you wished it to see him on top and for me to vanish.'[13]

Newman would not work as CMO for the salary offered. It had been agreed that he should retain his position as CMO to the Board of Education, but the salary package did not meet Newman's expectations for this double workload. He was especially conscious of his pay relative to that of Morant. The Ministry of Health Establishment File which covers these sensitive negotiations is packed with memos between Austen Chamberlain (1863–1937), Chancellor of the Exchequer at the Treasury, Addison at the Ministry and various official and personal communications from Newman to both of them on his dissatisfaction with his pay and consequent status.[14] Chamberlain's budget was being squeezed from all sides during this period of post-war austerity, and he initially refused Addison's request to increase the salary offered to Newman, despite his plea that:

> It is not at all uncommon in the public municipal service . . . to find professional men paid higher than the chief administration officers. The price in the market of first-rate professional men, whether engineers or medical men, is rapidly rising . . . the professional man who has administrative official experience has an enhanced value in the outside market.[15]

Addison persisted. Salaries of previous CMOs showed no progression for the post. Incomes of local Medical Officers of Health were often higher: those of Liverpool and Birmingham, for example ('together with fees they are probably making £3,000 a year'[16]).

Newman reluctantly settled for Chamberlain's token increase to £2,100 per annum (which included £100 for his post at the Board of Education). His

[12] MH 78/92. Ministry of Health Establishment File.
[13] Letter from Morant to Addison, 28.08.1919, in Addison Papers, box 53, folder 505 (Bodleian Library, University of Oxford). Cited in F Honigsbaum, 'Christopher Addison: a realist in pursuit of dreams', in D Porter and R Porter (eds), *Doctors, Politics and Society* (Amsterdam, Rodopi, 1993), p. 236.
[14] MH 78/92.
[15] Ibid., memorandum dated 31.01.1919 from Addison to Chamberlain at the Treasury.
[16] Ibid.

'ultimatum' to take his services elsewhere – he had offers to be Medical Officer of Health at London County Council at £2,000 per annum, and Chairman of George Cadbury's Daily News publishing group – did not work.[17] Chamberlain was impervious to this sort of blackmail, noting to Addison that 'if any civil servant is to be allowed to say that he will have this and he won't have that in respect of the organisation of the department in which he serves, the position of Ministers would be humiliating and impossible'.[18]

The promising Addison–Morant–Newman team was dramatically broken by Morant's death from influenza in March 1920. The obituaries recounted how Morant had described his long-term association with Newman as the 'Siamese twin arrangement' or 'the combine'.[19] He had given Newman the equal status and respect he wished, and formed one of the closest CMO–Permanent Secretary relationships possible. Morant's replacement at the Ministry, Arthur Robinson, was not so accommodating of Newman's ego nor of the special role of the medical staff. There was a complete breakdown in anything other than formal communication between the Permanent Secretary and the Chief Medical Officer.[20] Newman had to re-establish his right of access to the Minister, and to keep his salary up to that offered to the Permanent Secretary. He finally secured his £3,000 per annum in June 1921. Interestingly, this was exactly the same salary given to Charles on his appointment as CMO in 1950.[21]

With the departure of Addison as Minister in April 1921, Newman was left exposed to take the full criticism of the press and the medical profession for what they called the 'Newman Policy' at the Ministry. He was portrayed as a power-hungry bureaucrat who had manipulated Addison and Morant to achieve his personal ambitions. He had demanded the recognition for developing state medicine; now he was getting it.[22] Without a supportive Minister and Permanent Secretary, he was increasingly isolated at the Ministry and lacked the connections to promote his plans for 'preventive medicine'.[23]

Managing the tripartite relationship

Subsequent CMOs found that their relationship with their Permanent Secretaries had benefited from Newman's persistence on the job's status. Although the archives record that Newman's right of access to the Minister was *ad hominem*, all successors seem to have retained this concession without debate. It certainly made sense – there was no way that the Permanent Secretary could advise the Minister on 'all' matters, as Robinson had confidently predicted in 1921.[24] It was natural that medical advice should come direct from the CMO, without the filter (and consequent delay) of the Permanent Secretary.

The advantage which Permanent Secretaries have offered in Whitehall has

[17] MH 139/2. Newman diary, 01.08.1919; 02.08.1919; 14.06.1919.
[18] MH 78/92. Chamberlain to Addison, 06.02.1919.
[19] *British Medical Journal*, 20.03.1920, and correspondence from Knutsford to Newman in Newman diary (MH 139/3), March 1920.
[20] S Stacey, *The Ministry of Health* (Unpublished D Phil., University of Oxford, 1984), p. 108.
[21] However, as inflation was negligible during this period salaries were more stable.
[22] *The Times*, 04.04.1921, p. 10, col.3.
[23] See Stacey, *The Ministry of Health*, for a more detailed analysis of this period.
[24] MH 78/92. Robinson to Addison, 25.02.1921.

been their relative longevity in Departments, giving them an unrivalled opportunity to acquire specific knowledge. Fifteen men held this position from the formation of the Ministry of Health in 1919 (and its successors, the Department of Health and Social Security 1968–1990, thereafter the Department of Health) through to 1998. Their tenures have ranged from Morant (one year – died in post) through to Arthur Robinson (fifteen years), but most of them stayed for five to ten years (see Appendix 3). During this period they were matched by only eight CMOs and some 33 Ministers or Secretaries of State for Health.

The authority wielded by the Permanent Secretaries is legendary. These 'backroom boys' who claim to be content to develop policy and advise Ministers without any of the associated limelight have found their role at the centre of public attention through popular fictional accounts of Whitehall life such as the television series *Yes, Minister*, and through the illuminating accounts of commentators like Peter Hennessy.[25] Very occasionally, they have been persuaded to offer comment on the machinations of Whitehall, but have rarely broken the strict civil service code of conduct. Without autobiographical sources, it is tricky to account accurately for their influence with Ministers and their relationships with CMOs. The dry memoranda and Establishment Files consigned to the National Archives will only ever tell part of the story.

The smoking and lung cancer issue

If Newman and Morant offer a positive picture of how the relationship could work, the combination of a dominant Permanent Secretary and a relatively weak CMO illustrates the pitfalls. Such a coupling occurred in the 1950s, a turbulent period for British domestic policy, combining post-war economic recession with high public expectations of the new National Health Service. The background to John Charles' appointment as CMO in 1950 was set out in Chapter 2. He was the best of a rather mediocre pool of internal candidates and he had been hesitant about moving from his Medical Officer of Health post in Newcastle-upon-Tyne to join Jameson as Deputy CMO in 1944. He was aware that he lacked the confident public persona which the post demanded. However, he more than compensated for this through his intellectual abilities and behind-the-scenes diplomacy. Charles had one year with the outgoing Permanent Secretary Sir William Scott Douglas, the very effective partner to Jameson during the period of creation of the National Health Service. In 1951 Douglas was replaced by John Hawton (1904– 1982), who was to remain at the Ministry until his enforced retirement, coincident with Charles' departure in 1960.

Hawton was a classic civil servant, educated at St John's College, Cambridge. He was a Middle Temple Barrister who entered the Ministry of Health in 1927. He had been closely involved in drafting the National Health Service Bill and had been earmarked for the Permanent Secretary role from that point onwards. Once in that post, he dominated both the Ministry and Charles himself. This did not have to be a problem. In fact, it could have worked to Charles' advantage, leaving him time to develop his own style of working. It became a problem, however, because of the way in which Hawton attempted to usurp the medical advice role of the CMO on a seminal issue: the relationship between tobacco smoking and lung cancer.

[25] P Hennessy, *Whitehall* (London, Secker and Warburg, 1989).

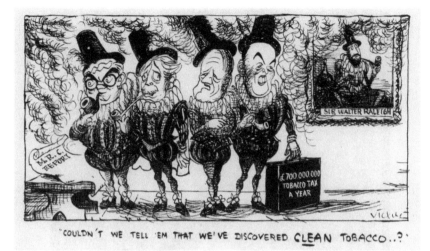

"COULDN'T WE TELL 'EM THAT WE'VE DISCOVERED CLEAN TOBACCO..?'

Figure 3.1 From right: Charles Hill, Harold Macmillan, RAB Butler and Peter Thorney-croft. On the potential impact of the MRC report on smoking and lung cancer on the tobacco revenue (*New Statesman*, 6th July 1957). © Solo Syndication. Reproduced with permission.

In 1950, the year that Charles became CMO, five reports were published which linked lung cancer and cigarette smoking. Prior to this, an informal Medical Research Council conference had been held in 1947 to discuss the increasing mortality rate from lung cancer. This was a sensitive issue – cancer was an undiscussed subject in society but there was a recognition that research was needed, if only to disprove the various causal theories, which included air pollution and radioactive dust. In the 1950s, some 85 per cent of British men were regular smokers, but tobacco was not initially a prime suspect. At that time, the tobacco industry was viewed by the public and government alike as just another commercial interest.[26] The industry was, though, a special case. The government received large revenues from tobacco duty – money which was desperately needed to match the spiralling costs of the new National Health Service.[27] As a result, a 'special relationship' had evolved between the government and the tobacco industry which Whitehall was under pressure to maintain.

At the Medical Research Council conference on lung cancer in 1947, Austin Bradford Hill proposed that a research programme on lung cancer be carried out by his Medical Research Council statistical unit, and the recruitment of Richard Doll. In 1951 the pair wrote to all 60,000 doctors on the Medical Register asking them to complete a questionnaire about their smoking habits. The *British Medical Journal* assisted, ensuring a near 100 per cent completion rate.[28] Their research

[26] M Hilton, *Smoking in British Popular Culture, 1800–2000: perfect pleasures* (Manchester, Manchester University Press, 2000).

[27] Ibid., p. 169. The government was receiving some £610 million p.a. from the tobacco tax.

[28] R Doll and AB Hill, 'A study of the aetiology of carcinoma of the lung', *British Medical Journal*, 1956, (II), 1271–86; R Doll and AB Hill, 'The mortality of doctors in relation to their smoking habits: a preliminary report', *British Medical Journal*, 1954, (I), 1451–2; R Doll and AB Hill, 'Lung cancer and other causes of death in relation to smoking: a second report on the mortality of British doctors', *British Medical Journal*, 1956, (II), 1071–81.

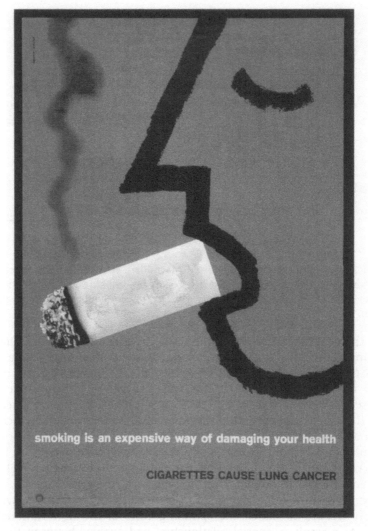

smoking is an expensive way of damaging your health

CIGARETTES CAUSE LUNG CANCER

Figure 3.2 Ministry of Health poster warning which linked the cost of smoking with lung cancer. © Wellcome Library. Reproduced with permission.

outcomes provided independent validation for similar research in the United States of America (USA) by Ernst Wynder and Edwin Graham which had proved for the first time an *association* between smoking and lung cancer.[29] Yet the publication of this research passed almost without comment in the British press. It did not, however, escape the attention of a member of the government's Standing Advisory Committee on Cancer and Radiotherapy – one of nine standing committees which had been formed through the 1946 National Health Service Act to advise the Minister and the Central Health Services Council. In 1949

[29] EL Wynder and EA Graham, 'Tobacco smoking as a possible etiological factor in bronchiogenic carcinoma: a study of 648 proved cases', *Journal of the American Medical Association*, 1950, 143, 329–36.

Horace Joules (a founding member of the Socialist Medical Association[30]) suggested that the Ministry of Health should conduct a publicity campaign about the possible dangers of tobacco smoking. But the Standing Advisory Committee, chaired by Sir Ernest Rock Carling (a lifelong heavy smoker), rejected the idea, pointing to the preliminary nature of the research and the difficulty of drawing such conclusions from it.

Charles wrote to the Medical Research Council in 1950 asking for details of Bradford Hill's research, but he failed to persuade the Standing Advisory Committee to advise the Minister (Iain MacLeod) to make a public statement. Bradford Hill initiated a follow-up project, while the Standing Advisory Committee was berated by Joules for its inactivity. They reluctantly drafted a briefing in 1952, following the death of King George VI, a heavy smoker, who had died after an operation for lung cancer. However, they wanted to word the briefing to suggest that the relationship was only proven between 'excessive smoking' and lung cancer.

At this point, the Imperial Tobacco Company (which had 80 per cent of the British cigarette market) contacted the Ministry of Health to try to stimulate research which would disprove the findings of Bradford Hill and Doll.[31] Through a series of meetings with the tobacco industry, the scientific worth of their own research and future projects was debated. Ironically, after these meetings, the Director of the Medical Research Council, Dr FHK Green, sent Bradford Hill a box of cigars to thank him for his sensitive handling of the tobacco companies.[32]

What was Charles doing while these discussions were going on? He followed a line which on the surface seemed reasonable. He determined to obtain further validation and to advise his Minister on the appropriate course of action. First, he asked Percy Stocks, Senior Research Fellow at the British Empire Cancer Campaign, to obtain independent referees for the conflicting research of Bradford Hill and the tobacco industry.[33] But by this stage (1953) there was interest in Parliament and in the press about the supposed link between smoking and lung cancer, and the Minister of Health, Iain MacLeod, was under pressure to make a public statement. Charles' next action was to amend the draft statement which the Standing Advisory Committee had prepared. He wanted it 'toned down a bit' – crucially changing the phrasing from 'there is an obligation . . . to warn young people' to 'it is desirable . . . that young people are warned'.[34] Another draft was prepared. Meanwhile the tobacco industry maintained its pressure on its contact

---

[30] J Stewart, *The Battle for Health: a political history of the Socialist Medical Association, 1930–51* (Aldershot, Ashgate Press, 1999).

[31] MH 55/2232. Cancer – smoking and lung cancer file. 09.03.1956 letter from Partridge of the Imperial Tobacco Company to Hawton; 25.07.1956 letter from Sir Alexander Maxwell, Chairman of Tobacco Manufacturers Standing Committee to Hawton.

[32] The letter reads: Dear Tony, I send you these cigars in grateful (if ironical) appreciation of your tactful handling of the tobacconists yesterday, and in gratitude also for your advice, help and hospitality over many years. I hope that they are tolerable and have sufficiently matured (I know little about such things). I hope much more of course, that they do not plunge you, of all people, into the equivocal but dangerous category of a 'heavy smoker' – but I hardly suppose there are enough of them for that. Yours ever . . . (letter quoted in D Pollock, *Denial and Delay* (ASH, 1999), p. 17.

[33] MH 55/1011.

[34] Pollock, *Denial and Delay*, p. 23.

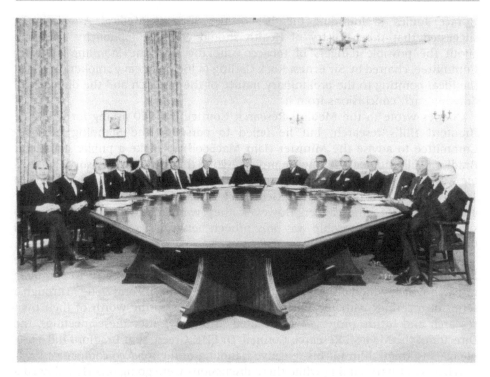

Figure 3.3 The Medical Research Council's 50th anniversary in 1963 (Godber is third from right). Note the ashtrays placed under the table for the photo.

Medical Officer in the Ministry, Neville Goodman, to rubbish the work of Bradford Hill and Doll.[35]

MacLeod finally decided he had to make a statement, and obtained the approval of the Treasury, as long as he did not make too big an issue of it. A press conference was held in February 1954, which explained the 'limited' research on a possible link between smoking and lung cancer. During this press conference, MacLeod chain-smoked four large cigarettes, lighting each one from the last. He was flanked by his CMO Charles (a non-smoker) and by Sir Harold Himsworth, Head of the Medical Research Council, who held his pipe in his hand but did not actually light it. The press coverage was prominent but not as excessive as some feared. This reflected perhaps the fact that this new information targeted one of the nation's most popular habits. It was not news that anyone wanted to hear.

For the next eight years, the Ministry of Health prevaricated and reassessed the smoking and lung cancer research. A health education campaign was not forthcoming, and much of this inactivity was exacerbated by the manipulation of the policy-making system by the Ministry's Permanent Secretary, John Hawton. Papers at the National Archives show that Hawton stymied new research and provided misinformation to the Standing Advisory Committee and Ministers.[36]

---

[35] MH 55/2232. Goodman to Charles minute, 21.08.1956.
[36] See, for example, the correspondence in MH 55/2232 between Hawton, the Treasury and Partridge of the Imperial Tobacco Company.

The explanation for this is not to be found in the official Whitehall archives – that would deprecate Hawton's considerable civil servant skills. But it is clear, from other 1950s key players in this story, that Hawton was under considerable pressure from both the Treasury and the tobacco industry – and that he had developed perhaps inappropriately close relations with the Imperial Tobacco Company. He was nearing the end of a long civil service career and was increasingly suffering from ill-health – some of it alcohol induced. Despite periods of sick-leave which in any other senior civil servant would have resulted in immediate compassionate retirement, he did not go until 1960, aged 56 years.[37]

Why did Charles not use his CMO authority to override Hawton's delaying tactics? This was after all about a medical policy issue, one which required the sort of sophisticated epidemiological skills which Charles had, and could have exploited in a direct approach to the Minister. The Ministry files strongly suggest that contact between the CMO and the Minister was mostly channelled through the Permanent Secretary's office.[38] Charles admitted that he was not a pushy person. He preferred a reactive rather than proactive approach to his duties. He was unlikely to have kicked up a fuss when Hawton subtly redrew the chain of command. Charles had instituted a reduced schedule of meetings within the Department, abandoning the weekly briefings which Jameson had held with his staff. He put little time or effort into forging relations with the medical profession, or with important stakeholders like the Medical Research Council.

George Godber, Charles' successor, recalled that Charles could be influential. He had successfully promoted the cause of child health and he applied pressure to create a chair for James Spence at Durham.[39] He also chaired a group investigating the development of consultant services. It is true that Charles was the first CMO really to bear the brunt of the new National Health Service workload, and his advisory role had been extended to include serving as CMO to the Home Office (in addition to the Ministry of Health and the Ministry of Education). Yet Charles' real interest was in international health. He was Chair of the Executive Board of the World Health Organization between 1957 and 1958, President of the World Health Assembly in 1959 and Chair of the Fourth Expert Committee on Public Health Administration in 1960. The clearest indication of his international leanings is that when he retired as CMO he became a World Health Organization senior adviser. He remained in Geneva until a few weeks before his death in 1971 aged 77 years. Godber's obituary captures the essence of Charles' strengths as well as weaknesses:

> The record of John Charles' achievements in some fifty years of public health work is unlikely ever to be surpassed. Perhaps few of his colleagues knew him really well, for he was essentially retiring and self-effacing. He was, in fact, intensely human, capable of warm friendship, a generous and delightful host, and an enduring friend. He set his own value far below his true worth, but to those who knew

---

[37] After a three-year break he became of Chairman of the British Waterways Board in 1963 and from 1968 he was Vice-Chairman until 1974. He died in 1982.

[38] MH 55/2232. Several minutes from Hawton and the junior civil servant Pater are explicitly marked not to be passed through the CMO's office during 1956.

[39] James Spence (1892–1954) was a pioneer in child health in the post-war period.

> him intimately he leaves the memory of intense wisdom, great
> kindliness, and essential humanity.[40]

But to return to the 1950s, the handling of the tobacco and lung cancer issue did
not reflect Charles' best side. The Ministry resisted demands for health education
programmes, even when confronted with Bradford Hill and Doll's definitive
research paper in the *British Medical Journal* in 1954. The Standing Medical
Advisory Committee tried to push the Minister, in 1953, to approve a campaign
to be run by the Central Health Services Council, and to get local authorities to
issue advice. These calls for action became stuck in the mire of Whitehall budget
negotiations. The Central Health Services Council finally rejected the Minister's
recommendation in 1955, citing the doubts which the latest Medical Research
Council research were casting on the supposed links.[41]

Hawton was now in frequent contact with (Ernest) John Partridge, the
Secretary of the Imperial Tobacco Company. The two held regular meetings at
which Hawton briefed Partridge on the latest research findings, and updated him
on the Minister's proposals. Partridge even consulted Hawton on the wording of
the Imperial Tobacco Company's annual report and attempted (unsuccessfully) to
fix up meetings between Dr Clarence Cook Little, Scientific Director of the US
Tobacco Industry Research Council, and 'leading medical correspondents' during
a visit to Britain.[42]

In March 1956 the new Minister for Health, Robin Turton, departed from his
predecessor's line on smoking and lung cancer in answer to a parliamentary
question. He stated: 'There is a causal connection between smoking and lung
cancer. That we know.' Hawton immediately had to fend off irate protests from
the Treasury and from Partridge.[43] He attempted to placate these interested
parties by portraying the Minister's words as nothing more sinister than 'an
oral slip', and not a change in Ministerial policy. However, the issue was now
interesting the Prime Minister, Sir Anthony Eden, who established a Cabinet
subcommittee – GEN 524.[44] This committee drafted an acceptable statement for
Turton to read in the House of Commons on 7 May 1956. The *Times* responded
angrily, claiming that Turton's statement 'added nothing to public knowledge and
subtracted nothing from public anxiety'. It demanded an end to 'ministerial
platitudinising' and declared that 'the time has come for his Ministry to
summarise the ascertained facts, put them into plain language and publish
them in a cheap and arresting format'.[45]

New mortality rates released in 1956 maintained the pressure on the Ministry
to begin a health education campaign. Deaths from lung cancer had increased
from 279 per million in 1950 to 389 per million in 1955.[46] The Medical Research

---

[40] Charles obituaries: *Lancet*, 17.04.1971, (I), 812–13 (to which George Godber contributed
an outstanding testimonial); *British Medical Journal*, 17.04.1971, (I), 173.
[41] MH 55/2232.
[42] MH 55/2232. Letter, Partridge to Hawton, 09.03.1956.
[43] MH 55/2232. Correspondence dated 13.03.1956.
[44] CAB 130/115. Draft memorandum by the Ministry of Health to the Cabinet Home
Affairs Committee on Tobacco Smoking and Cancer of the Lung, April 1956. There is no
mention of advice from the CMO, only from the Standing Medical Advisory Committee.
[45] *The Times*, 08.05.1956.
[46] MH 55/2232. House of Commons non-oral answer, 11.03.1957.

Council by this stage had drafted its own statement. Sensibly, the Council saw more than enough statistical evidence to rely on:

> The recognition of the risk of cancer run by chimney sweeps and tar workers, for example, came many years before the responsible carcinogenic agents were isolated, and it was action based upon purely the statistical and epidemiological investigations of Dr Snow which stamped out cholera epidemics in this country seventeen years before the infecting organism was first seen under the microscope . . .[47]

The Medical Research Council failed to convince the junior medical staff at the Ministry. Goodman, the Deputy CMO with responsibility for this issue, wanted more evidence, not a 'reappraisal' of existing material. He put all sorts of practical difficulties in the way of poster campaigns and deciding who the message should come from. The government could issue pamphlets, he suggested, but this would require a great deal of negotiation with the Treasury.[48]

Charles knew Goodman was negative. He tried to intervene with the Ministry's Deputy Secretary, Dame Enid Russell Smith, to push the idea of a pamphlet. She resisted, concerned that such an initiative would incite the wrath of the tobacco industry. It would certainly retaliate in kind, given that it already spent £2.25 million on press and television cigarette advertising. Russell Smith proposed instead that campaigns should be a local authority responsibility (subject to Ministry approval), which would have the double benefit of hindering the tobacco industry's retaliation and would also pass the costs on to local government. This, she suggested, would be a logical development, given that central control over publicity had been delegated to local authorities to manage and fund during the war. In the 1950s, departments like the Ministry of Health were not keen on taking this responsibility back.

The tobacco and lung cancer issue continued to appear intermittently in Parliament, with the Minister of Health fielding oral and written questions using a mixture of well-tried techniques. The discomfort caused by public attention is evidenced by Turton's letter to Macmillan at the Treasury in March 1956, reassuring him that 'Chapman [MP for Northfield], who has a question down on the 23rd [about research into smoking and lung cancer], has told me that he will postpone it at my request'.[49]

By June 1957 the Cabinet committee had agreed on a statement for the Minister of Health to deliver, although its release was delayed. It was felt advisable to show it to representatives of the tobacco industry that had financed some of the recent Medical Research Council research. This enabled the industry to prepare a considered response, released on the same day as the parliamentary statement, 27 June. Hawton's hand is again detectable in the editing and timing of this statement. The associated press conference was delegated to the Parliamentary Secretary JK Vaughan-Morgan, because the Minister of Health, Dennis Vosper, was in hospital. This neatly allayed fears of a repeat of MacLeod's 1954 press conference, at which he chain-smoked. Vosper (a smoker) had been advised not to smoke; thankfully Vaughan-Morgan was a non-smoker. The emphasis of

---

[47] MH 55/2232. Draft dated 08.03.1956.
[48] MH 55/2227.
[49] MH 55/2232. Turton to Macmillan, 29.03.1956.

the Ministry's statement was that it was an individual's responsibility to assess the risk from lung cancer, and that the Ministry could now step back, having fulfilled its advisory role. Thus, the issue had slipped through the hands of the CMO and was more than willingly despatched by Whitehall to the Central Committee for Health Education and local government.

Although there was no movement on the research front, the Ministry was still under pressure from the medical community to develop educational programmes to discourage smoking. In July 1957, Charles received a letter proposing research into why smoking appeared to be such a hard habit to kick.[50] He forwarded this to the Medical Research Council, only to find it bounced back as 'not within their field'. He passed it on within the Ministry, but failed to follow it up. A local authority circular was proposed in 1958, as a way of maintaining some token interest in the subject. However, Hawton advised the new Minister of Health, Sir Derek Walker-Smith, 'I am not sure whether you will think this a good moment to stir up this controversial subject again. A progress report would of course help to defend you against any criticism of 'not bothering', but the matter is so quiet now that it might be better to wait and see?'[51]

In the face of such concerted inactivity, the initiative finally came from George Godber, one of Charles' two Deputy CMOs (but not at this time with any direct responsibility for the issue). Unlike Charles, Godber was comfortable with cultivating networks within the medical community. In 1958, he had been approached by Charles Fletcher, a member of the Standing Medical Advisory Committee, with the suggestion that the two of them should lobby Robert Platt, the new President of the Royal College of Physicians, to suggest that it set up a committee on smoking and health. Platt, as an old friend of Godber's, was more than happy to assist, and Fletcher was appointed as Secretary.[52] Godber had a clear conscience over this as he had acted in his capacity as a member of the Royal College of Physicians Council. Once the committee was established, all the correspondence between himself and Fletcher passed openly through the Ministry files. Fletcher was an invited and welcome thorn in Godber's side. He used his frequent and explicit letters:

> to ask the Ministry of Health . . . what they are actually doing now in respect of the lung problem. In particular, what steps, if any, they are taking to assist local authorities with 'health education' and if the Ministry has any evidence of any effect of anything that they are doing.[53]

Godber needed the assistance of this sort of external pressure to carry weight with the Minister, but the Royal College of Physicians' involvement was also used by the Permanent Secretary as a delaying tactic – why not postpone Ministerial action until the Royal College of Physicians published its report?[54] The Scottish Health Department meanwhile had embarked on a detailed analysis of the impact

---

[50] MH 55/2224.
[51] MH 55/2224.
[52] Robert Platt (1900–1978), Professor of Medicine at Manchester University, had been elected as President in 1957 – the first provincial and the first academic to hold this prestigious post.
[53] MH 55/2226. CM Fletcher to Godber, 18.01.1960.
[54] Pollock, *Denial and Delay*, p. 69.

of tobacco advertising and the limited local government health education campaigns, and concluded that the latter was doomed to fail without substantial central government support. The Scottish CMO, Kenneth Cowan, who provided a strong lead in this research, could do nothing but sit and wait for Whitehall to issue instructions. The Permanent Secretary at the Scottish Health Department, Douglas Haddow, had been more proactive, preparing a detailed memorandum, which noted that Scotland had the highest rates of lung cancer in Europe (followed by England and Wales), and called for a £1 million anti-smoking advertising campaign and a 50 per cent increase in tax on cigarettes which he estimated would reduce consumption by 30 per cent.[55] He was resigned to his report disappearing into the Ministry of Health's files without action. This is not to say that it had not received attention. It had stimulated considerable anxiety among officials at the Ministry, which junior staff had attempted to deal with. It has even been suggested that this report was deliberately kept away from Godber, who had become CMO in 1960 on Charles' belated retirement.[56]

There was some external pressure during these years of Ministerial prevarication, notably from Medical Officers of Health in local government. In September 1960, Dr JA Scott, Medical Officer of Health for London County Council, wrote to Goodman at the Ministry enclosing an advertisement photograph clipping from the *Daily Telegraph* of 30 August:

> in which the services of a lieutenant, Royal Navy, and naval equipment appear to have been enlisted by the Imperial Tobacco Company for the purpose of advertising 'Export Woodbines'. I feel sure that you will wish to know more about it and I should certainly be relieved to know that participation by the armed services in tobacco advertising will not continue indefinitely.[57]

The Admiralty subsequently confirmed that they had had no involvement. The Imperial Tobacco Company had used a model and hired the helicopter and uniform, but this farce clearly illustrates that it took a public health professional from outside Whitehall to prick what had become a comfortable relationship.[58]

The Royal College of Physicians' report on smoking and health was finally published in March 1962.[59] It provided the heavyweight independent scientific confirmation of Bradford Hill and Doll's research that the Ministry so desperately needed. This let them off the hook with the Treasury and the tobacco industry. If the public now reduced tobacco consumption (which they did almost overnight), it would not be the Ministry's 'fault'. Enoch Powell, who had become Minister for Health in July 1960, received an advance copy of the report through Godber in

[55] Ibid.

[56] Pollock, *Denial and Delay*. Pollock claims that Godber was not aware of Haddow's report until he read the draft of Pollock's book.

[57] MH 55/2226. JA Scott to Goodman, 08.09.1960.

[58] A very similar complaint was made to the CMO's office in 1999 about the sponsorship of the Royal Airforce Benevolent Fund concert by a tobacco company.

[59] Royal College of Physicians of London, *Smoking and Health: report of the Royal College of Physicians of London on smoking in relation to cancer of the lung and other diseases* (London, Pitman Medical, 1962).

November 1961. His caustic response noted that the only effective action would be for the Treasury to raise tobacco duty:

> The publication of the Report will excite temporary interest and for weeks afterwards we shall have to answer a shower of tiresome questions about what the Government is not doing, but unless my colleague [Chancellor of the Exchequer] is prepared to use the fiscal weapon, I personally propose to indulge in as little humbug as I can get away with.[60]

Powell's irritated memorandum reflected the general mood at the Ministry, which in the lead-up to publication of the report was already defeatist. Officials could not generate any enthusiasm for an advertising campaign, and considered that the report had some worrying loopholes and would be too technical for the average man in the street to understand. Most crucially, there was still no conclusive evidence that smoking caused lung cancer, and until that was available, the tobacco industry could quite justifiably complain about any initiatives which might damage its business.

In the event, the Royal College of Physicians' report attracted considerable press attention. It had sold 33,000 copies by the autumn of 1963 and over 50,000 in the USA.[61] Although it was countered by the simultaneous publication of three documents by the Tobacco Advisory Committee and the Tobacco Manufacturers' Standing Committee for Research into the effects of smoking on health, the Royal College of Physicians' report appeared to produce a shift in sales from untipped cigarettes to filter cigarettes, cigars and pipe tobacco. Smoking cessation clinics were established by a number of local authorities and employers. The Ministry of Health even responded to pressure from its own staff and held lunch-time clinics at Alexander Fleming House.[62] As Powell had predicted, the Ministry was forced to respond to enquiries from the public and in parliamentary questions. Powell himself was interrogated on 12 March 1962 about the lack of resources for smoking prevention, the need to ban cigarette advertisements, and the lack of publicity campaigns.[63]

In the weeks after the launch of the report, the Interdepartmental Cabinet Committee was spurred into action by Lord Hailsham, who had been appointed by Macmillan to ensure an adequate response. Without Hailsham's personal anti-smoking enthusiasm it would undoubtedly have taken much longer to produce an integrated governmental response to this serious threat to health. Although television advertising of tobacco products was banned in 1965, it was not until 1971 that health warnings were put on cigarette packets – probably the first time that a large proportion of the British public became aware of the existence of the Chief Medical Officer.

The minutiae of the slow advancement of a health education campaign on the

[60] MH 55/2227. Powell minute, 11.11.1961.
[61] V Berridge, 'Science and policy: the case of post-war British smoking policy', in S Lock, LA Reynolds and EM Tansey (eds), *Ashes to Ashes: the history of smoking and health* (Amsterdam, Rodopi, 1998), p. 150.
[62] Hilton, *Smoking in British Popular Culture*, p. 174.
[63] Hansard, 1961–62, vol. 655. Written answers, 12 March 1962, p. 113; Oral answers – reply to Mr Lipton, p. 886.

dangers of tobacco smoking have been well-documented elsewhere.[64] We have shown how the CMO participated in, or rather, at times was excluded from, the development of health policy in this area. The cautious response of the Ministry to the new research at the beginning of the 1950s could be justified as an appropriate attitude to ongoing scientific investigations. Certainly any knee-jerk reaction would have been damaging to the then unsullied reputation of the tobacco industry. It is important also to remember that at this time sophisticated epidemiological modelling and lifestyle modification programmes were very new territory.[65] Yet Charles allowed Hawton to play this line for too long, and failed to insist that he, as CMO, should be involved in the assessment of the health risks of smoking. It took the Deputy CMO, Godber, to make the breakthrough by approaching the Royal College of Physicians to produce an independent report. This was the only way to circumvent the Treasury's opposition to an overt Ministry of Health attack on the lucrative tobacco duty.

The files on this episode, scattered between the Ministry of Health, the Cabinet Office and the Treasury, illustrate the power of civil service prevarication and of the dominance of the Permanent Secretary over the medical 'expertise' of the CMO. Part of this must lie in the personality factor – that Charles was rather more removed from the issue than one would expect.[66] His reliance on Goodman, the Senior Medical Officer at the Ministry with responsibility for cancer, to provide the medical input into the protracted discussions was convenient for the Treasury. Had Godber (an ardent non-smoker) been the nominated medical officer, he would not have allowed the matter to drag on for so long. That perhaps is precisely why he wasn't given this particular issue to deal with.

We return to the supposition that both Charles as CMO and Hawton as Permanent Secretary were persuaded to remain in their posts for longer than civil service codes of practice would normally require. Charles stayed an additional two years past the usual retirement age of 65 years, thus preventing the succession of Godber who would have quickly tackled the government on the smoking issue. In fact, it has been suggested that the civil service in the late 1950s actively sought an alternative to Godber as CMO because he was a threat to relations with the tobacco industry.[67] Whitehall's dogged determination to retain Hawton despite his clearly failing health lasted until 1960, when he was replaced

---

[64] For a detailed analysis of the issues around smoking and lung cancer, see S Lock, LA Reynolds and EM Tansey (eds), *Ashes to Ashes: the history of smoking and health* (Amsterdam, Rodopi, 1998). This edited collection is the result of a Wellcome Trust Witness Seminar which brought together many of the individuals who had first-hand experience of the developments of the 1950s and 1960s. See also C Webster, 'Tobacco smoking and addiction: a challenge to the National Health Service', *British Journal of Addiction*, 1984, 79 (1), 8–16.

[65] An example of the 'acceptability' of the tobacco industry in the late twentieth century can be seen in the appointment of a number of senior civil servants and politicians to industry positions: Clifford Jarratt (1909-1995) who had been Permanent Secretary at the DHSS (1964–70) became Chair of the Tobacco Research Council after his retirement (1971–78). Kenneth Clarke, Minister of Health (1982–1985) and Secretary of State for Health (1988–90), has been a Non-executive Director of British American Tobacco.

[66] CC Booth, 'Smoking and the gold-headed cane', in CC Booth (ed.), *Balancing Act: essays to honour Stephen Lock* (London, Keynes Press, 1991).

[67] Senior medical professional interview, 17.05.2000.

by Sir Bruce Fraser. This enabled the creation of a new, very compatible senior team at the Ministry of Health comprising Godber and Fraser with Powell as Minister between 1960 and 1963. They, too, had to counter the pressure of the Treasury, but, with Hawton gone, the tobacco industry had lost an influential ally.

Size matters: re-establishing a strong CMO

There is a high degree of consensus among the medical profession and senior civil servants that in George Godber the requisites for the post of CMO in the twentieth century were found in abundance. His tenure as CMO is within living memory (1960–1973) and this must enhance his reputation, but the epithets used by former colleagues all have a remarkable similarity: 'omniscient, encyclopaedic brain . . . huge capacity for work . . . has read everything before you have . . .'. When he retired in November 1973 the *British Medical Journal* commented that: '. . . it is no secret that his knowledge and fair judgement have brought him an influence on successive Ministers of Health that must be exceedingly rare.'[68]

He also had the necessary aura of authority. One junior colleague recalls that 'Godber was physically very imposing and very formidable looking. To a young civil servant he was actually quite a terrifying figure. He was a nice man to juniors but not above using his physical presence to intimidate people, and he would certainly intimidate administrators'.[69] Yet despite his fearsome intellectual reputation and the sense of awe he inspired in those he worked with, he retained a sense of humour. This is apparent in his recollections of the trials and errors of the new National Health Service, desperate for a modern image:

> I was with Ernest Brown (the Minister of Health) when he opened the new centre at the Scunthorpe Memorial Hospital. It was quite a nice little centre in the wrong place. There were one or two little snags about it. The day before he arrived to open it they found that they had not put in an electricity main which was rather essential for radiotherapy. The architect had planned a fine new system for a light lock in the diagnostic radiological department – a revolving door, but he had not measured the Sister-in-Charge and she got stuck with the door half way round on the morning before Ernest Brown arrived![70]

Godber was able to redress the balance within the Ministry of Health (which became the Department of Health and Social Services in 1968) between the administrative and medical branches. He reinstated the weekly TOTO (top of the office) meetings between the Minister, CMO and Permanent Secretary, and also the regular meetings with junior doctors which had been routine in Jameson's time. This reflected part of Godber's immediate strength as CMO: that he was ready to draw upon his 21 years of Whitehall experience, having joined the Ministry as a medical officer in 1939, with the ambition of shaping the development of a world-class healthcare system.

[68] *British Medical Journal*, 24.11.1973, (II), 442.
[69] Senior civil servant interview, 10.07.2000.
[70] G Godber, 'The MOH and the NHS', Second Duncan Lecture, University of Liverpool, 1984, published in *Community Medicine*, 1986, 8 (1), 1–14.

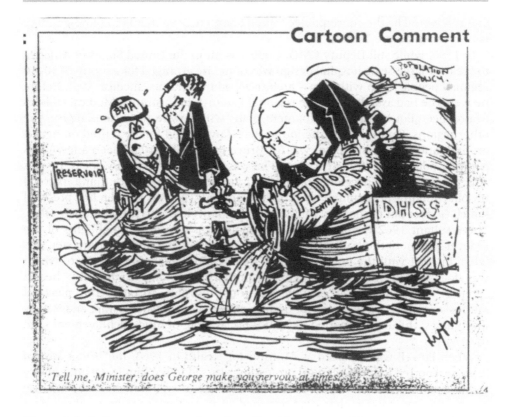

Figure 3.4 Godber's attempt to introduce fluoridation to Britain's water supplies (*The Practitioner*). © Wellcome Library. Reproduced with permission.

Godber had been brought in from the Ministry of Health's Nottingham region by Jameson (who had taught him on the Diploma in Public Health course at the London School of Hygiene and Tropical Medicine in the 1930s) to be his personal assistant for the National Health Service planning. From that point onwards, he was able to observe at first hand the dynamics and effectiveness of the senior team. In a post-retirement interview, he commented on how the various combinations of Ministers and Permanent Secretaries had functioned. In his opinion, the 1950s should have seen a much more proactive approach to National Health Service capital investment. He surmised that part of the explanation for the low capital investment was due to the lack of interest shown by Ministers: 'You felt that Iain [MacLeod] and Denis Vosper wanted to be where they were. But one never did feel that with Robin Turton. And there wasn't much creative input from him.'[71] Godber had been keen to point out, however, that the Ministers were reliant on their civil servants for the translation of ideas into policy: 'Maybe Turton wasn't adequately briefed upon the need, maybe more should have been done by the departmental staff themselves . . . [the Minister] should be told "if you could get a capital programme, this is how we could use it,

[71] Godber interview with Anthony Seldon, 27.06.1980. Wellcome Trust Contemporary Medical Archives Centre (GC/201/D.2), p. 15.

and this would be the consequence". Well I don't believe that kind of programme was ever put before Turton.'[72]

In 1960, while still Deputy CMO, Godber went to the United States of America to see how large-scale hospital design was done. He arranged for a group of 30–40 regional people to go with him – architects, administrators, medical staff. Before he went, he had asked two of the regional Senior Administrative Medical Officers to produce pilot hospital development plans which were then circulated to the other regions. On his return, he found that Hawton had finally retired on health grounds and that his successor was Sir Bruce Fraser. Fraser had been a few years behind Godber at Bedford School, and he was very receptive to new ideas. He was able to take Godber's regional plans and propose to the Treasury that a national hospital building programme was urgently needed. This was also the first proposal which Godber put to the new Minister, Enoch Powell, on his arrival in July 1960. The resultant 1962 Hospital Plan has remained as one of the highlights of the redevelopment of the National Health Service, but an equally important step was taken in 1961 with the publication of a Health and Welfare Services Plan, which was focused on the development of primary care and community health services.[73] This sustained activity was only possible through the personal enthusiasm and hard work of the Godber–Fraser–Powell partnership, and starkly illuminates the earlier period of 1955–60 as one of underachievement and inactivity.

When Powell was replaced as Minister for Health in 1963, the *British Medical Journal* reported that the medical profession was sad to see him leave after a very positive period.[74] The new Minister was Anthony Barber, but not for long because a general election in October 1964 returned a Labour Government. Godber's next two Ministers were both strong personalities – Kenneth Robinson served from October 1964 until 1968, during which time he successfully facilitated the general practitioner contract and less successfully produced the Green Paper on National Health Service reorganisation. As a general practitioner's son he was as steeped as Godber in the history and tradition of British medical care and he did not want to abandon the philosophy of a National Health Service. Then, in 1968, the unwieldy Department of Health and Social Security was created, absorbing the Ministry of Health. The Secretary of State position was demanded by, and given to, Richard Crossman.

Crossman and Godber already knew each other well. Both were at New College, Oxford in the late 1920s. That gave Godber a bravado which was rare amongst Crossman's many other associates. Godber relished the arrival of Crossman:

> Crossman was again a stimulus the Department needed. They had got on well with Kenneth. They understood him. He was a friend. They really needed to be shaken up. You know you get bedded down

---

[72] Ibid., p. 17.

[73] For a detailed discussion of the Hospital Plan, see D Allen, 'An analysis of the factors affecting the development of the 1962 hospital plan for England and Wales', *Social Policy and Administration*, 1981, 15 (1), 3–18.

[74] 'The Minister of Health', *British Medical Journal*, 26.10.1963, (II), 1012.

awfully quickly in a department. I don't mean that friction is a necessary part of a relationship between politicians and civil servants, but you can get stuck in your ways very easily. Well no one was going to get stuck in their ways with Dick around . . . I had rows with him the same as everybody else did. But it didn't bother me because our relationship was one that he deliberately wished to have – that I could answer back.[75]

David Ennals, Crossman's friend and Minister of State at the Department of Health and Social Security, was less charitable:

I suppose he didn't treat civil servants that much worse than he treated other people, but civil servants were not able to treat him as other people could treat him. No civil servant would ever answer back to a Secretary of State. Dick would complete their sentences for them and sometimes get it wrong, he would berate them implying that they were incompetent, that they hadn't thought, he would never let them finish their defence . . . he couldn't see that civil servants were at a disadvantage and he just exploited the position. Sometimes he would have a session with civil servants and they would almost fall out of the room as if they had been battered.[76]

Godber admitted that on occasions Crossman went too far, bullying those who were susceptible to his tactics and refusing to enter into constructive discussions. He sympathised with the difficult relationship which Clifford Jarrett, as Permanent Secretary, had with Crossman (which is painfully exposed through various entries in Crossman's diaries), but claims that these were par for the course at this level in Whitehall.

Godber was also very keen to allow the Chief Nursing Officer, Chief Dental Officer and Chief Pharmaceutical Officer to advise Ministers in their own right, rather than through the CMO. He hoped that this would set a good example for wider doctor–nurse relationships, even implying that the doctor shouldn't always be the leader of the professional team.[77] This was an ethos which Calman successfully revived when he became CMO in 1991. Perhaps it is an indication that these two CMOs felt relatively secure and confident in their positions compared to predecessors who often sought to maintain rigid reporting lines to maintain the standing of their post.

Whitehall in the post-Fulton period

How did the late twentieth century restructurings of Whitehall affect the role of the CMO? The move towards greater transparency, reduced anonymity for senior civil servants, tighter accounting practices, and the proliferation in contracted-out services meant that the CMO, along with the Permanent Secretary, headed up a

[75] Seldon interview, p. 27.
[76] 'Symposium: the Crossman diaries reconsidered', *Contemporary Record*, 1987, 1 (2), 22–30.
[77] Seldon interview, p. 35.

very different kind of department than that fondly depicted in the BBC television programme *Yes, Minister*.

The Fulton Committee, which sat in 1966, was a significant break point in the history of the civil service, although it was but one in a long line of inquiries which had taken place since the seminal Northcote–Trevelyan Report of 1854.[78] In the politically charged atmosphere of Britain's post-war economic decline, Fulton pointed the finger of blame at the mandarins of Whitehall, cataloguing a plethora of institutional weaknesses. Fulton found that the service was too elitist, with middle- and upper-class 'Oxbridge' people filling most of the senior positions. There was also a lack of systematic training with too much emphasis at senior levels on 'the cult of the generalist'.

Fulton's proposals were largely blocked by both Whitehall and Parliament, but some substantial advances were made. One of the key insights of Fulton was that Whitehall needed to be more efficient. A culture of 'administrative management' was projected as an essential prerequisite for this. Direct outcomes were the formation of the Civil Service Department in 1968 (abolished in 1981) and a Civil Service College in 1970. More significantly, in 1971, the administrative class (the mandarin élite) was merged with the executive and clerical classes in preparation for the full 'open structure' which came in 1972.

The biggest impact was in the early 1980s with the new Conservative Government. Margaret Thatcher brought Sir Derek (later Lord) Rayner into Whitehall from his position as Chairman at Marks and Spencer's as the Prime Minister's Efficiency Adviser, supported by a new Efficiency Unit. The ensuing scrutiny of all government departments forced considerable staff cuts. This was reinforced by the publication of an Efficiency Unit report in 1988: *Improving Management in Government: the next steps. Report to the Prime Minister*.[79] The report heralded the creation of executive ('Next Steps') agencies to work to clear performance targets and with a direct reporting line from the Chief Executive to Ministers. Three years later one of the last bastions of the Northcote–Trevelyan reforms was removed when the Civil Service Commission was reformed. Individual government departments now had greater control over the selection of their staff.

This sequence of change was frenetic. By 1994, some 97 executive agencies had been formed, accounting for nearly two-thirds of the civil service workforce. A new tranche of reforms emerged that same year through a White Paper (*The Civil Service: continuity and change*) which gave individual departments more autonomy over pay and conditions of service.[80] According to a *Next Steps* briefing note, by October 1994 some £2.1 billion worth of activities had been 'examined', resulting in an annual saving of £410 million and a reduction of 26,900 posts.[81] Ultimately, this drive towards greater devolution of powers from the centre (the Commission, the Civil Service Department, centrally managed pay and conditions) was a direct response to the greater *accountability* to which departments – and in particular the

[78] P Barberis, *The Whitehall Reader: the UK's administrative machine in action* (Buckingham, Open University Press, 1996), p. 1.
[79] Efficiency Unit, *Improving Management in Government: the next steps. Report to the Prime Minister* (London, HMSO, 1988).
[80] Cabinet Office, *The Civil Service: continuity and change* (Cmd. 2627) (London, HMSO, 1994).
[81] Barberis gives further details of the impact of staff losses in the various areas of the civil service: *The Whitehall Reader*, p. 11.

Next Steps agencies – were subject in relation to performance and efficiency. This was based on the premise that if you didn't control the inputs on efficiency, you couldn't sensibly be held to account for the output.

Selection of Permanent Secretaries

The selection of Permanent Secretaries (and this includes CMOs) had become a crucial factor in the successful operation of government. Some Prime Ministers took a greater degree of interest than others in these significant appointments. In 1945, Aneurin Bevan was able to choose a new Permanent Secretary to work with him at the Ministry of Health. He was given a choice of three names by Edward Bridges (Head of the Home Civil Service) and he opted for William Douglas. Foot recounts that Bevan had picked Douglas for qualities that were the opposite of his own. 'We can't have two Ministers of Health', Bevan had declared.[82] Ministerial attitudes were not always so rounded. Frank Cousins in 1964 refused to have Bruce Fraser as his Permanent Secretary at the Ministry of Technology. He told the Cabinet Secretary, Burke Trend: 'One, he doesn't like me, and two, I don't like him.'[83] Most Ministers, however, recognised that there was little room for manoeuvre at the top of Whitehall, and usually accepted the 'civil service man'.

In 1968, in response to the Fulton Report, a Senior Appointments Selection Committee was established. Through the head of the civil service, this offered candidates for particular posts for Prime Ministerial approval. It has increasingly adopted a 'job-centred' approach, in which the specific requirements of the post have been given priority rather than considering who is on the waiting list for civil service promotion.[84]

The Department of Health and Social Security was well-led during the turbulent years of reform in the 1970s and 1980s. Sir Patrick Nairne, who served as Permanent Secretary between 1975 and 1981, came to the Department from the Ministry of Defence with a good reputation. Barbara Castle was pleased to have him in her team:

> It fascinates me to watch how Pat Nairne is settling himself into his new job. In some ways his problem is the same as that of a new Minister: trying to assess the personal quality of the people with whom he has to work, ears open to all comments even gossip, but knowing that in the end he himself has to select the relevant. I like him enormously. I don't know whether it has anything to do with his long stint at Defence, but he clearly sees his job as to carry out orders; not to query the strategy, but to make sure it works – a welcome change from Philip [Rogers – the former PS] and Henry's [Yellowlees, CMO] soul-searchings. On this basis, a Minister is in business with his civil servants and can even carry a coward or two. Without this kind of approach from the top brass the doctrine of ministerial responsibility cannot work.[85]

[82] M Foot, *Aneurin Bevan: a biography* (London, McGibbon & Kee, 1973), pp. 42–3.

[83] G Goodman, *The Awkward Warrior: Frank Cousins – his life and times* (Nottingham, Spokesman, 1984), p. 409.

[84] Barberis, *The Elite of the Elite*, p. 129.

[85] B Castle, *The Castle Diaries, 1974–76* (London, Weidenfeld & Nicolson, 1980), p. 609.

Nairne was replaced in 1981 by Sir Kenneth Stowe. Patrick Jenkin (Minister of Health 1979–1981) had a tough three-month battle to secure Stowe's appointment as he had not been on the original list of the Senior Appointments Selection Committee's approved candidates. The civil service tried all sorts of tactics to divert Jenkin from his choice. Barberis suggests that it was only the personal intervention of Prime Minister Margaret Thatcher that did it.[86] Stowe worked hard during his five years at the Department of Health and Social Security to shore up the complex nightmare of social security as well as a rapidly changing National Health Service. His comment on social security in 1986 speaks volumes for the revolution in Whitehall and the impact of Raynerism on accountable management:

> We cannot go into liquidation, but neither can we dispose of unattractive subsidiaries or get out of the unrewarding markets we are operating in.[87]

Accountability

Since the rejuvenation of Parliamentary Select Committees in 1979, senior civil servants have had to account for the activities of each of the main Whitehall departments. The Fulton Report had eventually produced a mechanism which allowed civil servants a degree of recognition, if not responsibility, separate from that of Ministers (although technically they still appear on their behalf). This was quite a change. Herbert Morrison had famously said that Ministers were responsible for all the acts within their departments, even 'for every stamp stuck on an envelope'.[88] The system of accounting officers, responsible in their own right to the Commons' Committee of Public Accounts, has provided a stronger basis on which a civil servant can contradict a Minister, albeit over 'accountable management' issues rather than policy ones.

During the 1980s and 1990s, the Permanent Secretaries in the Department of Health faced an increasingly stressful regime. The National Health Service had come to dominate its raison d'être. The separation of health and social security into separate departments in 1988 helped ease the burden for the civil servants, but the spectre of crisis was ever present. As the Permanent Secretary, Sir Patrick Nairne, commented:

> All my time at the DHSS I felt you had to be ready as permanent secretary for one of those lightening strikes in the autumn . . . it was an extraordinarily difficult department to run . . . the benefit offices, the relationship with the NHS who were not civil servants, the social services administered by local authorities and the public health role.[89]

---

[86] Barberis, *The Elite of the Elite*, p. 127. Treasury and Civil Service Committee, *Seventh Report, Session 1985–86 – Civil Servants and Ministers: duties and responsibilities*, Vol. II – Annexes, Minutes of Evidence and Appendices, HC 92-II; Qs.486–7.
[87] K Stowe, 'Managing a Great Department of State', Royal Society of Arts, 21 April 1986, quoted in Hennessy, *Whitehall*, p. 423.
[88] House of Commons debates 1953/54, 5th series, vol. 530, col. 1274.
[89] Quoted in Hennessy, *Whitehall*, p. 421.

In addition to the onerous task of being an accounting officer, by the late 1980s the Permanent Secretary also had a greater degree of responsibility for a wide range of issues within his department. In an era which has seen unparalleled competition for funds, he or she was increasingly relied on to provide the critical policy statements and insider information from other rival Whitehall departments which his Minister could use to advantage when negotiating funding from the Treasury.[90] Justification perhaps for Tony Benn's quip that 'Britain is governed by the Prime Minister and the Permanent Secretaries'.[91] Barberis makes an additional useful point on the relative political influence which the Permanent Secretary can exert through his or her unique relationship with Ministers:

> . . . the first tremblings of a Ministerial career passing its meridian will often percolate through the Permanent Secretary – in the manner of nuance and subtlety rather than facile transmission. The Whitehall grapevine is never more efficient than when disseminating the political barometer.[92]

The Chief Medical Officers who have also held civil service rank of Permanent Secretary have not been immune from these reforms.

Conclusion

This chapter has focused on how the tripartite relationship between the CMO, Permanent Secretary and Minister has evolved. The frequency with which this 'team' changes means that the relationship is constantly being renegotiated. As Arthur Henderson (Ramsay MacDonald's Foreign Secretary) put it: 'The first 48 hours decide whether a new Minister is going to run his office or whether the office is going to run him.'[93] Godber's first encounter with Bevan was a classic example of how the 'chemistry' between the CMO and his minister could be sparked. In a meeting between the Ministry of Health officials and Bevan, concern was expressed by the former about the potential costs to the new National Health Service from the huge backlog of demands for eye tests and spectacles. Bevan heard the officials in silence and then remarked: 'That's all well and good, but I am not paying for monocles for toffs like you Godber.' When Godber mildly pointed out that he himself wore a monocle because he only had one eye and was short-sighted, Bevan was mortified and the two got on extremely well from that moment on.

There have been some Ministers, Permanent Secretaries and CMOs who stand out. Robert Maxwell modelled the 'success' of Health Ministers on four key characteristics: an ideal tenure of between three and five years; strategic vision and commitment; good selective judgement about priorities; and leadership. In his 1981 analysis of the 30 Ministers of Health or Secretaries of State for Health since the formation of the Ministry of Health in 1919, only a handful met these

---

[90] For a more detailed critique on the civil service of the 1980s and 1990s, see K Stowe, 'Good piano won't play bad music', *Public Administration*, 1992, 70, 387–94.
[91] Treasury and Civil Service Select Committee, Seventh Report, Session 1985–86 – *Civil Servants and Ministers: duties and responsibilities. Vol. II, Minutes of Evidence*, p. 491.
[92] Barberis, *The Elite of the Elite*, p. 31.
[93] E Clark, *Corps Diplomatique* (London, Allen Lane, 1973), p. 8.

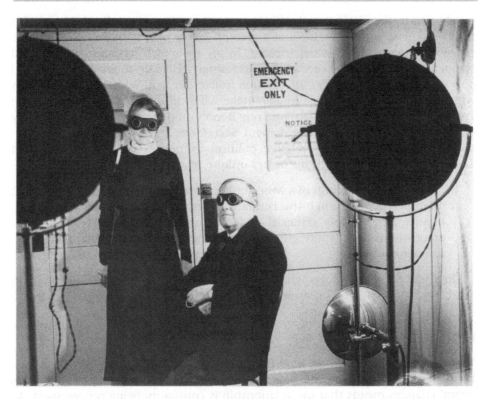

Figure 3.5 Sir Kingsley Wood, Minister of Health, receives artificial sun-ray treatment in 1936. © Hulton Deutsch Collection. Reproduced with permission.

criteria: Neville Chamberlain (as a legislator), Bevan (who gave shape and impetus to the National Health Service), Powell (for the hospital and local authority plans of the 1960s) and possibly Robinson (for negotiating with general practitioners).[94] It is perhaps no surprise to find that these Ministers were partnered by some of the more talented CMOs of this period such as Jameson and Godber.[95]

George Godber, in his address to the British Medical Association's 1981 annual meeting, concurred with Maxwell, but added other examples of Ministerial vision: Keith Joseph, who used his influence with private donors to secure endowments for chairs in some neglected disciplines in medicine, and David Owen for pushing through the introduction of the Resource Allocation Working Party which for the first time tackled the issue of regional resource allocation inequalities.[96] This is perhaps a more nuanced assessment, taking in wider politics such as the relative status of health in government and the financial regimes of the day. The view is substantiated by a recent reassessment of the Conservative's

[94] RJ Maxwell, 'On Ministers of Health', *Lancet*, 27.06.1981, (I), 1412–14.
[95] Charles Webster gives a very useful overview of the Ministerial successes and failures in *The Health Services Since the War, Vol. II* (London, HMSO, 1996), pp. 731–52. See for example how he highlights the relative weak performance of David Ennals and his failure to develop health policy.
[96] GE Godber, 'Doctors in government', *Health Trends*, 1981, 1 (13), 1–4.

'sacrifice' of NHS resources in the period 1951–1964.[97] There is little doubt that there have also been some periods in which the circumstances for being CMO have been more favourable than others.

Despite the enduring image of a fairly rigid Whitehall etiquette, there have been exceptions which bent the formal rules of access and communication. Aneurin Bevan, as Minister of Health (1945–51), frequently wandered unannounced into the offices of junior staff at the Ministry, with the tacit approval of his Permanent Secretary, William Douglas.[98] In 1994 easier internal communications were one of the aspirations acknowledged within *The Civil Service: continuity and change* document, which sought to enable direct access to Ministers and heads of department for officials down to assistant secretary level.[99] Also, as Whitehall opened up to the influence of special advisers, the flow of advice became more fluid, although remaining within the parameters set by the civil service. Permanent Secretaries became policy managers rather than policy initiators – better described as 'brokers' – or, as Barberis neatly puts it, to ensure that 'however many shafts of light there may be, they are projected onto the one canvas'.[100]

Permanent Secretaries had a wealth of Whitehall experience – more crucial than ever when 'external' CMOs were brought into the post. The majority of Permanent Secretaries had more than a quarter of a century in Whitehall before they reached the top.[101] But there is also the counter-argument that the maximum tenancy of Permanent Secretaries should be five years. In fact, calculations made for the period 1979–1994 indicate that the post has become self-limiting, with average incumbency 3.7 years.[102] This left a reduced window of opportunity for maximum effectiveness, particularly if we accept Nairne's hypothesis that Permanent Secretaries require a 'running-in period', and recognise that many Permanent Secretary posts latterly were filled by departmental transfer rather than internal, experienced promotions.[103]

The position of the CMO was strengthened by these developments, since with a longer average incumbency, he provided a valued degree of stability at the 'top of the office'. Godber famously would stand at the lift waiting to greet a new Minister as he or she arrived in the Department with the line 'you are the nth Minister/Secretary of State whom I have had the honour to serve'.[104] Acheson

---

[97] C Webster, 'Conservatives and consensus: the politics of the National Health Service, 1951–1954', in A Oakley and S Williams (eds), *The Politics of the Welfare State* (London, UCL Press, 1994), pp. 54–74.

[98] M Foot, *Aneurin Bevan: a biography. Vol. II: 1945–1960* (London, Davis Poynter, 1973), pp. 40–3.

[99] Cabinet Office, *The Civil Service: continuity and change* (Cmd. 2627) (London, HMSO, 1994), p. 38.

[100] Barberis, *The Elite of the Elite*, p. 42.

[101] For a useful example of how a Permanent Secretary can dominate the development of policy, see M Beloff, 'The Whitehall Factor: the role of the higher civil service, 1919–39', in G Peele and C Cook (eds), *The Politics of Reappraisal, 1918–1939* (London, Macmillan, 1975), which examines the impact of Sir Warren Fisher who was Permanent Secretary at the Treasury from 1919 to 1939.

[102] Ibid., pp. 184–5.

[103] P Nairne, 'Managing the DHSS elephant: reflections on a giant department', *Political Quarterly*, 1983, 54, 243–56.

[104] Senior medical civil servant interview, 16.02.2000.

likewise had a very strong sense of his role and position within government and Whitehall, and began his tenure as CMO by gaining admission to Permanent Secretaries' meetings chaired by the Cabinet Secretary. He even wrote to Margaret Thatcher to put his case for unrestricted access to brief her on anything he considered in the interests of the health of the public.[105]

The CMO can be viewed as a linchpin between medium-term senior civil servants and often very short-term Ministers. Once again, however, this chapter has shown that personality, and personal ability to influence the Whitehall machine and medical networks, has been critical to the success of health policies, and to the inherent authority of the CMO.

---

[105] Senior civil servant interview, 04.04.2000.

Chapter 4

Making advice count

Writing in 1936, the sixth CMO, Arthur Newsholme, said that there was:

> . . . an honest belief, common to many government departments, that technical advice is advice not to be given until called for by the secretariat who, it is assumed, are entirely competent to decide whether such advice is needed. Second, when such advice is on record, it is assumed that it can be safely reapplied in what are regarded by the secretariat as analogous circumstances.[1]

The CMO post is unusual within the senior levels of government. All the incumbents have had extensive professional training, in-depth experience of public health or clinical practice, and considerable technical expertise. They have also commanded large networks of professional, practitioner, scientific and academic contacts at home and internationally. The most senior administrative civil servants do not have this breadth and depth of professional expertise. There are others with a scientific and technical background but they tend to be in more junior grades.

The work of the CMO has involved drawing together research evidence, clinical views and expert opinion. How this information is sought, what choices are made about where to seek advice, how much to rely on internal sources rather than external, and how advice is synthesised to form a balanced view, are crucial to the influence and integrity of the CMO's role.

This chapter seeks to establish the internal dimensions of the post. We examine the fluctuating fortunes of the medical civil service, its status and security within Whitehall. More specifically we look at the impact during the latter period of the study of the rationalisation of the civil service support available to the CMO. The commissioning of external advice, and specifically how this impinges upon the relationship between the government and the medical profession, is covered in Chapters 5 and 6.

Valuing expertise in Whitehall

The word 'expertise' first came into use in the 1860s. Through its progressive consolidation with the process of legislation, it became part of the wider movement identified as 'professionalisation of government' in the nineteenth century.[2]

[1] A Newsholme, *The Last Thirty Years in Public Health* (London, George Allen and Unwin, 1936), p. 62.
[2] O McDonagh, 'The nineteenth century revolution in government: a reappraisal', *Historical Journal*, 1958, I, 52–67; R MacLeod (ed.), *Government and Expertise: specialists, administrators and professionals, 1860–1919* (Cambridge, Cambridge University Press, 1988); H Perkins, *The Rise of Professional Society: England since 1880* (London, Routledge, 1989).

In Chapter 1, we have shown how John Simon conjured up medical staff for his department at the Privy Council. Despite the growth of local public health expertise (there were 1,771 Medical Officers of Health by 1899), it was imperative to maintain a surveillance and advice system to ensure consistency of reform and the dominance of central government ideology. Simon tried to augment his limited staff to fulfil these expectations. His resignation, in 1876, was ostensibly the result of being denied three additional inspectors.

Seaton became CMO with a much more circumscribed role: ' . . . arrange as to the inspections to be undertaken under the direction of the Board by the Medical Inspectors, to examine their reports, and advise the Board upon them, to superintend generally the medical staff, and all matters relating to vaccination'.[3] With only nine inspectors to support him, Seaton's personal workload was intolerable. When asked to administer the scientific grant (Simon had done this with additional payment and clerical support), he protested in the strongest terms permissible within the etiquette of the civil service:

> To impose this further duty upon me without remuneration for it, would appear to me a great hardship and if I may without offence say so, a departure from an understanding on which I relied.[4]

Pressure of work undoubtedly precipitated Seaton's ill-health and untimely death in January 1880. His successor, George Buchanan, pursued the thankless task of getting extra medical staff. Chronic understaffing was now a critical issue. A backlog of routine sanitary and vaccination inspections, as well as a lack of capacity to conduct special inquiries, were major concerns. Fieldwork such as Power's investigation of the 'aerial spread' of smallpox from the Fulham smallpox hospital and the regional surveys of scarlet fever were postponed indefinitely.[5]

Civil service medical staff were regularly at the mercy of Treasury parsimony. Buchanan's repeated requests to the Treasury through the President of the Local Government Board for extra staff, and for higher salaries for his existing staff, were rebuffed. The workload continued to increase:

> . . . for the last year or two the daily work of the Department has had to be done at too high speed to be done properly, more and more of it has been postponed, and more and more has been left undone. At the same time other departments within the Board, other departments of Government, and all local governments have been inconvenienced by the delays and errors that arise.[6]

This explicit memorandum was typical of George Buchanan. His obituary noted that he 'was not always at pains to conceal his impatience with politicians who failed to realise the importance of [his] work'.[7] A letter he wrote to Charles Dilke, then President of the Local Government Board, in November 1883 pulled no punches either:

[3] MH 19/212. Lambert to Treasury, 06.04.1876.
[4] MH 19/212. Seaton to Lambert, 21.12.1877.
[5] RM McLeod, 'The frustration of state medicine', *Medical History*, 1967, XI, 19.
[6] T 1/8298A/6204/1887. Buchanan to Treasury, 06.08.1883.
[7] Buchanan obituaries: *Lancet*, 11.05.1895, (I), 1224–5; *British Medical Journal*, 11.05.1895, (I), 1066–7.

It would be a disaster to sanitary progress as well as a serious misfortune to the Board, if your Medical Officer should, by any reason of his utter preoccupation in routine business, lose sight of the true aim of his office, and cease to guide his department by the only trustworthy principles of sanitary reform.[8]

The spectre of disaster did appear, in November 1883, when epidemic cholera advanced through Europe. Buchanan used this to force the Treasury to pay for six temporary inspectors, but when the epidemic failed to materialise in Britain the staff were withdrawn. The Medical Department was reviewed in 1884 and 1887. Each time, no justification was found for increases in staff or salaries. One internal promotion to an Assistant Inspectorship was granted, but the Treasury stipulated shorter inspectors' reports, greater devolution of work to local sanitary officers, and that local authorities should pay for the inspection of their own districts.[9]

The research programme bore the brunt of the Treasury's tight regime. This valuable initiative had been established by John Simon. In the 1880s developments in bacteriology opened up new opportunities for research of great practical value. For example, it became possible to study zoonoses transmitted through milk. However, the Medical Department had to reduce its already small research budget from £1,900 to £1,100 per annum. Buchanan's warning resonates chillingly with findings of the Phillips Inquiry into the bovine spongiform encephalopathy (BSE) crisis a century later:

> However people may be satisfied to disbelieve medical theses, they will not be content that Farmers and Dairymen should forfeit business valued at thousands of pounds. The Government ought to be able to say that investigation of such disease in its veterinary aspects was being undertaken by the Agricultural Department, and that it was in its later relations being studied by your Medical Department, the two acting in concert and having all proper resources at their disposal. The Government will not be able to say so . . .[10]

In Whitehall, Buchanan had overstepped the mark. He had ordered inquiries into subjects which were considered 'speculative' and 'always under discussion in the medical world'. He was rebuked by a civil service superior, who accused him of attempting to create a 'Department of State Medicine', and he was told to confine his work to the agreed limits. For example, the maximum annual number and type of inspections were specified. He had to decline an invitation to give the first Milroy lecture on 'State Medicine and Public Health' in 1887.[11] At loggerheads with the Treasury, and to some extent, the Local Government Board, he was in sympathy with the widespread dissatisfaction within his own Medical Department. He made a final plea for an adequate pension:

> It is to your good offices that I look for the arrears of living in reasonable comfort and of doing in a modest fashion my duty for

---

[8] T 1/8298A/6204/1887. Buchanan to Sir Charles Dilke (President of Local Government Board), 17.11.1883.

[9] McLeod, 'The frustration of state medicine', p. 24.

[10] MH 19/217. Buchanan to President (Charles Ritchie), 26.01.1887.

[11] Royal College of Physicians Archives, 1021/4 letter Buchanan to Pitman, 27.04.1887.

the next few years towards my family, a duty which I could assuredly have discharged if, in giving my services to the public, I had not given them to Her Majesty's Government. You will probably be sensible that it is not to the interests of the Government to exhibit to men of ability desirous of entering the Medical Service of the Government, such an end to their careers as the Treasury is proposing for me – the Principal Medical Officer of your Medical Department.[12]

Buchanan's successor, Richard Thorne Thorne, had an equally hard time with the Treasury. He had himself resorted to a form of blackmail to get his own CMO salary maintained. He refused to accept the promotion if it involved a 'further lowering of the status of the office'.[13] His deputy, William Power, also successfully used this tactic. He only accepted promotion on condition that he could submit a memorandum protesting against the government's treatment of Medical Officers.[14] The work of the Medical Department was still outstripping the capacity of its staff. In 1891 over 200 correspondence files directed to Thorne Thorne were unopened and local inquiries were being severely delayed. Smallpox vaccination inspection was very poor – some 686 districts had not been inspected for two years or more, and the number of unvaccinated children was increasing.[15]

What irked Thorne Thorne and his medical colleagues at the Local Government Board most was that the lay secretariat, and the Treasury in particular, did not understand the nature of their work nor the need to be proactive in combating new disease threats. Indeed, they were viewed as creating unnecessary work to raise their value within Whitehall:

It was made clear to the Committee [of 1887] that the Medical Officers could relieve themselves by ceasing to invent all sorts of recondite investigations which they had been in the habit of undertaking without any authority from the Board. Lord Basing [Sclater Booth] told us that the practice was wholly wrong and thus the best way of stopping it was to let the Inspectors have their time well-filled up by the work they were ordered to do.[16]

The number of medical staff had increased to fourteen by 1892, but this brought little relief for the existing staff, and there were no salary increases. In that year, Thorne Thorne wrote to Owen, the Permanent Secretary, warning of impending nervous breakdowns if the threatened cholera reached Britain:

Both Mr Power and I have arrears of work which we see no present prospect of overtaking and this although we both regularly take home work at night. [sic] And apart from ever increasing current work, special questions involving much labour and time are always arising. Thus, at the present time, two Royal Commissions have intimated to me that they desire us to give evidence before them. I have not had any time to make preparations for this, nor have I even unpacked the

[12] T 1/8640/5732/1892. Buchanan to Ritchie, 13.06.1892.
[13] MH19/219. Minute, Ritchie, 03.08.1892.
[14] T 1/8660C/12060/1892. Memorandum, Power to President, 16.07.1892.
[15] MacLeod, 'The frustration of state medicine', p. 29.
[16] T 1/8660C/12060/1892.

voluminous papers submitted to me several months ago by one of the Commissions for perusal and study before giving evidence. Mr Power and I (notably Mr Power) have for years past foregone much of our allotted period of leave of absence . . .[17]

Thorne Thorne used this evidence of overwork to refuse to take on any additional duties (unless they were accompanied by appropriate resources). He refused to contemplate taking over responsibility for the Poor Law medical services and thus prolonged the division in central government medical duties. More damning still, he testified to the 1898 inquiry that he had even opposed Britain's involvement in the Paris and Vienna International Health Conferences of 1892 and 1894, because he could not attend personally and feared that if the Colonial and Foreign Offices sent their own medical representatives all cohesion in national health policy would be ruined.[18]

Thorne Thorne had limited success with the 1898 inquiry. His salary was increased to £1,500 (but this was still £500 less than Simon had received), and he was given some additional temporary staff to clear the backlog of work. However, there remained fundamental problems in the central Medical Department. It was very difficult to persuade suitably qualified medical staff to apply for temporary vacancies, not surprisingly, as the deficiencies of the Medical Department had been aired extensively in the *British Medical Journal*.[19]

Yet the Treasury could not keep on blocking expansion plans at the Local Government Board. By the end of the nineteenth century, public health was a very different concept even to Simon's vision of the 1850s. Bacteriology was a powerful new tool for the diagnosis of disease. It also helped inspections of water and food supplies. All this required specialist staff and laboratories, which were expensive. The state began to acknowledge that it had a broader responsibility for protecting the health of the public. Although Thorne Thorne died in December 1899, after months of illness exacerbated by overwork, the pressure on Power as his successor, and on his medical staff, continued unabated.

Power took a new approach. He persuaded the Treasury to appoint non-professional 'roving' inspectors, who were well-educated but cheaper than medical staff. Royal Commissions reporting on tuberculosis, venereal diseases, water supplies and sewerage disposal ensured that the Treasury did not stifle new initiatives completely. Power's successor, Newsholme, was equally resourceful, and successfully updated the functions of the Medical Department. He was instrumental in developing many new health services, including schemes for tuberculosis, venereal disease and infant welfare. As a long-serving Medical Officer of Health (1884–1908), he knew how to use a staged process of development for new projects, shaping it in the light of feedback from local implementation.

Yet despite some improvements in capacity, Newsholme and his team found themselves playing 'catch-up' on policy making as the underlying philosophy of government changed. Many policies had their origins outside Whitehall.[20] Lloyd

[17] Cited in MacLeod, 'The frustration of State Medicine', pp. 34–5.
[18] Report of the Departmental Committee on the Clerical Staff and Secretariat of the Local Government Board, 1898 xl. (C.8731) Mins. Evid. Q.1196.
[19] *British Medical Journal*, 1898, (I), 711.
[20] J Eyler, *Sir Arthur Newsholme and State Medicine, 1885–1935* (Cambridge, Cambridge University Press, 1997), p. 383.

George in particular developed a very personal interest in policy making, using his own preferred advisers on new projects such as national health insurance. It is testimony to Newsholme's sense of team spirit, or perhaps, resilience, that he did not take umbrage at being marginal to much health policy formulation. It was a dynamic and creative period for him otherwise and he led many innovative programmes.

Was the salvation of the medical civil service found in the creation of a dedicated department, free from subjugation to the Local Government Board, as many historians have seen it?[21] Simon certainly saw this as a solution to safeguarding the health of the nation. Yet when a Ministry of Health was finally created in 1919, it was a flawed concept. Newsholme undoubtedly achieved more in his period at the end of the time of the Local Government Board than did his successor Newman at the new Ministry of Health.

The market value of the CMO

At the dawn of the Ministry of Health in 1919, the question of the CMO's financial value again reared its head. Newman's pay and rank were matters not just personal to him. Other medical staff at the Ministry, and the medical profession more generally, watched closely every stage of the negotiations. Addison, the Health Minister, was at fault. He had 'publicly announced and a copy [of the details of Newman's rank and pay] in writing was furnished to all medical staff as evidence of the new position of medicine in the civil service established by the creation of the Ministry of Health'.[22] Newman's salary re-evaluation took it from the initial £2,100 to £3,000. This was significant because it defined his status relative to the wider medical profession. The post of CMO would only command respect if it was seen as the pinnacle of the profession and remunerated accordingly.

The medical staff at the Ministry fought their own battle for salaries commensurate with other civil servants' posts. Newman noted in his diary that the atmosphere at the first meeting between Addison and the medical staff was 'v[ery] cold and discouraging'.[23] The Medical Staff Association at the Ministry (of which Newman was not a member) later sent a deputation to Addison to tell him of the tension between themselves and administrative staff created by the lack of pay parity.

The Permanent Secretary, Morant, attempted to bridge the gap between Newman and Addison, and tried to address the imbalance between the medical and administrative hierarchies. He tried to placate Newman over his concerns whilst reassuring the medical staff that 'the fullest possible weight' would be given to the 'medical point of view'.[24] Morant knew about other developments within Whitehall, in particular the recommendations of the Whitley Council,

---

[21] F Honigsbaum, *The Struggle for the Ministry of Health 1914–19*. Occasional Papers in Social Administration No.37 (London, G Bell, 1970); F Honigsbaum, *Health, Happiness and Security: the creation of the National Health Service* (London, Routledge, 1989).

[22] MH 78/92. Newman personal letter to Addison, 11.11.1920.

[23] MH 139/3. Newman diary, 07.07.1919.

[24] MH 107/26. Memorandum 'The organisation of the medical staff of the Ministry of Health'.

which ruled that technical officers should not be graded in the same way as senior civil servants. However, he also wanted a fully integrated Ministry free of rigid divisions between medical and administrative staff.[25] He predicted privately that this would produce medical dominance, but the structure that he and Newman devised established two separate but parallel hierarchies.

Chamberlain, the Chancellor of the Exchequer, also attempted to exploit the Whitley Council ruling in the Treasury's favour, refusing to concede that the post of CMO was comparable with the Solicitor to the Treasury. The latter was a departmental manager, not just a specialist under the control of a departmental head. Chamberlain suggested that fairer comparison for Newman was the post held by Sir Douglas Hall, technical adviser to the Ministry of Agriculture. The Chancellor's overriding concern was probably the state of departmental budgets, but it illustrates the contemporary government's determination and persistence to redress the balance in favour of rank and file 'generalist' civil servants. When Newman threw down the precedent set by John Simon for CMO parity with the Permanent Secretary, Chamberlain testily replied:

> I do not propose to argue with you the precedent which you and Fisher think you have found. I do not recognise its applicability, and it is in any case nearly fifty years old.[26]

Newman got his pay rise but at a salary equivalent to a Permanent Secretary's deputy. By 1965, the CMO (George Godber) was earning £2,200 per annum, while the Permanent Secretary (Arnold France) was earning £3,000.[27] Part of the explanation for this can be found in the general view of the position of technical experts in the civil service: that they should be 'on tap but not on top'.[28]

Experts may have had relatively low Whitehall status, but in certain areas of government work the complexity of the issues meant that they had become essential. In 1931, the Tomlin Commissioners estimated that there were some 10 000 engineers, scientists, doctors and other specialists employed in the civil service.[29] There were benefits. The technical expert had a degree of relative freedom within his department which the 'generalist' did not. He was often able to 'initiate and, by judiciously cultivating the legal adviser and Permanent Secretary, submit measures which greatly extended government activity'.[30] Kitson Clark noted in 1959:

> The work of a government department nowadays has the same proportions as an iceberg: one third of it, if so much, is above water in the daylight world of party politics and public controversy, two-

[25] MH 78/92. Morant to Barter (his Private Secretary), 15.02.1919.

[26] MH 78/92. Chancellor of the Exchequer's response to a Board of Education memorandum, February 1919.

[27] EW Cohen, *The Growth of the British Civil Service, 1780–1939* (London, Frank Cass, 1965), p. 206.

[28] A Newsholme, *The Last Thirty Years in Public Health* (London, George Allen & Unwin, 1936), p. 50. Newsholme was reporting the comments of an unnamed Minister.

[29] Report of the Royal (Tomlin) Commission on the Civil Service, (Cd. 3909), 1931. Paras. 171 and 172.

[30] McLeod, *Government and Expertise*, pp. 12–13.

thirds of it, if not more, is below in the dark important technical world which the public cannot see.[31]

Managing the National Health Service

With the creation of the National Health Service (NHS) in 1948, the Ministry of Health for the first time had direct control over a comprehensive medical service.[32] Health, and its delivery through the NHS, became increasingly politicised during the 1950s and 1960s, partly because of ongoing disputes over function and financing. This brought a new dimension to the role of the CMO: a corporate role, as part of the senior management team of the NHS. Although Newman and MacNalty were involved in the planning and delivery of medical services (especially the Emergency Medical Service from 1938), it was Wilson Jameson who transformed the CMO into an integral part of the Ministry's senior team on health services as well as public health. His role in the establishment of the NHS is discussed in detail in Chapter 5.

In 1948 there was no massive expansion in either administrative or medical staff in Whitehall to oversee the new NHS. A review in 1951, established partly in response to worsening economic forecasts, reduced Ministry of Health staff from 5,300 to 2,724. The Ministry retained 21 officials of the rank of Assistant Secretary and above to manage the fourteen regional hospital boards, 377 hospital management committees, 138 executive councils and 145 local health and welfare authorities.[33] It was not a clear-cut case of reducing numbers. There was support from the Acton Society Trust surveys and from the 1955 Guillebaud Report (into the cost of the NHS) for a better research department and for more statisticians and economists within the Ministry.[34] As Webster notes, many of the structural problems experienced by the Ministry of Health in the 1950s had at their heart poor relations between the administrative and medical branches, something that had reached crisis point during Newman's era.[35] Furthermore, the image of the Ministry as a civil service career backwater was a chronic problem.[36]

There has also been criticism of the way in which the Ministry of Health developed its external relations, especially with local government (which retained control of a wide range of health and welfare services). Griffith, in

[31] G Kitson Clark, '"Statesmen in disguise": reflexions on the history of the neutrality of the civil service', *Historical Journal*, 1959, II, 38.
[32] See C Ham, *Health Policy in Britain: the politics and organisation of the NHS* (Basingstoke, Palgrave, 1999) for a good overview of the development of health policy within the NHS.
[33] C Webster, *The Health Services Since the War. Vol. I. Problems of Health Care: the National Health Service before 1957* (London, HMSO, 1988), p. 238.
[34] The Acton Society Trust, funded by the Rowntree Social Service Trust and the Nuffield Provincial Hospitals Trust, was set up in 1955 to promote economic, political and social research. The Trust carried out a series of studies, under the direction of TE Chester (later professor at Manchester University), into the organisation and administration of hospitals in the NHS. The first report was published in 1955, and subsequent reports in 1956, 1957, two in 1958 and the last one in 1959. Great Britain, Ministry of Health and Scottish Home and Health Department, *Report of the Committee of Enquiry into the Cost of the National Health Service.* (Chairman: CW Guillebaud) (London, HMSO, 1956). Cmd. 9663.
[35] Webster *Health Services, Vol. 1*, p. 239.
[36] M Kogan, 'Social Services: their Whitehall status', *New Society*, 21.08.1969.

1966, highlighted the Ministry's narrow interpretation of its role, in ensuring that local authorities and Medical Officers of Health followed government policy.[37] His view – that the Ministry had a 'relatively relaxed attitude' to what happened locally – was a point with which Godber concurred.[38]

The wider local government and health functions of the Ministry of Health were separated in January 1951. This was a logical redistribution of the machinery of government, but health lost housing. This had come to dominate Ministerial planning and budgets, but it carried weight. The loss of housing reduced the governmental influence of the Minister of Health, once the Ministry of Housing and Local Government was established. Without direct Cabinet representation, it was harder to progress a National Health Service capital programme. Less ambitious health service developments also suffered. In 1949, for example, the Ministry had wanted to provide a chiropody service, but because of Treasury restrictions permission was not given to establish this as a local authority service until 1959.[39]

After the split in 1951, the NHS dominated the life of the Ministry of Health, but the CMO was not always closely involved in this area of business. Newman's wider vision for a Ministry of Health as the locus of 'preventive medicine' appeared to have been subsumed within a clinically dominant culture. The declining fortunes of the discipline of public health were mirrored by its stagnation within the Ministry of Health. The arrival of Godber, in 1960, with his Diploma in Public Health and passionate belief in wider health responsibilities, went some way to redressing the balance. The NHS had evolved into a moloch, feeding greedily on the time and energy of the senior medical staff.

Relations between the Ministry of Health and local government were further strained by disputes over the contested territory of public health services. As Ann Cartwright's classic 1967 study of general practitioners highlighted, doctors resented the Ministry's support of local authority health services (e.g. health visitors and district nurses). In their eyes, they should have belonged to them, not the Medical Officers of Health.[40] Such tensions made life difficult for the CMO who was expected to be supportive both of the Medical Officer of Health role and of general practitioners.

The Department of Health and Social Security

> 'Dealing with the doctors is even worse than negotiating with the French.'
>
> (Senior DHSS official, 1976[41])

The massive Department of Health and Social Security, affectionately known by its staff as the 'Department of Stealth and Total Obscurity', was created in 1968 by

---

[37] JAG Grifftth, *Central Departments and Local Authorities* (London, Allen & Unwin, 1966).
[38] J Welshman, *Municipal Medicine: public health in twentieth century Britain* (Oxford, Peter Lang, 2000), p. 256. Godber's comments were made in an interview by Welshman in 1994.
[39] Ibid., p. 263.
[40] A Cartwright, *Patients and their Doctors: a study of general practice* (London, Routledge and Kegan Paul, 1967).
[41] Quoted in P Hennessy, *Whitehall* (London, Pimlico, 2001), p. 421.

Harold Wilson as a large empire to satisfy Richard Crossman's ambitions.[42] Although the two Ministries merged in name, there was only minimal effective integration. Each 'Ministry' kept its own Minister and separate staff. Wilson admitted, in 1976, that he had made the wrong decision:

> When . . . after consulting the civil servants, I merged the two – Health and Social Services – I think that was probably the wrong step. In fact, soon afterwards – I take full responsibility for it – they were saying to me that they were not sure they ought not to have advised me to merge Social Services with the Home Office . . .[43]

The problems caused by this merger were still rumbling on in 1970. Crossman discovered that some of his senior civil servants had been involved in discussions on the future of the Department for Employment and Pensions and the Department of Health and Social Security without his knowledge: 'I realised once again that I still have two Departments carrying on as though they are independent Ministries'.[44] By the late 1960s, there was also a realisation within both Whitehall and the medical profession that the structure of the NHS, in place since 1948, was no longer fit for purpose.

Godber departed as CMO when he reached the then civil service retirement age of 65 years in 1973, immediately before the first NHS reorganisation was implemented. Three Ministers of Health had tried to produce an effective blue-print for NHS reorganisation. Kenneth Robinson (1964–68) put out the first Green Paper in 1968.[45] This was subsequently worked up by Richard Crossman (1968–70) with limited assistance from a Royal Commission on Local Government (1969). The resulting 1973 National Health Service (Reorganisation) Act was a weak, half-hearted attempt at restructuring, significant only for its abandonment of the tripartite NHS structure.[46] Crossman's plan was finally implemented with only minor amendments by the incoming Conservative Minister, Keith Joseph (1970–74), in April 1974.

Godber had strongly championed the creation of a two-tier system of regional and district health authorities, known colloquially by Department of Health and Social Security staff as the 'Godber bricks' of the National Health Service. He did not want NHS regional boundaries to be coterminous with those of local government (a risk of a 'thin end of the wedge' towards a local government-controlled health service). However, Godber did push for a local electoral base to the reformed health service, which would reflect community demands and link with wider social services. He was influential with Robinson, but lost ground with Crossman, who inserted a third tier of area health authorities.

The post-1974 NHS continued to dominate the Department of Health and

[42] D Owen, *Time to Declare* (London, M Joseph, 1991), p. 226.
[43] *Eleventh Report from the Expenditure Committee, Session 1976–77*, 'The Civil Service', vol.II, part II., p. 786.
[44] R Crossman, *The Crossman Diaries* (London, Hamilton, 1979), p. 833. 24 February 1970.
[45] *National Health Service. The Administrative Structure of the Medical and Related Services in England and Wales* (London, HMSO, 1968). See C Webster, *The Health Services Since the War. Vol. II: Government and Health Care, the National Health Service, 1958–1979* (London, HMSO, 1996), pp. 321–73 on Labour plans for health service reorganisation.
[46] National Health Service Reorganisation Act 1973, cap.32.

Social Security after the retirement of Godber. His successor, Henry Yellowlees, majored on 'medical manpower planning' in an attempt to cope with the rapidly increasing staff demands of the health service. One medical civil servant who was assigned to this task saw it as 'a futile exercise – like designing a car for Ford which would not be marketed for 20 years: how could anybody expect to anticipate forward demand to that extent?'[47] Medical staff within the Department of Health and Social Security had been redeployed following a 1972 report by civil servants and management consultants from McKinsey & Co., so as to closer align them with the anticipated new structure of the NHS.[48]

In the 1970s, there was a perception that the Department of Health and Social Security was struggling to define its role and that of its staff. This was reflected in a special issue of *Health Trends* in 1976. Entitled *'Functions of the Medical Staff of the Department of Health and Social Security'*, it was devoted to clarifying their position for the benefit of medical staff in the NHS and other health agencies.[49] It explained such functions as: the cycles of inspection which medical civil servants carried out for general practitioners; the increasing range of European Economic Community (EEC) agreements; responsibilities under the 1968 Medicines Act; and the creation of a new separate medical division dedicated to the health aspects of chemical contamination of food and environmental pollution.

During the 1970s, medical civil servants carved out a new niche for themselves in commissioning and evaluating medical research. Although Simon had a small grant for medical research, it had failed to flourish within the Medical Department, particularly after the creation of the Medical Research Committee in 1913. The Committee was renamed the Medical Research Council in 1919, and continued to maintain a useful autonomy from the Ministry of Health. Direct funding of medical research by the Ministry was minimal. Although the 1946 National Health Service Act had authorised the Minister to conduct or assist research 'into any matters relating to the causation, prevention, diagnosis or treatment of illness or mental defectiveness', it was not until 1962 that a small research division was established. In 1966–67 its annual expenditure on commissioned research was £750,000, by 1973–74 this had risen to over £16 million and the programme was co-ordinated by a Chief Scientist (first appointed in 1973).

Wider medical expertise within Whitehall was also increasingly being recognised and integrated within the Department of Health and Social Security. Yellowlees fostered the development of links with medical civil servants in the Department of the Environment, the Ministry of Agriculture, Fisheries and Foods, the Home Office and other Departments. He saw this horizontal co-ordination of medical expertise within Whitehall as one of his most satisfying achievements. Through this 'open door' approach he could augment the depleted expertise of the 145 medical staff he controlled in London. Although Yellowlees stimulated some of this, part of the motivation for improved interdepartmental communications had come in 1980 through a damning Social Services Committee investigation into policy making at the Department of Health and Social Security. This

[47] Senior medical civil servant interview, 28.08.02.
[48] Department of Health and Social Security, *The DHSS in Relation to the Health and Personal Social Services: review team report* (London, HMSO, 1972).
[49] *Health Trends*, 1976, 8 (3).

prompted the creation of a Policy Strategy Unit and ultimately underpinned subsequent wide-ranging reviews of health policy and service delivery.[50]

The impact of Whitehall reviews

As Klein and others have noted, the domination of the Department of Health and Social Security by the NHS was causing increasing concern.[51] We have already highlighted (in Chapter 3) the 'new broom' ethos which the Conservative Government imposed from 1979, which peaked in the culture of management efficiency in the 1980s. It initiated a progressive purge on Whitehall staff and resources. The Department of Health and Social Security and its later incarnations, as one of the biggest Departments, suffered heavily. A rolling series of reviews was initiated in 1979. These investigated the medical as well as the administrative divisions, thereby requiring the CMO explicitly to justify his staff. Acheson, who bore the brunt of some of the most detailed reviews as CMO between 1983 and 1991, later complained of the impact this had on his work:

> I was being submitted to intense scrutiny and requirement to reduce my resources . . . it was almost continuous and took away from me much of my energy and intellectual resources doing something which was not actually my job.[52]

In April 1979 there were 21 senior medical posts. A Whitehall-wide review was conducted early in the Conservative administration by Sir Geoffrey Wardale. His report in 1981 recommended a continuous and systematic review of Senior Open Structure posts. One of the four Deputy CMO and three other posts were lost in 1982 following the Wardale review, reducing the number of senior medical posts to seventeen.[53] During 1982 the Treasury-sponsored review of Department of Health and Social Security medical staff used the Wardale criteria to judge the appropriate level of staffing. This review resulted in the loss of a further three posts, reducing the number of senior medical staff to fourteen.

Further reviews included the Moseley Review of the senior medical posts in the DHSS (1986); the Benner Godfrey Review of the Deputy Chief Medical Officer posts (1988); the 'Trefoil Report' by Heather Gwynn on the functions and structure of the Department of Health (1990); the Herbecq Review of the Senior Open Structure (1990), Alderslade's scrutiny of the Department of

[50] See Ham, *Health Policy in Britain*, for more information on policy making at the Department of Health and Social Security.

[51] For a detailed study of the NHS, see R Klein, *The New Politics of the NHS* (New York, Prentice Hall, 4th edn, 2001); G Rivett, *From Cradle to Grave: fifty years of the NHS* (London, King's Fund, 1998) – an updated version of this text is maintained at www.nhs.history. com. The two-volume official history of the NHS is by C Webster, *The Health Services Since the War: problems of health care. The National Health Service before 1957* (London, HMSO, 1988) and *The Health Services Since the War: government and health care. The British National Health Service, 1958–1979* (London, HMSO, 1996).

[52] BSE inquiry, oral transcript of evidence from Sir Donald Acheson, 06.11.1998, p. 121.

[53] The Deputy CMO post which was lost had been held by Dr John Evans. He was appointed instead as Deputy Secretary, covering similar areas of work to those he had previously.

Health Medical Division (1990), which recommended integrated teamworking for medical and administrative divisions; the Greenfield and Hale Report on the future organisation of the Health and Social Services Divisions (1991) and the Functions and Manpower Review (1993), which focused particularly on the regional structure of the NHS. Most of these reports were commissioned with the fundamental purpose of reducing expenditure. However, they all commented on the need to retain doctors as civil servants.

A new Department of Health

It took 20 years fully to acknowledge the Department of Health and Social Security's structural problems and to find a solution. On 26 July 1988 the Department was split along the natural fault line into separate Departments of Social Security and Health. The Permanent Secretary at the time was Sir Christopher France, who had joined the Department in 1984 as Deputy Secretary (Health). France became second Permanent Secretary in 1986 and succeeded Sir Kenneth Stowe as Permanent Secretary in March 1987. When he was asked to lead the Department from the social security side, contrary to established practice, France expressed his dissatisfaction with the unwieldy structure, specifically: 'To my mind this new arrangement was not satisfactory and I had made clear my opposition to it. But having been asked to do the job in that way, I had no option but to devote much of my time to social security matters, delegating the administrative lead on health to a Second Permanent Secretary [Michael Partridge], who dealt with health issues until July 1988.'[54]

When the Department for Health and Social Security was divided the NHS was amidst an ongoing review, initiated by John Moore, who was the last Secretary of State for Social Services. Following the division of the Department, John Moore continued as Secretary of State for Social Services and Kenneth Clarke, who had previously been Minister of State for Health under Norman Fowler, was appointed Secretary of State for Health. Sir Christopher France, in his witness statement to the BSE Inquiry in 1998, commented on the lack of warning and haste with which the decision was made:

> It is worth pausing on the creation of the DH [Department of Health], since it is a useful example of the practicalities of briefing incoming Ministers and illustrates the realities of running a large Department. I was told at 9.15 a.m. on the day in question that the DHSS (with some 80,000 staff) was to be split and that an additional Secretary of State and two other Ministers would be arriving that afternoon, when Parliament was to be informed of the existence of the two new Departments. So my staff and I had four or five hours to inform the Department(s) and tell people how the process was actually going to be managed and provide accommodation, telephones, Private Secretaries and so on for three new Ministers. In the circumstances, there was no question of preparing special briefings for incoming Ministers. My recollection is that they received a selection of existing papers

[54] BSE Inquiry, witness statement of Sir Christopher France. No. 275B, p. 5.

bearing on current problems and extensive oral briefings from senior officials.[55]

Further to France's comment on the political impetuosity behind the division, Peter Hennessy lists the activities of the reformatted Department of Health in 1989, which provide a clear indication of the sheer scale of activity and financial responsibility which Clarke had to manage. With a budget of £21,691 million (1988–89) and a staff of 8,789 (excluding NHS staff), the Department oversaw the issue of 1,400 new drug product licences, 6.6 million hospital in-patients in England, 37.5 million hospital out-patients in England, 5 million childhood immunisations, 32 million courses of dental treatment and some 335 million prescriptions dispensed.[56] Even this downsized Department dominated government activity.

Reviews of senior medical civil servants

The CMO and Deputy CMO posts in particular were scrutinised no less than eight times between 1981 and 1994 to establish whether the numbers and grades of staff employed accurately matched the work requirements. The Deputy CMO function was critical within the pyramid of overall responsibility, taking a large share of delegated duties from the CMO, whilst also managing specific services. The 1982 Treasury Review had suggested that Deputy CMOs should be given titles, which would serve to clarify the specific areas for which they had responsibilities. It also justified the reduction in Deputy CMO posts from four to three. This now appears to have been the 'thin end of the wedge' for senior medical civil servants.

The Moseley Report, published in April 1986, had been commissioned by Sir Kenneth Stowe, the Department's Permanent Secretary, in October 1985 as part of the first three-yearly programme of reviews recommended by the Wardale Report.[57] Sir George Moseley's team investigated the workload of the CMO and remaining three Deputy CMO posts in the context of the support available to the CMO and their other duties. It commented specifically on the responsibilities of the CMO:

> The sheer scale of personal responsibility seemed to us to have dimensions which distinguish it even from some of the highest posts of all within Whitehall. The occupant of the post has statutory responsibilities in his own right; he is adviser to a number of Ministerial Heads of Department around Whitehall as well as to the Secretary of State for Health and Social Services; he is a recognisable 'public' figure, regarded by the media as speaking with an independent and professional authority. Add to this the CMO's responsibilities for

[55] BSE Inquiry, witness statement of Sir Christopher France. No. 275B, p. 5. Such was the haste of the split that Michael Partridge had to be tracked down by the French police on the second day of his holiday to be recalled to take charge of the new Department of Social Security as Permanent Secretary.

[56] Hennessy, *Whitehall*, pp. 419–23.

[57] George Moseley (1925–) had been Permanent Secretary to the Department of the Environment between 1981 and 1985.

ensuring the proper and timely input of professional medical advice to health policy making within the Department, together with the very heavy representational role which he bears . . .[58]

It recommended that more systematic support should be provided for the CMO by his deputies, but that a saving could be achieved by cutting the Deputy CMO posts from three to two, although acknowledging that the two posts that would remain if the reduction was implemented were already fully loaded. This was never going to be a popular suggestion:

> We had an opportunity of discussing these conclusions with the CMO [Acheson], and we believe it right to record that he would be strongly opposed to any reduction in the number of DCMO [Deputy Chief Medical Officer] posts and indeed challenges the conclusions we have drawn from the material we collected during the review. In particular the CMO believes that the medical group has been unduly reduced in its senior grades since 1979 by comparison with the administration group; that the range and sensitivity of medical issues on which senior members of the group have to advise Ministers has significantly increased over recent years; and that there already exist certain deficiencies in the capability of the group to serve Ministers adequately that can only be exacerbated by a reduction in the number of DCMO posts.[59]

This was the first serious attack Acheson sustained during his time as CMO on his support network, although the loss of the Deputy CMO post in 1982 had been seen as a sign of things to come. Incoming Conservative Ministers had made known early in the 1980s their intention to reduce the number of medical staff in the Department of Health and Social Security.[60] The Moseley proposals were of a different order and explicitly provoked by the government's desire to reduce public administration expenditure. In the event, the Deputy CMO posts remained until 1992, and several other Moseley suggestions, including that of having a Deputy CMO replacement for the CMO on the National Health Service Management Board, were not implemented (though later one of the two Deputy CMOs was also designated as 'Medical Director' of the National Health Service Executive Board).

In 1988, a further review, this time specifically of the Deputy CMO posts, was carried out by Mr Patrick Benner and Dr Malcolm Godfrey.[61] It was found that there was ample work to justify three Deputy CMOs, but that since the move to

---

[58] Report on the Review of the Senior Open Structure, DHSS (April 1986), hereafter cited as the Moseley Report, p. 29–30.

[59] Ibid., p. 31.

[60] Mrs Thatcher is reputed to have known the exact number of doctors working in the Department of Health and Social Security in 1979 and to have told Patrick Jenkin, the new Secretary of State, that one of his objectives should be to send many of them 'back to the NHS to do proper medical jobs'.

[61] *Review of the Deputy Chief Medical Officer Posts in the DHSS*, report by Mr Patrick Benner and Dr Malcolm Godfrey, August 1988. Benner had just retired from his Deputy Secretary post at the Department of Health and Social Security where he was seen as Ken Stowe's most trusted and dependable colleague. He had masterminded with Stowe the handling of the nurses' strike in the mid-1980s.

Richmond House in 1988, they and the CMO had lost some support from their junior staff who remained at the Elephant and Castle. The report also drew attention to long-standing recruitment problems to medical posts within the Department of Health, and the lack of adequate crisis management planning. It found that since the Moseley Report (April 1986) there had been a discernible increase in the amount of work undertaken by the medical staff, and that with the predictions for AIDS and reform of the NHS, this would undoubtedly increase in the foreseeable future. The report also acknowledged that a substantial part of the CMO function required the personal input of the CMO, especially attendance at international meetings. While these duties could not always be effectively delegated to Deputy CMO level, the 1988 report urged that other duties, for example representation in medical organisations, should be reallocated to relieve the burden on the CMO.

The Benner–Godfrey Report also considered the CMO's position on the National Health Service Management Board, which required his attendance at two sets of fortnightly meetings and also at regional reviews. They noted, however, that 'since he is often prevented by other duties from being present at Board meetings and is very rarely able to attend the other meetings and reviews, it has been agreed that a Deputy CMO should attend all the meetings'.[62] Duplication of attendances (when the CMO did attend) was seen as unsatisfactory, and '(particularly in the National Health Service) the status of the Deputy CMO is capable of being misunderstood'. They proposed therefore that a Deputy CMO should become a member of the National Health Service Management Board in their own right, with the CMO retaining the right to attend meetings as and when he was able, 'particularly for presentational reasons'.[63]

Benner–Godfrey also recommended that the CMO could usefully be relieved of the overall management of the medical side of the Department, including recruitment, staff movements, career development and continuing education: 'Most of them are time-consuming; and failure to tackle them effectively is potentially damaging to morale and efficiency, and, in the longer run, to the ability to retain and recruit staff. It seems to us that it is becoming increasingly difficult for the CMO to give these personnel matters the time they require . . .'[64] Although this report also failed to stimulate a reorganisation in the CMO's responsibilities, the proposal from the 1982 Treasury Review that the three Deputy CMOs should be given titles to reflect their responsibilities was finally implemented in 1990.

Following the separation of the National Health Service Management Executive, the rest of the Department of Health became known as the 'Wider Department', and was managed from Whitehall through parallel hierarchies reporting to the CMO and the Permanent Secretary, respectively. Paired divisions were created in October 1991 to cover all the main non-NHS aspects of the Department's work, but significant duplication of management remained: 'Unnecessary tension is caused by artificial links between pay and grading.'[65] A

---

[62] Dr RM Oliver was the Deputy CMO with this function.
[63] *Review of the Deputy Chief Medical Officer Posts in the DHSS*, report by Mr Patrick Benner and Dr Malcolm Godfrey, August 1988, p. 12.
[64] Ibid., p. 13.
[65] *Banks Review of the Wider Department of Health* (June 1994), p. 8.

number of NHS administrative staff were recruited to the 'Wider Department'. A more recent study by Rudolf Klein and Patricia Day (as part of a larger Whitehall research project) suggested that, as an exercise in remodelling policy and management divisions, this reform did not work well, partly because of the clash of NHS managerial and civil service cultures.[66]

In April 1991 a small reduction of workload for the CMO was achieved through the establishment of the Medicines Control Agency as a 'Next Steps' agency. Acheson retired in September 1991 and was succeeded by Kenneth Calman. In 1992 the Moseley proposals to reduce the number of Deputy CMOs to two was implemented on the retirement of Michael Abrams, whose duties had been for the 'Wider Department' and were merged with those of Jeremy Metters. The other remaining Deputy CMO post, held by Diana Walford, had already been retitled as Deputy Chief Medical Officer and Medical Director of the National Health Service Management Board. When Walford was appointed as Director of the Public Health Laboratory Service in 1992, a period of several months followed when Calman had the support of a single Deputy. During this interval senior medical cover in the Department of Health was very thinly spread.

The 1994 Banks Review

The most fundamental restructuring took place in April 1995, following the review of Department of Health senior management in 1994 by the retired civil servant Mrs Terri Banks, who had previously been Director of Health Authority Finance at the Department of Health and Social Security.[67] The review included two commissioned studies, one by management consultants from Coopers and Lybrand on business processes within the Department, the other by the School for Advanced Urban Studies (University of Bristol) on the external contacts of the 'Wider Department'. The report identified a considerable workload relative to other government departments. In 1993, for example, the Department had answered 25,560 letters from MPs, 58,600 letters from the public, provided speeches and briefings for more than 130 parliamentary debates and answered an average of 28 parliamentary questions each sitting day.[68] Through a series of interviews with the Ministers who formed the Department's main 'customer' base, it found that they were generally happy with the quality of advice they received from the CMO and his staff. The report made several recommendations, some of which were reiterations from earlier reviews, particularly on the need to reduce the CMO's workload and ensuring that he retained sufficient support from medical staff within the Department.

With specific regard to departmental organisation, Banks recommended that policy and implementation functions should be as closely aligned as possible. This went against the 1990 Trefoil Report by Heather Gwynn, which in the light of the move of the Department of Health's National Health Service Executive Division to Leeds in 1992, had recommended a clear distinction between policy and implementation. To facilitate this, Banks suggested that a small high-level

---

[66] D Day and R Klein, *Steering but not Rowing? The Transformation of the Department of Health: a case study* (University of Bristol, 1997).
[67] Gillian Teresa Banks, Department of Health and Social Security civil servant, 1972–1985.
[68] *Banks Review* (June 1994), p. 32.

policy management group should be created to support the Departmental Management Board. The group would assist with priority setting and reduce non-urgent work. Other recommendations included tighter allocation of work to relevant grades to avoid 'grade skipping', more explicit criteria for the retention of committees, and a move away from calendar-driven meetings towards issue-driven meetings.[69] One result of the National Health Executive's transfer to Leeds was that medical staff working there felt distanced from the CMO and their other medical colleagues in London.

At the time of the Banks Review in 1994, almost all doctors in the 'Wider Department' were grouped into three medical divisions with their own management hierarchy (excluding those in specialist agencies such as the Medicines Control Agency). Banks advised merging the medical and administrative 'paired' divisions, ending the separate system of professional reporting lines which had been in place since the formation of the Ministry of Health in 1919. The aim of the reorganisation was to enable the Department to operate more effectively and efficiently. The proposed 'teamworking' ethos was intended to encourage greater flexibility and improved job satisfaction. This reflected a wider Whitehall sympathy with more fluid organisational structures, which had included the development of Job Evaluation for Senior Posts (JESP) scores to estimate job weighting. Teamworking facilitated a transition from formal civil service grades to a more flexible allocation of duties. Within the Department of Health, this had implications for the relative status of medical and administrative staff. Banks anticipated that:

> The need to pay professionals sufficient to recruit and retain good quality people should not necessarily translate into an assumption about their place in the hierarchy. It should be possible for people to be managerially accountable to somebody who is paid less than them.[70]

The restructuring also fulfilled a wider motivation. As the Permanent Secretary, Sir Graham Hart, noted: 'It made a substantial contribution towards the large reductions in Departmental running costs which Ministers required of the Department over the period from 1994.'[71] Banks had proposed that the number of external medical and scientific committees could be 'pruned and rationalised', resulting in further internal savings as the related work of administrators and professionals could be proportionately cut. An additional review was commissioned at the same time as the Banks Review from a former Deputy CMO, Dr John Evans.[72] This focused on how expert advice was obtained by the Department, and recommended, as Banks had, more reliance on external sources, even though in future this might have to be paid for.

As a result of the 1995 reorganisation, medical and administrative staff were

---

[69] Ibid., p. 38.

[70] Ibid., p. 26.

[71] BSE Inquiry, witness statement of Sir Graham Hart. No.180, section 22.

[72] *A Review of the Department of Health's Arrangement for Obtaining Medical and Scientific Advice* (March 1995). John Evans had at one stage been 'groomed' as a potential CMO himself, and had been moved from the medical division into the administrative division by the Permanent Secretary Ken Stowe to give him a wide range of experience. This did not endear him to the current CMO, Henry Yellowlees. Senior medical civil servant interview, 22.07.2002.

integrated, producing stronger reporting lines to the Permanent Secretary. Although some medical staff now managed administrative staff, the reality for the survivors of the cull was in the loss of their *esprit de corps* and, for those working on their own in administrative-led branches and divisions, the erosion of readily available senior medical advice.

The 1995 restructuring also involved the creation of a Public Health Group Board within the Wider Department of Health, comprising the Permanent Secretary, the CMO, Deputy CMO, Chief Nursing Officer, Finance Director and the two Heads of Divisions in the Public Health Group. This met monthly, and provided a mechanism through which wider issues could be discussed and referred. It gave the CMO an additional useful channel of influence at a time when his staff and resources were diminishing.

However, the new integrated hierarchy was not popular. The retired CMO, Acheson, used the 1998 BSE Inquiry to make his views on the consequences of the 1995 restructuring of the Department clear:

> Since the subsequent integration of the Department, which I under-stand has left the CMO with hardly any staff for whom he is manage-rially accountable, it is difficult to see how this responsibility [for the quality of medical advice] can be discharged effectively or indeed how he could successfully insist, against opposition, on any necessary changes to address any new problems or emergencies. This is, I believe, a unique penalty for a person working at this level of responsibility, whether in the public or private sector, and risks compromising the independence of the CMO which is so important to the protection and improvement of health in this country.[73]

The restructuring fell during the tenure of Kenneth Calman (1991–98). Although he remained as head of the medical civil service staff for professional matters, he lost his direct line management of over 100 medical and 40 scientific personnel. This had implications for the prioritisation and allocation of departmental work, and budget allocations for CMO projects.

In 1990, while still CMO, Acheson had expressed his concerns for the integration of the parallel hierarchies after the Alderslade 'experiment'. At that point, his comments were confidential, but in 1998, through his inquiry evidence, they became public, thereby a useful circumvention of the civil service bar on post-retirement disclosure. Acheson's criticism of integrated hierarchies was not repeated publicly by Calman, who, despite having also retired as CMO by the time he gave evidence to the BSE Inquiry, did not touch on this issue in his statements and evidence. Yet, between April 1995 (when the recommendations of the Banks Report and Evans Review were implemented) and the production of the BSE memorandum in 1998, there was a 21 per cent reduction in staff and a 27 per cent reduction in departmental running costs: a financial vindication of Whitehall's drive for efficiency through the abolition of separate medical and administrative hierarchies.[74] Although compulsory redundancies were avoided, many junior doctors were moved into jobs in 'Next Steps' agencies, the NHS and

[73] BSE Inquiry, witness statement of Sir Donald Acheson. No. 251, section 18.
[74] BSE Inquiry memorandum, 'The structure of the Department of Health between 1985 and 1996' (DH2/98).

non-departmental public bodies (such as the National Radiological Protection Board and the Public Health Laboratory Service). More senior doctors were eligible for the generous redundancy package, but those that remained suffered a difficult period when medical staff morale plummeted.

The National Health Service

How did the CMO's responsibility within the National Health Service alter during this period of intense restructuring? An appreciation of the broader management changes in the NHS is relevant here. Following the 1983 inquiry into the National Health Service by Roy Griffiths, Managing Director and Deputy Chairman of the supermarket chain Sainsbury's, the Department of Health and Social Security increasingly moved away from day-to-day management. A National Health Service Management Board was established on 1 April 1985, consisting of a Chairman (Second Permanent Secretary);[75] six executive members (the Directors of Financial Management, Health Authority Finance, Operations, Personnel, Planning, and Information Technology and Health Authority Liaison) with three non-executive members, (the CMO, the Chief Nursing Officer and a senior NHS officer).

In 1989 policy making for the NHS was separated from the main Department of Health through the creation of a National Health Service Policy Board (including the CMO) and a separate National Health Service Management Executive, led by a Chief Executive. Its relocation to Leeds in 1992 was another significant shift in the arrangement of medical staff within the Department of Health. The National Health Service Management Executive was further rationalised in 1993 and renamed the National Health Service Executive, which 'remained within the central government framework as an integral part of the Department of Health'.[76] The National Health Service Executive also directed the work of the teams in regional health authorities led by regional general managers. In 1996 the regional health authorities were abolished and their management teams absorbed into the Department of Health as eight regional offices of the National Health Service Executive. This gave Calman as CMO a new opportunity to draw on the expertise of the Regional Directors of Public Health.

In theory, the new NHS management structure could have helped to reduce the CMO's workload. Several of the reviews, as discussed earlier, suggested that his seat on the Executive Board could be usefully delegated to a Deputy CMO. However, although Diana Walford and (later) Graham Winyard, as Deputy CMOs and Medical Directors of the National Health Service, were members of the Board, both Acheson and Calman also attended regularly. This was important in symbolising the direct relevance of the work of the CMO to the NHS.

In this chapter, we have demonstrated that the CMO's direct management of doctors has only ever extended to a small group of medical civil servants directly employed within his department in Whitehall. Its size has fluctuated considerably during this 143-year period. Surely Calman's reported comments in 1998 – that his staff now consisted of a secretary and a mobile phone – would have resonated with

---

[75] This post was initially held by Victor Paige, until his resignation in 1986, when he was succeeded by Len Peach with the new title of Chief Executive.
[76] *Banks Review*, p. 11.

his nineteenth century predecessors at the Local Government Board?[77] This reality is contrary to popular perception of the CMO, who is often mistakenly seen as in charge of all doctors in Britain, both within the NHS and all other health concerns.

Yet, as Acheson noted in his evidence to the BSE Inquiry, the CMO has never had a management line or any power of direction over public health doctors: Medical Officers of Health or their successors, the Directors of Public Health. They were free to accept or reject his advice: 'At best the CMO may be seen as *primus inter pares*.'[78] His authority within the wider medical profession was therefore critically dependent on his performance as the government's medical adviser and his personal credibility.

The importance of location

Health was located in the centre of Whitehall in the nineteenth century. Simon initially worked from the Privy Council Offices, and subsequently maintained a room in 8 Richmond Terrace, ensuring a continuity of close proximity to government Ministers and officials. When the main part of Simon's post moved to the Local Government Board in 1871, he took his department into larger Whitehall premises. The new Ministry of Health formed in 1919, in essence a renamed Local Government Board, remained in Whitehall until 1951 when the

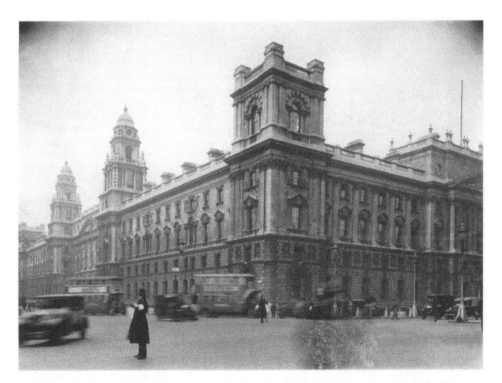

Figure 4.1 The Ministry of Health, c. 1930. © Wellcome Library. Reproduced with permission.

[77] 'Staff cuts would leave CMO stranded', *British Medical Journal*, 1998, 317, 232.
[78] BSE Inquiry, witness statement of Sir Donald Acheson. No.251, section 13.

Ministry lost its responsibility for housing and local government, and with it the Whitehall offices. New premises were acquired in Saville Row. There the Ministry of Health stayed until relocated, in 1968, south of the Thames to the new purpose-built Alexander Fleming House at the Elephant and Castle.

When Crossman took up his appointment as Secretary of State for Health and Social Security, in 1968, he determined to retain his room at the Privy Council Office in John Adam Street, from which he co-ordinated the newly merged department. He complained about the dismal location of the main Ministry of Health offices:

> I made my first visit to the collection of huge modern glass blocks that was custom-built for the Ministry of Health at the Elephant and Castle. It is on a ghastly site and Kenneth Robinson told me they chose it for its cheapness. It cost only half as much as normal sites for government buildings but a great deal of the money they saved is now being spent on air-conditioning and double glazing because the building stands right on top of an underground railway which makes the most dreadful din. It's also appallingly inconvenient because, though it's only three-quarters of a mile from Westminster and though from his

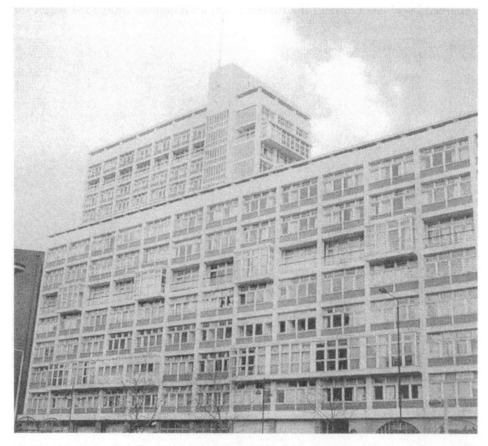

Figure 4.2 Alexander Fleming House, designed by the Hungarian-born architect Ernö Goldfinger for the Department of Health and Social Security in 1968.

room at the top of the twelve-storey block the Minister can see the House of Commons, he may take anything from three to twenty minutes to get there through the traffic. It was hoped that one effect of plonking the building down there would be to improve the area and attract other government buildings. It hasn't happened and the Ministry stands there isolated and terrible.[79]

However, by August 1968, it had become clear that there was insufficient space at John Adam Street for five Ministers, their offices, Permanent Secretaries, Deputy Secretaries, Under Secretaries and others. Despite a desperate search for better offices, on the pretext that they would be closer to Westminster, Crossman was left with no choice but to move in with 'the hordes' at the Elephant and Castle.[80]

Crossman had the option of having his main base away from the Elephant and Castle but the CMO was not so fortunate. Yet Godber took little interest in his surroundings: he moved his camp bed from Saville Row to Alexander Fleming House without comment. His successor, Yellowlees, detested the building, as he unfortunately and unwittingly informed its architect, Ernö Goldfinger, at a dinner.[81] He tried several times to move out, but only in 1987–88 were senior staff moved into the newly built Richmond House at 79 Whitehall.[82]

By the 1980s health was once again 'central' to Whitehall, both geographically and politically. Even on a smaller scale, the physical proximity of the offices of the CMO, Permanent Secretary and the Ministers has been important for good communications within the Department (as is clear from our interviews, as well as from evidence given to inquiries such as that on BSE). The frequent, daily contact at the 'top of the office' was easier at times when there were adjacent offices. Even in the age of email, face-to-face business is still valuable.[83]

Conclusion

In this chapter we have explored a further significant function of the CMO: managing a government department. This has complemented his position as the government's medical adviser. While the CMO was himself a technical 'expert', the increasingly complex world of medical science has required the construction of a permanent team of specialist advisers within Whitehall. The CMO has been supported in his duties by this team, but has also acquired a leadership and management role. The associated issues of sufficient medical staff, their status and their integration within the mainstream Whitehall system have been recurrent

---

[79] R Crossman, *The Crossman Diaries. Vol. III: Secretary of State for Social Services, 1968–70* (London, Hamish Hamilton, 1977), p. 17.

[80] Ibid., p. 175.

[81] Interview, 14.07.1999. Yellowlees called the prize-winning Alexander Fleming House 'the most horrible building I've ever been in'.

[82] It was reputedly Norman Fowler who secured Richmond House for the Department of Health and Social Security. The building had been intended for the Overseas Development Agency, but a row between No. 10 and the Foreign Office, who had campaigned to have the Agency 'across the road' from their main building, enabled Fowler to successfully argue for the transfer of the Department of Health and Social Security back to Whitehall.

[83] Sir Graham Hart, admitted during the BSE Inquiry that email contact with Calman was useful, but that he could not personally use it, leaving it instead to his private office staff.

themes since the appointment of John Simon in 1855. The power of any CMO partly lies with his deputies – he has to be very sure that at the level below him there are people who can cope with crises. In the 1980s, for example, Acheson relied on Michael Abrams to handle the Chernobyl radiation incident, and on Ed Harris to deal with a wide range of food scares including botulism found in hazelnut yoghurt and the contamination of Mars bars by their plastic wrappers.

There is a discernible sophistication in the politics of expertise over this period. The freedom which experts enjoy because of their unique role and knowledge has acquired a form of administrative semi-autonomy. This was at its most apparent during the 'golden age' of the mid-nineteenth century, before the expert became enmeshed within 'departmental structures which compelled him to rely on secretarial sanction, formal procedures and codes, and which finally constrained him to terms of reference not of his choosing or design'.[84] Also, from the 1880s, there was increasing use of the 'bureaucratic brake'. Innovations in science, medicine and technology became mired in a new legalistic culture of government, facilitated by the rapid expansion in the civil service – from 50,000 civil servants in 1881 to 280,000 by 1914. The technical experts found themselves subsumed within larger government departments and their policy-making role downgraded to that of 'adviser'. The CMO's position within this system has had to be constantly re-secured.

The quality of medical civil servants has also fluctuated – linked to the image of technical experts within Whitehall and their status as viewed through salary levels – relative to both the mainstream civil service and to medical professionals outside Whitehall. This is visible not only for the formative period of the medical civil service in the 1870s, but also to a lesser extent in the 1970s, when the medical hierarchy appeared to stagnate within the wider bureaucracy of the Department of Health and Social Security. The attractions of working in the medical civil service have never been great: long hours and non-existent private practice have dissuaded many from making the move from clinical medicine. A significant number of those who entered the Department after the formation of the National Health Service had already worked in other areas of medicine: 're-treads', as one such medical civil servant described himself. For many, it was a second stab at finding the right medical career, often undertaken in their thirties and forties. After the initial instability of the Local Government Board, the medical civil servant came to be seen within the wider civil service as more secure, having a job for life. Yet job security has not always been the prime motivator and many doctors come to Whitehall with a passionate belief in the state's responsibility for health and healthcare.

We began this chapter by discussing how medical expertise has fitted into Whitehall, concentrating specifically on the experts within the system, the state's employees. They are the 'human' link between the government and the public, 'the repository of central knowledge, wisdom and tradition . . . a skilled adviser, a beneficial mediator as well'.[85] The CMO led this group by example. His personal dedication, and ability to withstand attacks upon the group's size, function and credibility, have played a large part over the years in the recruitment and reputation of the medical civil service.

[84] McLeod, *Government and Expertise*, p. 15.

[85] JS Harris, *British Government Inspection: the local services and the central department* (London, Stevens, 1955), pp. viii–ix.

Chapter 5

A doctor's doctor?

The medical profession has always been interested in the appointment of the CMO, beginning with Simon's appointment as Principal Medical Officer in 1855. In Chapter 2, we discussed how the profession critically commented on, and increasingly became actively involved in, the selection process for a new CMO. Why has this remained an important issue for the profession? Here, we examine how the medical profession has worked with and through the CMO to ensure that their professional interests are protected and advanced. We look in detail at the strategic deployment of Jameson (the ninth CMO) to bring the medical profession into the planned National Health Service in 1948, and at the difficulties experienced by Yellowlees as he sought to maintain the trust of both the government and the profession during the 1974 pay beds dispute. The state and the medical profession have always been uneasy bedfellows, as Lloyd George put it in 1911:

> I had two hours' discussion with the medical men themselves the other day. I do not think there has been anything like it since the days when Daniel went into the lions' den . . . but I can assure you they treated me with the same civility as the lions treated my illustrious predecessor . . . except these lions knew their anatomy.[1]

The underlying tension, in this narrative, arises from the changing nature of the relationship between the medical profession and the state. Medicine has become central to a modern society, yet the role of the state in the direct provision of healthcare has demanded that this relationship is properly adjudicated. Even the first CMO in post, John Simon, was exploited by the medical profession for his access to Ministers, and, likewise, Ministers expected him to hold the confidence of the profession.

In the early years of our history, the state also acknowledged the risk to the health of the public from unqualified doctors. The establishment, in 1858, of a Medical Register for qualified practitioners, which was to be maintained by an independent General Medical Council (GMC), helped to crystallise the professionalisation of medicine and its engagement with the state. The 1858 Act did not 'outlaw' unorthodox medicine, but made it illegal to practise as a doctor without qualifications from a recognised medical school.[2] Furthermore, the Act required that all 'public' medical posts in hospitals, clinics and the Poor Law medical services could only be held by people on the Medical Register. CMOs have since

[1] David Lloyd George speech in Birmingham, 11.06.1911, recounted in David Owen, *Time to Declare* (London, M Joseph, 1991), p. 234.
[2] 1858 Medical Act. 21 & 22 Vict. c.90.

played a prominent role through the GMC in ensuring the quality of medical care.[3]

A good example of the linchpin role of the CMO can be seen in 1970, at the height of the British Medical Association's (BMA's) revolt over the GMC's refusal to modernise.[4] The regional branches of the BMA threatened to advise members to withhold the proposed annual £2 registration fee in protest at the failure of the GMC to review its functions and structure, specifically the lack of representation for registered doctors. The BMA went further, to suggest that if the GMC did not modernise then the Medical Register should be moved to the Department of Health and Social Security, thus effectively eroding medicine's professional independence from the state. Godber, as CMO, brokered a solution by convening a working party consisting of representatives from the medical Royal Colleges, the universities and the BMA, which was chaired by a lay member of the GMC (Sir Brynmor Jones). Only the CMO had the governmental authority and professional integrity to direct this response.

After several years of discussion, the resultant 1978 Medical Act expanded the GMC from 46 to 93 members, and altered the balance to provide a majority of elected members over nominees.[5] However, the right to a seat for the CMO was not, as expected, enshrined by the Act. Although most CMOs (after John Simon) had been members of the GMC as Crown nominees, there was no 'safe seat' for them. After 1978, there was an extra-legislative agreement that the English CMO would always be nominated, and that the three other territorial CMOs would take it in turn to hold a seat.[6] Following the 1983 Medical Act, which consolidated the Medical Acts of 1956 and 1978, the GMC's composition again changed, and Ken Calman was the last CMO to be a nominated member of council.[7] Since Calman's term of office on the council expired on 16 September 1996, the CMO has attended as an observer. In more recent years, the CMO has been proactive in translating political concerns over medical regulation, especially in the area of medical malpractice, into pressure on the GMC to implement reforms.

The emergence of 'state medicine'

Beginning with the employment of Poor Law medical officers in the early nineteenth century, the state steadily took direct control for a wide range of medical and health-related services. Some of these were provided by doctors on a contractor capitation basis, but the efficient solution was directly to employ full-time doctors. Inevitably this encroached into the domain of self-employed 'regular' medical practitioners. Before the 1930s, however, there had only been a smattering of suggestions that the state should employ all medical practitioners. The Labour Party's Advisory Committee on Public Health published a report in

---

[3] John Simon was Crown Member of the General Medical Council after his retirement from Whitehall. He filled the vacancy left by the death of Alexander Parkes, and served on the GMC from 1876 until 1895.

[4] M Stacey, *Regulating British Medicine: the General Medical Council* (Chichester, John Wiley, 1992), p. 37.

[5] 1978 Medical Act. c.12.

[6] Ibid., p. 72.

[7] 1983 Medical Act. c.54.

1919 entitled *The Organisation of the Preventive and Curative Medical Services and Hospital and Laboratory Systems under a Ministry of Health*.[8] This advocated a salaried medical service, which included the hospital consultants. Yet, Sidney Webb was at pains to reassure doctors that the Labour Party had not committed itself to a full-time 'state army of salaried clinicians'.[9]

There is no discernible, precise point at which the relationship between the profession and the state changed (that would assume the existence of a single voice for the medical profession). Yet there have been points in time when medical practitioners have been more united, mostly as a response to threats to livelihood or professional autonomy from the state provision of medical services. The BMA, although now seen as the most high-profile 'trade union' body for doctors, has by no means always represented them all. Its traditional core of support has been with the general practitioners. In 1918, the BMA had around 15,000 members, out of a total of 43,000 on the Medical Register. By 1945, 50,000 of the 69,003 registered practitioners had joined the BMA.[10] The reason was the imminent arrival of the National Health Service, effected through the NHS Act of 1946 and operational from 5 July 1948.[11]

When the Ministry of Health was formed in 1919 the government tacitly gave a higher priority to health services. The Ministry, in theory, should have provided a centralised administration to integrate existing services. In reality, it failed to capitalise on its potential power within government and had to content itself with directing services through other organisations, usually under the control of local government. The only real control over the health activities of local authorities was the 'stick' of withholding substantial grants.[12]

The 'medical profession' in its various forms lobbied the government through the Ministry of Health during this inter-war period. By the time that George Newman came into post, in 1919, the medical profession firmly regarded the CMO as its spokesman within Whitehall.[13] Newman had already proved his value through health initiatives pursued whilst he was CMO to the Board of Education. These had included the establishment of the school medical inspection system, which had the potential to increase work (and therefore income) for general practitioners. At a new dedicated Health Ministry, Newman hoped to extend his influence. The medical profession expected to be alongside him.

Newman's vision was to establish 'Preventive Medicine' (invariably capitalised) as a concept wider than simply 'public health' with its infectious disease connotations. He defined it as 'the removal of the occasion of disease and physical

---

[8] The Labour Party, memorandum prepared by the Advisory Committee on Public Health, *The Organisation of the Preventive and Curative Medical Services and Hosptial and Laboratory Systems under a Ministry of Health* (London, July 1919).

[9] Quoted in B Abel-Smith, *The Hospitals, 1800–1948* (London, Heinemann Books, 1964), pp. 286–8.

[10] H Eckstein, *Pressure Group Politics* (London, George Allen & Unwin, 1960), pp. 44–5.

[11] 1946 National Health Service Act. 9 & 10 Geo. VI. c.81.

[12] For a concise analysis of the new duties of the Ministry of Health and how it related to other government departments, see A Newsholme, *The Ministry of Health* (London, Putnams and Sons, 1925). Although Newsholme never directly discusses or criticises his successor Newman, he uses this publication to highlight the failure properly to arrange the healthcare of children.

[13] He received regular deputations from the medical Royal Colleges.

inefficiency, combined with the husbanding of the physical resources of the individual'.[14] He presented it as the foundation stone of medicine: 'In fact it is not so much a separate subject of the curriculum that is required as a pervading influence, but an attitude of mind, permeating and guiding all clinical study and practice.'[15] As a pragmatist, he recognised an opportunity to effect an integration of services not under his direct control, whilst appealing to the needs of a cash-bound government and to the sectional interests of the medical profession.

Newman's holistic approach, invoking a much older Hippocratic tradition, sought to reconcile the conflicting interests of the state, the medical profession and, above all, the patient.[16] He welcomed the involvement of general practitioners in preventive medicine. He had already given evidence to the Royal Commission on the Poor Laws in 1910, which approved the Webbs' plan to bring insurance doctors under the control of public health authorities.[17] Newman's handling of a potentially explosive union between the state and the medical profession was more astute than his predecessor. Arthur Newsholme had riled the leaders of the BMA, especially Dr Alfred Cox and Sir Henry Brackenbury, by failing to quash rumours about the balance of power in such a relationship. His blindness to the realities of medical politics effectively meant that his days as CMO were numbered.

Preventive Medicine also opened up the potential for expanding the already significant cadre of 'auxiliary' services, which included by 1914 some 600 health visitors and a similar number of infant welfare and maternity centres. These initiatives had been a response to the need for domestic rather than public health reform: a persistently high infant mortality rate at the end of the nineteenth century seemed immune to conventional sanitary reform strategies. Health visiting thus developed the role of local councils. From the 1890s, they began to employ women (usually middle class) to visit working-class mothers in their own homes, giving advice on hygiene and infant care.[18]

Newman played out his views publicly and quite deliberately so. He wished to recruit as many medical practitioners as possible to his crusade for integrated health services. He was not an isolated voice calling for reform, but his vision did not chime with those of other, equally influential figures, notably Lord Dawson of Penn.[19] As Chair of the Minister of Health's new Consultative Council on Medical and Allied Services, Dawson's report, in 1920, *Future Provision of Medical and Allied*

---

[14] R Cooter, *Surgery and Society in Peace and War: orthopaedics and the organisation of modern medicine* (London, Macmillan, 1993), p. 165; G Newman, *An Outline of the Practice of Preventive Medicine: a memorandum addressed to the Minister of Health* (London, HMSO, 1919), p. 6.

[15] Newman, *Outline*, p. 126.

[16] For a detailed critique of Newman's view on Preventive Medicine, see S Sturdy, 'Hippocrates and state medicine: George Newman outlines the founding policy of the Ministry of Health', in C Lawrence and G Weisz (eds), *Greater than the Parts: holism in biomedicine* (Oxford, Oxford University Press, 1998), pp. 112–34.

[17] Royal Commission on the Poor Laws, *Minutes of Evidence, vol. 9* (PP 1910, Vol. 49), pp. 262–88.

[18] J Lewis, *The Politics of Motherhood: class and maternal welfare 1919–1939* (London, Croom Helm, 1980).

[19] Bertrand Dawson was a consultant physician who developed close connections with the government. B Dawson, 'The future of the medical profession: the Cavendish Lectures', *British Medical Journal*, 1918, (II), 23–6, and 1919, (II), 56–60. For a good biography, see C Webster, 'The metamorphosis of Dawson of Penn', in D Porter and R Porter (eds), *Doctors, Politics and Society* (Amsterdam, Rodopi Press, 1993), pp. 212–28.

Services, is now considered one of the foundation stones of the British welfare state.[20] He called for preventive and curative medical services to be integrated (music to Newman's ears) and for the creation of a network of primary and secondary health centres, under the co-ordination of area health authorities. But Dawson, as a leading consultant physician, also had a hidden agenda to protect the interests of the medical practitioners by ensuring that they stayed independent of government control.

Despite the power of its vision for the future, Dawson's report was shelved. The Ministry of Health did not have the funds to finance such an ambitious scheme during an economic recession. The Consultative Council did not meet again. Newman did not give up, but his approach was subtle. He never declared an intention to bring doctors into a salaried system and he avoided providing detailed plans for an integrated health service. Therefore, he never fell out with the medical profession. His approach to the reform of clinical teaching was similar. His enormous respect for the high-ranking consultants meant that he preferred to accommodate them if possible, and he leant heavily on sympathetic consultants like Clifford Allbut and Thomas Barlow (President of the Royal College of Physicians), trusted allies from his Board of Education days.[21]

Medical Royal Colleges

The two oldest medical Royal Colleges – the Physicians and the Surgeons – along with others more recently founded, operated very effectively in influencing at the highest levels of government. Their leaders have been some of the most eminent people in medicine, elected for their individual clinical expertise, but also increasingly for their diplomatic skills and ability to communicate the interests of their organisations. The state has found the Colleges willing partners in discussions on the development of medical services – a useful way of integrating the views of many of those who actually deliver the goods.

In 1918 the Royal Colleges of Physicians and Surgeons in London formed a joint committee to work with Addison, who was then Minister for Reconstruction, to plan the proposed Ministry of Health.[22] Addison's subsequent Consultative Council on Medical and Allied Services was also composed largely of senior members of the Royal Colleges. Throughout the lead-up to the formation of the NHS, the Royal Colleges exerted influence, as did the BMA, on the Ministry. Their specific remit was to protect and promote the interests of consultants, which often conflicted with those of the general practitioners and public health doctors.

Newman's diaries show him as a regular first point of contact between the Royal Colleges and the Ministry. This role, as intermediary, increased his value both to Whitehall and the medical profession. Subsequent CMOs have consolidated these relationships, both formally and informally. Godber, for example, made excellent use of his friendships at the Royal College of Physicians, where he was a member of Council, to get around the Ministerial impasse on the smoking and lung cancer issue, as discussed in Chapter 3.[23]

[20] *Interim Report on the Future Provision of Medical and Allied Services* (Cmd. 693, 1920).
[21] Sturdy, 'Hippocrates and state medicine', p. 133. Fn.57.
[22] For correspondence and minutes of this committee, see MH 78/68.
[23] This is discussed in detail in Chapter 3.

Another good example of the CMO's interaction with the medical profession concerned orthopaedics services in the early 1920s. This was the early, optimistic period at the Ministry of Health and provides an illustration of how the medical profession played their avenues of influence through both Newman and Dawson. In May 1919 Newman received a pre-publication copy of a proposal by Robert Jones and Gaythorne Girdlestone for a national scheme of treatment centres for crippled children. Significantly, he was not sent this copy directly: it came to him via Dawson. This 'mistake' was undoubtedly a deliberate ploy by Jones and Girdlestone to buy Dawson into their proposals in the hope that he would integrate them into the recommendations in his forthcoming report. Perhaps they judged that Dawson would be more sympathetic to their cause than Newman.

The orthopaedic surgeons then paid two visits during 1920 to Newman at the Ministry of Health to consolidate their campaign. Newman's ideas for 'holistic' approaches to healthcare gave them hope that he would persuade the Minister to act on their proposals. Yet Newman was pessimistic: the Ministry had few funds for capital projects and the onus for service development was still very much on local government. His suggestion that they redirect their requests to local authorities, despite his offer to publicise their scheme in his annual report for 1923, must have done great damage to the image of the CMO as an all-powerful and influential 'gatekeeper'.[24] These events must surely also have filtered through to the medical profession. Was this a one-off incident? Bynum charts a similar decline in Newman's international health policy influence. He was part of the Rockefeller 'scene' in the early 1920s, but their contacts were later made through significant British doctors such as Walter Morley Fletcher, TR Elliott, Henry Dale, Francis Fraser and others in organisations such as the Medical Research Council.[25]

The British Medical Association and the National Health Service

By the early 1930s the existing systems of medical care and healthcare in Britain were in a mess. The hospital system was fractured into municipal and voluntary organisations. There was little attempt at regional co-ordination. There was no integration with other components of healthcare such as the panel doctors (who provided treatment under the National Insurance Act of 1911) and the remainder of general practitioners. The government and the medical profession recognised that a fundamental restructuring of the healthcare system was long overdue. The ideas being debated at this time were not in the same league as subsequent radical plans proposed by William Beveridge for a welfare state, nor their transformation through Aneurin Bevan into the comprehensive state medical service; but, though less ambitious, they were significant.

[24] For a full analysis of these events, see Cooter, *Surgery and Society*, pp. 157–9, 164–71. His study of orthopaedics in Britain in the inter-war period provides a valuable insight into how policy developments were delicately balanced between the government, medical profession and charity organisations.

[25] WF Bynum, 'Sir George Newman and the American Way', in V Nutton and R Porter (eds), *The History of Medical Education in Britain* (Amsterdam, Rodopi, 1995), p. 43.

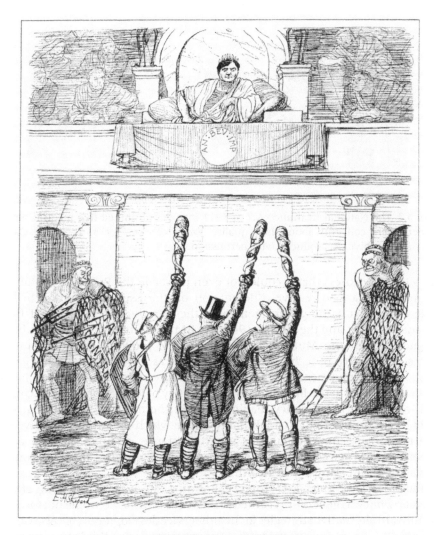

MORITURI TE SALUTANT.

Figure 5.1 Members of the British Medical Association, represented as gladiators, conceding the introduction of the National Health Service to Aneurin Bevan, represented as Nero. Drawing by EH Shepherd for *Punch*, 3rd April 1946. © Punch Cartoon Library and Archive. Reproduced with permission.

In the inter-war period the BMA came to embody 'meso-corporatism', whereby a more powerful professional group defended a sectoral monopoly interest against weaker consumer interests. In essence, politics became medicalised and medicine politicised.[26] In 1904 the BMA had called for the Local Government Board to be reorganised to give the Medical Department more influence. It is a sign of the

[26] Anne Digby, 'Medicine and the English state, 1901–1948', in SJD Green and RC Whiting (eds), *The Boundaries of the State in Modern Britain* (Cambridge, Cambridge University Press, 1996), p. 216.

THE EXPRESS PANEL DOCTOR.

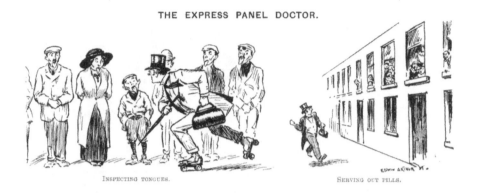

INSPECTING TONGUES.

SERVING OUT PILLS.

Figure 5.2 The National Insurance Act of 1911 introduced limited free medical services, but there were concerns about their quality. *Punch* cartoon, 1913. © Punch Cartoon Library and Archive. Reproduced with permission.

BMA's then weakness that it could not even persuade the President of the Local Government Board to receive a deputation on the issue. In addition to high-profile clashes with the government over the introduction of National Health Insurance in 1911, and the NHS in 1948, the BMA was in more or less continuous dialogue through the Ministry of Health on the provision of public medical services, as a source of technical knowledge and as a way of mobilising general practitioners' involvement in state policies.[27] More significantly, it had lobbied hard in the run-up to the formation of the Ministry of Health for advisory councils which could be given a policy-making role. Furthermore, it insisted that there should be a statutory right to publish any advice which the Minister received but chose to ignore.[28] But, despite this proactive stance, at times of 'high policy' creation, the BMA was forced to join the queue of powerful interest groups to negotiate with the Ministry of Health.

Arthur MacNalty, the CMO from 1935 until 1940, was part of some of these discussions, but was generally regarded as a reactive CMO, who would not forcefully push forward alternative strategies for health service development (see also Chapter 2). MacNalty's name appears in few discussion papers during this formative period, and in only a handful of articles in the medical press.[29] The government saw his retirement as an opportunity to bring in a more dynamic person, with the ability to contribute to policy development, and, more critically, with the skill to deliver the support of the BMA and the Royal Colleges when necessary.

MacNalty was replaced by Wilson Jameson, who, as discussed in Chapter 2, had once spurned the Ministry of Health's attempts to recruit him, likening the atmosphere there to a 'poorly run girls' school'. Second time around, in 1939, the persuasive tactics of the Minister of Health, Malcolm MacDonald, were successful and a highly able new CMO was appointed at a critical time for the development of a National Health Service.

[27] Eckstein, *Pressure Group Politics*, pp. 46–8.
[28] MH 78/80. Notes of a meeting between Addison and the medical lobby, 10.10.1918.
[29] MH 80/24. Memorandum on 'Provision of Specialist Services by the CMO', 15.03.1937; A MacNalty, 'Medicine and the public health', *British Medical Journal*, 1948, (II), 6–9.

Engaging with the doctors' trade union

Although the BMA had its own plans for a reformed health service, the severe economic recession of the 1920s and 1930s left the government with little room for manoeuvre in the inter-war period. Dawson's report had been shelved, mainly for funding reasons, in 1920. However, the financial crisis within the voluntary hospital sector kept up the pressure for reform and for alternatives to the existing insurance and Friendly Society funding methods for these institutions. The Cave Committee, in 1921, recommended increased regional co-ordination of voluntary hospitals through local committees, but this would not solve the financial crises. In 1924 a Royal Commission on Health Insurance was established, chaired by Lord Lawrence. It reported, in 1929, advocating a comprehensive medical service, supported not by health insurance but from general public funds. This, too, was destined to be shelved because of the implications for public expenditure.

The Local Government Act, passed in 1929, removed the stigma of Poor Law medical treatment by enabling the Poor Law medical services to be taken over by local authorities.[30] This was progress. It gave the local Medical Officers of Health a greater opportunity to co-ordinate preventive and curative services within their districts, although many found that they lacked the staff and resources fully to take advantage of this legislation.

There was increasing debate in Britain on health service reform. The influential Political and Economic Planning (PEP) think-tank produced a report in 1937, although no strong proposals emerged from it.[31] The BMA, aware of a ground swell of discontent, conducted its own studies of healthcare reform. In 1930, it published *The BMA's Proposals for a General Medical Service for the Nation*, and a related document entitled *Health Policy*.[32] It later revised this and reissued it in 1938. By the time the Second World War began in September 1939, the government had recognised that a substantial restructuring could be delayed no longer.[33]

Jameson, whilst still Dean at the London School of Hygiene and Tropical Medicine, already had a keen interest in reforming the health services. In September 1939 he had formed the 'Gas Bag' Committee, a small group of influential colleagues, including Edward Mellanby, Allen Daley, George Pickering, WWC Topley, Ernest Rock Carling, Landsborough Thomson and Harold Himsworth. This group met regularly on Saturday mornings for a year at the School. There was no formal agenda, but the multidisciplinary strengths of this group meant that they discussed a wide range of topical health issues.[34]

[30] 1929 Local Government Act. 19 & 20 Geo. V. c.17.

[31] PEP, *Report on the British Health Services* (London, PEP, 1937).

[32] *The British Medical Association's Proposals for a General Medical Service for the Nation* (London, British Medical Association, August 1930).

[33] For a detailed analysis of the pre-NHS discussions, see D Fox, *Health Policies, Health Politics: the British and American Experience, 1911–1965* (Princeton NJ, Princeton University Press, 1985); C Webster, *The Health Services Since the War, Vol. I* (London, HMSO, 1988).

[34] Jameson was also instrumental in the formation of a later monthly non-political discussion group called the Keppel Club, also based at the London School of Hygiene and Tropical Medicine from 1953 to 1974. Membership was by invitation and included Brian Abel Smith, John Fry, John Brotherston, Walter Holland, Jerry Morris, Stephen Taylor, Richard Titmuss and Michael Warren. G Rivett, *From Cradle to Grave: fifty years of the NHS* (London, King's Fund, 1998), p. 52; J Fry, 'The Keppel Club (1952–74): lessons from the past for the future', *British Medical Journal*, 1991, 303, 1596–8.

Discussions took on a slightly more formal nature in 1940 when the Nuffield Provincial Hospitals Trust formed a Medical Advisory Council. This met quarterly in the boardroom at the Radcliffe Infirmary in Oxford with Sir Farquhar Buzzard in the chair. Jameson (while still Dean) attended, along with other influential people, including John Pater, a senior civil servant at the Ministry of Health. Some of the other parties interested in hospital reorganisation – especially the County Councils Association and the Association of Municipal Corporations – resented what they viewed as preferential treatment for the Nuffield Provincial Hospitals Trust, and feared that this would push the Ministry further away from a municipally controlled hospital system. Certainly it appeared to be easier for senior medical figures like Buzzard to access the civil servants. The BMA by this stage was also gearing up to make a contribution: it established a Medical Planning Commission in 1940 which met regularly throughout 1941, with 73 representatives from all the main interest groups within the medical profession.

The government, under pressure from such organisations, issued a statement through the Health Minister, Ernest Brown, on 9 October 1941, announcing a hospital survey with a view to regionalisation of services. The first covered the London hospitals, but by 1945 the whole country had been surveyed. The Nuffield Provincial Hospitals Trust was a co-sponsor of this work. This further antagonised the municipal organisations, who suspected (wrongly) that the Trust was privy to the Ministry's decision-making process.[35] The ten regional hospital surveys were completed between 1941 and 1944. They covered all types of hospital – municipal, voluntary and even mothballed emergency isolation facilities. Collectively they became known as the 'Domesday Book' of British hospitals. They exposed the grim reality of a grossly inequitable distribution of hospital beds, equipment and medical staff. George Godber, as a junior Ministry of Health doctor, had undertaken the survey for the Sheffield and East Midlands region – an invaluable experience which informed his subsequent hospital planning as CMO.

The BMA's Medical Planning Commission issued its interim report in June 1942, advocating regional hospital boards with strong national co-ordination.[36] Jameson had had nothing to do with this, but used his Harveian Oration in October 1942 to welcome the BMA's initiative towards the better 'utilisation of medicine by the state'.[37] In November 1942, William Beveridge's White Paper *Social Insurance and Allied Services* was published and provoked an amazing public demand for copies.[38] It went much further than Beveridge's initial brief, and proposed the creation of a National Health Service, free at the point of delivery for everyone. Once accepted by the government, the medical profession was aware that a fundamental restructuring of its work was unavoidable. Consultations on the form of the medical profession's participation began almost immediately, and Jameson was a key player.

Jameson's unique position made him invaluable to the government in the ensuing negotiations, especially with the BMA. He had direct access to the Minister and had developed a good working partnership with the Permanent

[35] Fox, *Health Policies*, p. 98.
[36] As Webster notes, this plan was so close to Dawson's vision in 1920 that it must have irked him to see it plagiarised. However, he appeared to willingly participate in the Medical Planning Commission and pressure groups despite failing health. Webster, 'The metamorphosis of Dawson of Penn', p. 222.
[37] W Jameson, 'War and the advancement of social medicine', *Lancet*, 1942, (II), 475.
[38] *Social Insurance and Allied Services*, Cmd. 6404 (London, HMSO, 1942).

Secretary (Sir John Maude, later Sir William Douglas). Crucially, he was well-known and well-respected by the medical profession. Thus throughout the twelve-month consultation period leading up to the White Paper of February 1944, Jameson helped the government by 'flying kites' with the medical profession. As the CMO had no executive powers, Jameson was allowed to broach ideas which the government could later disclaim as merely tentative suggestions. This was the mechanism by which Charles Hill, Deputy Secretary of the BMA, secured Jameson's permission to release the idea of a fully salaried medical service to a mass meeting of the Metropolitan Counties Branch of the BMA in March 1942. The reaction was hostile, but because of the way the information had been released, the government was able to reassure the House of Commons that this was only an exploratory proposal.

In August 1944 the BMA balloted its members on the main proposals in a White Paper that proposed the establishment of a National Health Service.[39] The results showed general practitioners as less supportive of the plans than the profession as a whole. The biggest obstacle which the new Minister of Health, Henry Willink, had to overcome was to local authority control over the new system. Both Jameson and Maude initially maintained their position that any comprehensive health service should be controlled by local government, but Jameson increasingly recognised that there had to be some reconciliation between his desires and the opposition of the medical profession.[40] Jameson worked closely with the various interested parties – not only doctors but dentists, pharmacists and opticians. Through meetings and a press conference he sought to allay fears over the crucial issues of regionalisation and medical independence: 'All I would like to do at the present time is to give some sort of assurance that, as a doctor in the Ministry of Health, I really believe that this scheme has in it a great deal that will benefit not merely the medical profession but the British public as well.'[41]

The BMA held a 'Panel Conference' in the autumn of 1944 to formulate views on the components of a National Health Service, and how doctors should be employed. Suggestions that doctors would become salaried employees within a local authority controlled system were roundly condemned. Negotiations began in earnest, but in July 1945 a general election brought in a Labour Government with Aneurin Bevan as Minister of Health. Jameson found him an enthusiastic partner in the search for a solution to the problem of bringing the medical profession on board without creating major divisions. They worked well together. Jameson was an integral part of the small team which Bevan formed to construct a Bill, which was presented to Parliament in March 1946, only eight months after he became Minister of Health.[42]

[39] Ministry of Health, Department of Health for Scotland, *A National Health Service*, Cmd. 6502 (London, HMSO, 1944).

[40] MH 77/26. Second meeting with the Representative Committee of the Medical Profession, 15.04.1943.

[41] N Goodman, *Wilson Jameson: architect of national health* (London, George Allen and Unwin, 1970), p. 119.

[42] The team also included Godber, who had been asked by Jameson in 1944 to act as 'odd job boy' during the week at the Ministry. It was characteristic of Godber's commitment and appetite for work that he travelled back to Nottingham at the weekends to maintain his regional duties. Other members of the team included the Deputy CMO John Charles, Permanent Secretary Sir William Douglas, Deputy Secretary Sir John Hawton, Deputy Secretary Arthur Rucker and Under Secretary John Pater.

The change of Minister shifted the balance in policy making within the Ministry away from the civil servants at a crucial point in the negotiations. Some of the recent Health Ministers, especially Elliot, MacDonald and Brown, had stepped back from drafting policy, reacting instead to papers produced by Sir John Maude, the Permanent Secretary. It has even been suggested that Maude showed the Ministry's doctors' salary plan to outsiders, including Anderson at the BMA, before his own Minister (Brown) got to see it.[43] Bevan would never tolerate this type of civil service behaviour, and Maude was moved from the Ministry of Health before he arrived. The new White Paper which accompanied the Bill explained the fundamental restructuring which Bevan's small team had designed. Two main initiatives differed from Willink's draft: the nationalisation of all hospitals and their management through regional hospital boards, and the contracting of doctors to local executive councils. This was not quite the comprehensive salaried service which the BMA vehemently opposed. Jameson and other key civil servants had experience of managing the wartime Emergency Medical Service which had employed consultants within a regionalised hospital system. From this, they knew that Bevan's plans were feasible.[44]

During the ensuing parliamentary debates, the hospital consultants promoted their views through Lord Moran, President of the Royal College of Physicians.[45] The hospital issue was resolved and the Bill received royal assent on 6 November 1946. The appointed day for the new National Health Service was fixed as 5 July 1948. However, the BMA was not convinced that the Act represented the best interests of its members. A plebiscite was held on whether to proceed with negotiations, and the negative motion was carried with a majority of 5,000 votes. It was not until February 1947 that the BMA returned to the negotiating table, aware that the government had continued to talk to the consultants through the medical Royal Colleges. After a year of protracted negotiations, stalemate was reached in January 1948: 90 per cent of the vote of BMA members was against the Act.

In March another BMA special representative meeting decided not to enter the service unless the conditions were completely revised in its favour. At the eleventh hour Bevan adopted a more conciliatory tone, and a third BMA plebiscite achieved the result required for the general practitioners to join the NHS. When 5 July 1948 dawned, the whole medical profession supported the NHS. Jameson's role in the previous eight years of negotiation had proved vital. Bevan publicly paid tribute to his contribution in the House of Commons and in a speech at a King's Fund dinner to mark the tenth anniversary of the NHS.

Professional organisations, such as the BMA, had been constrained by their inability to provide one voice for the profession. Bevan had been able to negotiate separately with the consultants (through the medical Royal Colleges) and the

---

[43] F Honigsbaum, *Health, Happiness and Security* (London, Routledge, 1989), p. 217.
[44] JE Pater, *The Making of the National Health Service* (London, King Edward's Fund, 1981), pp. 178-9.
[45] For a more detailed account of the negotiations with the Royal Colleges and the BMA, see C Webster, *The Health Services Since the War, vol. I* (London, HMSO, 1988). Dan Fox, in *Health Policies, Health Politics*, p. 134, also recounts an anecdote from Brian Abel Smith, who had been close to Bevan in the 1950s. He claimed that Bevan chose to do much of the negotiating with Moran over dinner at Prunier's Restaurant.

general practitioners (through the BMA).[46] Jameson was instrumental in this, able to exploit his long-standing friendships and connections within the Royal College of Physicians and the London medical establishment. Although Bevan had begun his Ministry with a charm offensive, dining at various medical Royal Colleges, there was a limit to his availability and willingness to socialise with the medical profession. Jameson became his eyes and ears in such informal encounters, allowing him to retain some degree of separation from the people with whom he had to negotiate. Given his infamous after-dinner quip about having to 'stuff their [the consultants] mouths with gold' to bring them on board the NHS, Bevan quickly lost the 'clever and charming' epithets which the *British Medical Journal* had initially accorded him.[47]

Despite the massive accomplishment of establishing the NHS in 1948, the divisions within the medical profession, particularly between primary and secondary healthcare, continued to cause concern to the Ministry of Health and necessarily to the CMO.

Jameson served only another two years before retiring aged 65 years in 1950, but he had played a major part in making the NHS operational. He continued to be involved from his post-Whitehall retirement position at the King's Fund. He went into retirement with his stature high in the medical world. This is perhaps surprising because he was the first CMO to have had a major role as an agent of government in achieving a key goal (i.e. the establishment of a National Health Service). Forty years later, Acheson took soundings on the possibility of standing for election as President of the Royal College of Physicians after his retirement as CMO. He was left in no doubt that he would not be successful because he was perceived as having been too close to government (in this case during the NHS internal market reforms of the Thatcher government).[48] Bevan did not emerge quite so well as Jameson in the opinion of the *British Medical Journal*:

> His vicious attacks on the profession, his attempts to sow discord, and his rudeness in negotiation would never be forgotten. He never rose above being a clever politician and at critical moments failed to become the statesman. He had done his best to make himself disliked by the medical profession, and, by and large, he had succeeded.[49]

Post-NHS relationships

In 1918 the Haldane Report on the machinery of government had recommended the use of expert advisory committees by the various Boards and Ministries. Although Addison had formed the Consultative Council on Medical and Allied

---

[46] Webster, *Health Services Since the War*, pp. 116–19; R Stevens, *Medical Practice in Modern England: the impact of specialisation and state medicine* (New Haven, Yale University Press, 1966), pp. 77–9, 92–3.

[47] *British Medical Journal*, 1945, (II; suppl.), 63; 1943, (II), 119.

[48] Senior health professional interview, 16.02.2000.

[49] 'Aneurin Bevan', *British Medical Journal*, 1960, (II), 203–4. It should be stressed, however, that the *BMJ* has complete editorial freedom from the British Medical Association. The *BMJ*'s line on Bevan mellowed considerably, and by the time of his death in 1960 it had recontextualised the struggle for the NHS.

Services in 1920, this disintegrated shortly afterwards. An *ad hoc* Medical Advisory Committee, created in 1930, performed a partial function, but cannot be considered as an adequate formal mechanism of the type suggested by Haldane. This became a major debating issue in discussions on the creation of the NHS, with the local authorities seeking a permanent consultative arrangement.

The 1946 National Health Service Act had also established the Central Health Services Council, which appeared to satisfy local authority demands, although the medical profession niggled that its own authority would be diminished with such a strong lay membership. The Central Health Services Council, which did not meet until 27 July 1948, had 41 members, of whom 21 were medically qualified. The Ministry of Health had solicited lists of candidates from related organisations. In the event it chose fifteen general practitioners from the BMA's list. The Presidents of the medical Royal Colleges and two others were *ex officio* members, and there were also representatives for mental health, voluntary hospitals, dentists and local government.[50]

The standing subcommittees of the Central Health Services Council were more useful than the main committee, which met only quarterly and proved to be somewhat unwieldy. (These Standing Advisory Committees are touched on in more detail in Chapter 3 on the tripartite relationship and in Chapter 6 on policy formation.) Bevan submitted 30 questions to the Central Health Services Council during its first eighteen months of operation and also received unsolicited advice on a further twelve topics.[51] An eclectic mix of issues reflected the virgin territory of a national comprehensive health service, from care for the elderly through to the prescribing practices of general practitioners and the development of cancer services. The CMO played a facilitating role, ensuring that issues which he wished to be progressed were provided as briefing papers for Standing Medical Advisory Committees, and then waiting for their clinical advice to become available to Ministers.

Another mechanism by which the government sought to establish easier communications with the medical profession was the Joint Consultants Committee. This was formed in 1948 to allow the medical Royal Colleges and the BMA to speak for the consultant body with one voice. At this stage there were about 4,500 consultants, and many specialties were massively understaffed. The Joint Consultants Committee has since played a significant role in formalising the profession's views on issues such as the maintenance of standards of professional knowledge and skill, and the development of specialist hospital services. With representatives from the medical Royal Colleges (usually their Presidents), and from the consultants and junior doctors' committees of the BMA, it has proved a strong channel for dialogue, and the focal point for contact has remained the CMO.[52] The relationship between the CMO and the Joint Consultants Committee has not been free of tension. The Committee's quarterly meetings have often

[50] C Webster, *The National Health Service: a political history* (Oxford, Oxford University Press, 1998), p. 242.
[51] G Rivett, *From Cradle to Grave: fifty years of the NHS* (London, King's Fund, 1998), p. 50.
[52] For an example of the type of representation the Joint Consultants Committee has made to the government on the subject of increasing consultant numbers, see: Memorandum by the Joint Consultants Committee, Select Committee on Health, 1998–99, Appendices to Minutes of Evidence. Electronic copy at: www.parliament.the-stationery-office.co.uk/pa/cm199899/cmselect/htm.

been quite combative with the CMO being asked to explain or justify government policies that the medical profession were unhappy about. One senior official has described the position of the CMO and other Department of Health officials who attended the meetings, at times, as 'like ducks in a shooting gallery'.[53]

One of Godber's key interests was the development of medical specialties. He was involved in negotiations on this issue while Deputy CMO in the late 1950s, and as CMO he chaired the Advisory Committee on Consultant Establishments in which the Joint Consultants Committee was actively involved. This examined all applications for consultant posts to ensure that they were allocated to the regions with greatest need and that less popular specialties received support.[54] Godber also involved the Joint Consultants Committee in his working party on medical management, the outcome of which were the 'cogwheel' reports of the late 1960s.[55]

The CMO was sometimes required to adjudicate on some trivial issues. In 1965 the Joint Consultants Committee complained about the Ministry of Health's proposals to make junior doctors eat in the main hospital canteens along with nurses and other staff. Godber negotiated a compromise in which a part of the main canteen would be sectioned off for the exclusive use of doctors, to which the Joint Consultants Committee finally agreed. Hardly a matter of life and death, but illustrative of the way in which the medical profession expected the CMO to liaise with the Ministry on its behalf.[56]

In April 1974, following a proposal from the President of the Royal Society of Medicine, a 'Conference' of the medical Royal Colleges was formed with a Standing Joint Committee of sixteen members. In 1996, this became the Academy of Medical Royal Colleges. A constitution and articles of association were drawn up and charitable status given later that year. The formation of the Academy was partly a response to ensure that the views of smaller Royal Colleges were heard by government and to provide a single point of contact for the government and others who wanted a Royal College view on matters of policy.

In the first few years of the NHS the BMA continued to be the main representative of the general practitioners, and maintained several of its pre-NHS structures, including the General Medical Services Committee. The rifts which the NHS had opened within the medical profession continued to widen during the 1950s. This was part of the reason for the establishment of a new College of General Practitioners in 1952, which within four years had 22 regional faculties and around 4,000 members.[57] It was awarded a royal charter in 1972. The College ensured the professional representation of general practitioners within negotiations between the wider profession and government, a role which the BMA could only partially fulfil.

For Godber, the 'Janus' issue – being able to 'face two ways at the same time' – was central to his integrity as CMO. He consciously drew on his observation of

---

[53] Private information.

[54] G Godber, 'Trends in specialisation and their effect on the practice of medicine', *British Medical Journal*, 1961, (II), 841–7.

[55] Ministry of Health, *First Report of the Joint Working Party on the Organisation of Medical Work in Hospitals* (London, HMSO, 1967). This report and its successors were nicknamed the 'cogwheel' reports because of the images used on their covers.

[56] British Medical Association Archives. E/2/41/1 Policy File 2 (2) 2 (38) 11: Joint Consultants Committee correspondence, 11.06.1965.

[57] Rivett, *From Cradle to Grave*, p. 91.

Jameson's delicate role in the negotiations for the NHS, and balanced his responsibilities towards the Department of Health and Social Security with those to the other Departments where he served as CMO, and to the medical profession. He recognised that there was a fine line between loyalty to one's Minister and to the profession:

> . . . but that loyalty should never extend to saying what's comfortable. And he must be prepared to put down on paper the consequences of a particular course that seems to him wrong and will be for these reasons damaging and he can't agree with it. In the extreme case, that might be so serious that he would have to say, 'I can't continue.' But he reaches that point, I think, only when he feels that the ministerial course proposed is one he would not be able to defend outside.[58]

Crossman records in his diaries only one instance when Godber used this ultimate threat: 'If the Cabinet takes that decision, I shall have to go'. This was over the issue of doctors' pay in January 1969. Crossman then duly translated this threat to Wilson and the Cabinet so that, as Godber puts it, 'I reckon I was used as the head of the battering ram'.[59]

We have already examined in Chapter 3 the sensitive relationship between CMOs, civil servants and Ministers. Godber was more than comfortable handling the irascible Crossman, and confident in his own secure position between Whitehall and the medical profession. Crossman's diaries reveal numerous instances in which Godber's advice was apposite and well-received. Only rarely does one get the feeling that Godber's true authority, and capacity to side with the medical profession against the government, is acknowledged by Crossman:

> . . . I had a long meeting with the Joint Consultants Committee, a very high-grade committee of the eight leading men in the medical profession. They wanted to talk to me about the Green Paper but Godber had warned me that in his view the medical profession was going to explode about various things, in particular my reaction to Ely [critical report on the Ely Mental Hospital in Cardiff]. So I passed him a message that I wanted to discuss this, and after quite an easy consultation about the Green Paper I said, 'Now we come to Ely', and told them about the inspectorate. What interested me was that they had got a completely false impression . . . the more I talked the more the JCC felt they had been mis-briefed. And by whom? Nobody except Godber and the Ministry. In the course of that hour and a half I had to overcome the impression which the Ministry had been sedulously creating and I think it went pretty well.[60]

[58] Godber interview with Anthony Seldon, 27.06.1980. Wellcome Trust Contemporary Medical Archives Centre (GC/201/D.2), p. 33.
[59] Seldon interview, p. 33; R Crossman, *The Crossman Diaries, Vol. III: Secretary of State for Social Services, 1968–70* (London, Hamish Hamilton, 1977), p. 335. 'I dropped it to him [Wilson] that I had just left George Godber, who had made it clear that if this was rejected or referred to the Prices and Incomes Board he would have to resign, and the fact that perhaps one of the most prominent civil servants would go duly registered with the PM. After half an hour it became clear that, unless Harold was deceiving me, he would back me.' (22.01.1969)
[60] Ibid., p. 464. (29.04.1969)

Of course Crossman was providing his own take on events, but it is a unique insight into life at the Ministry and in particular how he used his CMO in 'scene setting' with the medical profession. But Godber's strength in his contacts with the profession occasionally worked against him in the partisan eyes of Crossman, for example when Godber attempted to block a staff move:

> I must now bring in Clifford Jarrett [Permanent Secretary] and work out how to lever Baker away from the CMO, because I can't break with Godber. He is a very powerful man in the Department and people never like acting against his wishes. He is away half the time around the world, advising the World Health Organization, in America, lecturing. He is remote, out of touch now, I think, except with the lord high panjandra and the physicians in the Royal Colleges in London. He knows all the top people but nothing about ordinary life, yet on the other hand he is radical and left wing. I don't want to quarrel with him.[61]

Godber's reputation within the medical profession was never questioned. He was seen as a 'socially committed and deeply principled' man who could judiciously use his considerable authority to steer the profession towards his goals.[62] Godber's long-standing public commitment to general practice was welcomed by the specialty.[63] It also allowed him to make some less favourable remarks in the security of knowledge that they would not be misinterpreted, as in his Pickles Lecture to the Royal College of General Practitioners when he drew attention to what he called the 'long tail' of poor practice which was dragging the reputation of that specialty down.[64]

Godber had a consistent interest in promoting general practice. He used his influence with Sir Isaac Wolfson to persuade him to fund a chair in general practice at St Thomas's Medical School, and with Bernard Sunley to fund the appointment of Peter Higgins as Professor of General Practice at Guy's.[65] These two posts were a significant advance in the establishment of academic general practice, and could not have been achieved without Godber's influence.

One of Us? Castle, Yellowlees and the pay beds dispute

The delicate position of the CMO between the medical profession and the government of the day was most acutely apparent during the 1974 pay beds

[61] Ibid., p. 665. (04.10.1969)

[62] Senior medical professional interview, 28.08.2002.

[63] One interviewee suggested that Godber did general practice a service by nominating an increasing number of GPs for public honours, thus raising the status of the specialty. However, he refused to put John Hunt forward for an honour because of his private practice – which Godber could not personally reconcile with his commitment to the NHS. Senior medical professional interview, 04.04.2000.

[64] G Godber, 'Change and Continuity' (William Pickles Lecture, RCGP), *Journal of the Royal College of General Practitioners*, 1985, 35, 320–5.

[65] Sir Isaac Wolfson (1897–1991) developed the Great Universal Stores and used his fortune to create the Wolfson Foundation for the advancement of health, education and youth activities, and also to found Wolfson College at the University of Oxford. Bernard Sunley (1910–1964) was an entrepreneur who founded Bernard Sunley and Sons Ltd.

dispute. By this stage, the NHS had become increasingly politicised. The Labour Government which came into office in February 1974 also brought in Barbara Castle as Minister of Health for two very turbulent years. The medical profession had been pressing for a massive injection of cash into the NHS for some time, and when the new Labour Government came in, the BMA, particularly through its Secretary Derek Stevenson, demanded an additional £500 million (at a time when the annual budget of the NHS was £3 billion) and a Royal Commission. Stevenson proposed a variety of ways to increase funding, including charging for general practitioner appointments, top-up insurance and lottery-type schemes. He declared that in the NHS 'morale has never been lower'. As Timmins succinctly puts it: 'It was into this already heady brew that Labour stirred the final ingredient needed to make gunpowder. It had determined to phase pay beds out of the NHS.'[66]

Pay beds, the private domain of consultants within NHS hospitals, had remained intact since the creation of the NHS in 1948. Despite an initial decrease in private health insurance after 1948, from the 1960s there was a steady trickle of new business, mainly from British United Provident Association (BUPA) which was the biggest of the health insurance providers. Part of the explanation for this lies with the more expensive surgical procedures which were now possible, but it was mainly due to the expansion in company schemes – an attractive bonus for workers at a time when wage increases were economically difficult. By 1970 almost two million people were covered by private health insurance. When the Labour Government came into office in 1974 this figure had increased to 2.4 million (four per cent of the population), two-thirds of whom were in company schemes. Insurance patients were treated in some 3,700 beds in small private hospitals, but also increasingly in pay beds in NHS hospitals which could offer access to high-technology operating facilities.

This row had rumbled around Parliament for some time. A Commons Expenditure Committee in 1971 had investigated complaints of queue jumping, inappropriate use of NHS equipment and consultants skimping on their NHS patients, although it found (much to the dismay of the Labour opposition members) that there was insufficient evidence to substantiate these pervasive claims.[67] Yet there is rarely smoke without fire, and there was substance to some of the accusations. The fees paid to the NHS were gross approximations of the actual cost of private patients and there was also an element of inequity in the system, as the nurses and junior doctors involved in the provision of treatment did not share in the consultants' private patient income. The Labour Party saw this as ripe material for a manifesto promise, hence the 1974 pledge to 'phase out private practice from the hospital service'.

David Owen, a Junior Health Minister on Castle's new team, recalls that the manifesto pledge caused alarm in Whitehall, and that Sir Philip Rogers, the Permanent Secretary, had tried to warn them off this idea:

> Sir Philip deployed a strong case against our taking any action. He
> warned us that the mood of the medical profession was very brittle and

[66] N Timmins, *The Five Giants: a biography of the welfare state* (London, Fontana Press, 1996), p. 333.
[67] Fourth Report from the Expenditure Committee, NHS Facilities for Private Patients (London, HMSO, 1972).

said that the considered judgement of himself, the Chief Medical Officer [Yellowlees] and all the top officials was that, in the best interests of the National Health Service, we should avoid a confrontation with the doctors on this issue. Rather movingly he insisted that if the Secretary of State [Castle], having heard him out, came to a different conclusion then that was the last that she would hear of it and everyone in the Department would carry out her policy faithfully and to the best of their abilities.[68]

Castle, after listening to Rogers' advice, pressed ahead with her plans to phase out pay beds.

The 'gunpowder' was finally ignited in June 1974, when members from the National Union of Public Employees refused to service patients in the two private wards at the new Charing Cross Hospital, known locally as the 'Fulham Hilton'.[69] The ensuing ten-day dispute attracted considerable media attention and forced a showdown between the Department of Health and Social Security and the BMA. Although a local settlement was reached (which allowed for unused beds in the private wards to be given to NHS patients), the timing of the dispute was unfortunate, coming when negotiations (chaired by Owen) were already taking place on a consultants' contract. Castle was tempted to use more stick than carrot in persuading some consultants to accept whole-time contracts with the NHS, threatening only to give merit awards to whole-timers. By December 1974 some consultants were 'working to contract' in protest, claiming that Castle's proposals in total amounted to the extinction of private medicine in Britain. Walpole Lewin, Chairman of the British Medical Association's Council, declared in *The Times*, 'We are fighting for the independence of the profession'.[70]

The year 1975 opened with a sixteen-week working-to-contract protest by consultants, swiftly followed by disagreements with the junior doctors over their promised reduced-hours agreement. The general practitioners were also threatening mutiny, collecting 16,000 unsigned and undated resignations to be used if Castle reneged on the forthcoming pay award. The BMA expressed concern about lengthening waiting lists and possible harm to patients. In the face of an obdurate Minister of Health, it appealed to the Prime Minister, Harold Wilson, to intervene. He declined, and Castle pressed ahead, issuing her paper, *The Separation of Private Practice from National Health Service Hospitals*, in August 1975.[71]

The medical profession put aside internal differences and united, claiming that the NHS was facing a crisis on a scale unseen since its formation in 1948. By December 1975 the junior doctors had joined the consultants in all-out industrial action, forcing casualty and other departments to close in hospitals throughout the country. Wilson finally succumbed to pressure and telephoned the distinguished solicitor, Arnold Goodman, to arbitrate between the medical profession and Castle. Goodman already had experience in the disputes, having been engaged in August by BUPA to advise on the pay beds issue, and he soon became seen as the medical profession's saviour.

[68] D Owen, *Time to Declare* (London, Michael Joseph, 1991), p. 232.
[69] Timmins, *The Five Giants*, p. 334.
[70] *The Times*, 31.12.1974.
[71] Department of Health and Social Security, The *Separation of Private Practice from National Health Service Hospitals: a consultative document* (London, DHSS, 1975).

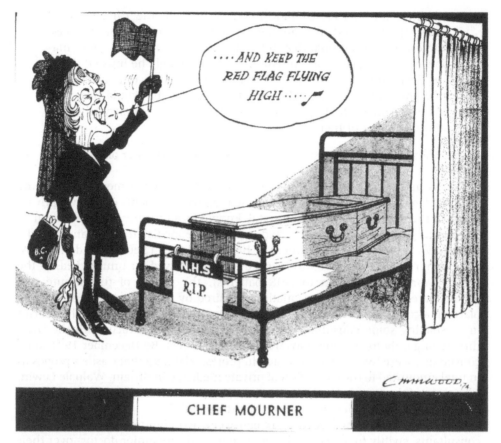

CHIEF MOURNER

Figure 5.3 Barbara Castle's role in the 1974 NHS crisis (*Daily Mail*, 10th July 1974). © Solo Syndication. Reproduced with permission.

Castle, one presumes to save face in the Cabinet and to attempt to solve the problem herself, initially met with Goodman in private and on her own. In the subsequent negotiations, she took along her Health Minister David Owen, her Political Adviser Jack Straw, her Private Secretary Norman Warner and her Permanent Secretary Patrick Nairne. This close team excluded the one obvious 'link' with the medical profession – the Chief Medical Officer, Henry Yellowlees. In his biography, Owen later commented that:

> . . . Dr Yellowlees, though a pleasant person, was not tough enough either with us Ministers or with the BMA. His predecessor, Sir George Godber, had been a commanding figure of quite exceptional character and had stood up even to Dick Crossman.[72]

Although Yellowlees disputes his characterisation in Owen's memoirs, and suggests that it was perhaps a retrospective rationalisation, another person who was also closely involved in the pay beds crisis offered this explanation:

[72] Owen, *Time to Declare*, p. 236.

This was as much about Labour Party politics as it was about medical politics and part of the trouble was that Henry didn't have enough political awareness.[73]

For ten days the negotiations between the government and the BMA took place quietly in Goodman's flat. The CMO was excluded from the discussions from the outset. The result was an agreement to phase out pay beds using an independent board, which would ensure that the pace of change would be compensated for by new developments in private hospitals. Yellowlees, to his dismay, learnt that an agreement had been reached, not through his own Department, but from a senior medical colleague at one of the medical Royal Colleges the day after the deal had been done. He returned to the Department 'white with anger . . . we were all concerned that he was going to have another heart attack'.[74] The exclusion left a deep impression on Yellowlees.

> Mrs Castle had been told by Labour members that she must be careful of the doctors in the Department – that they worked for the profession – and nothing made me more angry than this gross slur on my loyalty. I was outraged at covert suggestions that the Secretary of State might have given some credence to these accusations and excluded me from the Goodman discussions as a consequence. Whatever the real reasons might have been it was not so much the fact of the exclusion, for Secretaries of State can do what they like in such matters, but the way in which it was carried out which so affected me as CMO. That the CMO needs to maintain his credibility with the leaders of his profession had apparently not been considered. I was furious and deeply hurt and the relationship with the Secretary of State was severely strained. For several months I avoided attending many of her meetings. The matter was resolved when she was replaced by David Ennals.[75]

Yet the damage, as Yellowlees suspected, had been done. A senior doctor within one of the medical Royal Colleges who had been involved with the 1974 issues commented that Yellowlees seemed to him to be 'a charming man, but from the College perspective he didn't really feature on our radar as a significant person to deal with'.[76]

Yet there were other occasions on which Yellowlees was used as a negotiator with the profession and he continued to be the conduit for negotiations between the hospital consultants and the Department of Health and Social Security. He used to keep a framed ticket on his desk for a missed performance of Handel's *Messiah* at the Albert Hall to remind him of the occasion when he was forced to abandon the concert to participate in an all-night negotiating session with the medical profession. As he said, there are more important things in life than work.

[73] Politician interview, 10.07.2000.
[74] Politician interview, 10.07.2000.
[75] Yellowlees interview, 14.07.1999.
[76] Senior medical professional interview, 28.08.2002.

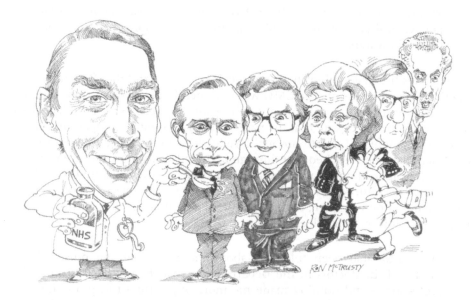

Figure 5.4 Henry Yellowlees with the Secretaries of State for Health he served: Norman Fowler, Patrick Jenkin, Barbara Castle, David Ennals and Keith Joseph. The cartoon was specially commissioned by the BMA GPs committee as a retirement gift for Yellowlees. Property of Henry Yellowlees. Reproduced with permission.

Conclusion

The professional integrity and position of the CMO of the day as intermediary has become increasingly tense during the long period of development of state medical services. His personal medical knowledge made him the only person within Whitehall who could accurately assess the demands of his colleagues for better medical services, and, to a lesser extent, their demands for better remuneration for their work. In maintaining the confidence of the profession, and of the government, the CMO has had to tread a fine line. As the case studies in this chapter illustrate, CMOs have occasionally fallen foul of the niceties of the etiquette of medical politics or the wider forces of large-scale political crises.

Most of the key disputes between the government and the medical profession have money or professional autonomy in their various guises as the common cause. From the BMA's lobbying to protect the rights of doctors to determine their own incomes in the inter-war period, to the place of private medicine within the NHS in the 1970s, the position of the CMO in these episodes has been to try to articulate to both sides the health impact of the planned developments. Thus it could be suggested that Yellowlees really had no cause to be involved in the 1974 disputes, which were essentially about doctors' pay.

By the 1980s, the era of cost containment had dawned. The politicisation of health service financing had reached a new peak and was transgressing formerly established boundaries to enter the realm of the independence of general practitioners.[77] For example, Acheson clearly saw Fowler and Clarke's 'limited list' proposals in November 1984 as having deeper implications for patients, in addition to its envisaged impact on prescription costs.[78] The idea that general practitioners would be constrained to prescribe from an authorised list of cheaper generic drugs was perceived by the profession as an attack on the very heart of medical autonomy. However, Clarke had seen the success of the Health Maintenance Organizations in the USA in controlling pharmaceutical costs. His plan aimed to correct a chronic systems fault in British social policy. The government refused to consult with the BMA, which in turn expressed its anger to the CMO. Acheson suffered 'acute distress' because of the increasingly unpleasant exchanges between Ministers and the medical profession.[79] He vented his own anger at the profession's refusal to accept the Ministerial line, most notably in one meeting with representatives from the Royal College of Physicians. After his outburst, Bryan Rayner, one of the Permanent Under Secretaries, was sent by Norman Fowler to 'mend the fences'.[80]

Although he received the brunt of the Ministers' frustration, Acheson emerged more secure in their confidence. The medical profession, despite an unlikely alliance with the Labour Party and the pharmaceutical industry, had to accept a compromise. As punishment, according to one observer, they 'cold-shouldered' Acheson for some time because of his perceived failure to support their cause.[81] In February 1985 the government agreed that the drugs list would be extended from 30 to 100 items and that the profession would be consulted on its composition and participate in a new Advisory Committee on National Health Service Drugs. As Rudolf Klein puts it: 'It was an accidental rather than deliberate trial of strength with the medical profession – the limited list episode proved to Ministers that it was possible to take on the doctors without getting a bloody nose.'[82] Acheson's relationship with the BMA in the later period of his office never really recovered. Between 1987 and 1991 there was virtually no contact between the CMO and the general practitioners' branch of the BMA, and as one closely involved doctor put it: 'It took several years to restore the relationship.'[83]

Taking on the medical profession has invariably proved more complicated, given its assumption that the CMO should be 'one of us'. Yet some CMOs have been willing to tackle unpalatable issues. Calman, in particular, in recent years made considerable progress, utilising a problem with European Law as an opportunity to modernise a rather antiquated system of postgraduate medical education. On the problem of poorly performing doctors, an issue which was emerging publicly in the early 1990s, it was more awkward for Calman to take a line without risking his reputation with the profession. His tactic was to give an

---

[77] For more information, see B Rayner, 'The development of primary health care policy in the 1980s: a view from the centre', in P Day (ed.), *Managing Change and Implementing Primary Health Care Policy* (Centre for the Analysis of Social Policy, Bath, 1992).

[78] Fowler and Acheson were both relatively new arrivals to the Department of Health and Social Security (Fowler became Secretary of State for Social Services in June 1983, and Acheson became CMO in December 1983).

[79] Government Minister interview, 11.07.2000.

[80] Senior medical professional interview, 28.08.2002.

[81] Health commentator interview. 08.06.2000.

[82] R Klein, *The New Politics of the NHS* (New York, Prentice Hall, 2001), p. 140.

[83] Senior medical professional interview, 19.11.2002.

advance warning to the profession that it had to adopt appropriate standards through a system of appraisal and revalidation. He followed up on this friendly advice with the revelation that if the profession did not put its own house in order, that the government would do it for them.[84] His report in 1994 on 'Maintaining Medical Excellence' was seen by some as stepping on the toes of the General Medical Council, and did not win him friends within the BMA, yet many inside these organisations privately acknowledged that reform was needed.[85]

Invariably, some of the success or failure in these situations is determined by personality and established profile. It is difficult at the senior level, at which most critical negotiations and discussions take place, to eliminate the need for personal credibility. Jameson observed how Bevan worked on the medical profession over dinners in London clubs and restaurants. One closely connected adviser noted that Godber and Robert Platt, President of the Royal College of Physicians, used to share car journeys and that many useful decisions appeared to emerge from these rides. Godber used a similar tactic with John Richardson, Chair of the Joint Consultants Committee: although they would sometimes put on a show of active debate in committee meetings, it was clear that a deal had already been done during the preceding car journey.[86] Another senior medical civil servant commented that despite Yellowlees' unfortunate pay beds crisis, he 'spent an awful lot of time looking after the Joint Consultants Committee and the Royal Colleges and massaging egos'.[87]

More recently, the balance of influence has shifted yet again with the progressive use of independent 'special advisers' in government. In 1995–96 there were 38 special advisers; by 1998–99 this had increased to 72.[88] Some, such as Brian Abel-Smith (1926–1996), who was a special health adviser in the 1960s and 1970s, were already closely involved with policy formation, but more recently their instalment in Whitehall has served to displace some of the traditional lobbying routes of the medical profession, and, necessarily, the perceived value of the CMO as mediator. Thus when Roy Griffiths was developing his plans for reforming the NHS in the early 1980s, he did not include Acheson in his select 'sounding board'. He preferred instead to hold private meetings every two or three weeks at the Sainsbury's headquarters with a group of health professionals.[89]

In the final years of our history, 1997 and 1998, a new Labour Government had been elected and it was inevitable that new channels of influence would come into play. The new Ministers' personal networks (developed in opposition)

---

[84] Senior medical professional interview, 19.11.2002.

[85] Senior medical professional interview, 28.08.2002.

[86] Senior medical civil servant interview, 22.07.2002.

[87] Senior medical civil servant interview, 17.05.2000.

[88] D Richards and MJ Smith, *Governance and Public Policy in the United Kingdom* (Oxford, Oxford University Press, 2002), p. 219.

[89] This group included Brian Creamer, Dean of Medicine at United Medical and Dental Schools of Guy's and St Thomas's; Walter Holland, Professor of Health at the London School of Economics; Barry Jackson, later President of the Royal College of Surgeons (1998–2001); David Morrell, Professor of General Practice at United Medical and Dental Schools of Guy's and St Thomas's, with Cliff Graham, a senior civil servant, in attendance as secretary. Health professional interview, 14.02.2000.

widened the inputs to policy development. So, too, did a more substantive cadre of special advisers than had existed in the past. Some saw this as a healthy, external 'breath of fresh air' for a government department that had become set in its ways. Others feared that mainstream civil servants would be marginalised. Permanent Secretary Graham Hart met with senior members of the Department weekly without the Minister. It was clear to those who understood Whitehall that new channels of influence were being developed, not to displace civil servants but to reduce Ministerial dependence on them as an exclusive source of advice.[90]

It was truly a new era as an unprecedented turnover of the senior management of the Department of Health took place. Within that two-year period, the roll-call of those who left for retirement or pastures new included: Sir Graham Hart (Permanent Secretary), Sir Alan Langlands (Chief Executive of the NHS), Dame Yvonne Moores (Chief Nursing Officer), Dr Graham Winyard (Medical Director of the NHS and Deputy CMO), Sir Herbert Laming (Chief Inspector of Social Services) and, the fourteenth Chief Medical Officer, and the last in our history, Sir Kenneth Calman.

[90] Senior civil servant interview, 11.09.2002.

Chapter 6

Engaging external expertise

Health in Britain has probably been subjected to more conscious 'policy forma-tion' than almost any other area of government activity.[1] Policy, like 'expertise', is a relatively new word in the English language, originating in the nineteenth century as a derivation of 'police'. The two concepts of expertise and policy formation fit naturally together. Over the years many CMOs have been skilled practitioners of both, employing personal expertise and that of selected advisers to the formation of appropriate strategies for the security and development of the nation's health. In this chapter, through the examples of acquired immune deficiency syndrome (AIDS) and bovine spongiform encephalopathy (BSE), we attempt to understand the significance of the CMO's position within Whitehall, and between the government, the medical profession and the public. We show how his personal authority has been critical in the success of specific health policies.

It has not been the role of the CMO to decide policy. That is a Ministerial privilege. However, the line between being the initiator and architect of an important new policy and being responsible for introducing it has often been a very fine one. A Minister has the personal responsibility for the actions taken by his or her department, but as the business of government became increasingly complicated, Ministers often ventured beyond their civil servants for advice. Various mechanisms have been used to generate alternative perspectives, most notably political advisers and 'think-tanks'. This development has not always been popular with civil servants, as Crossman noted in 1970 when he wished to set up a 'working group':

> Into 21a [Crossman's office] there came rather sheepishly Clifford Jarrett, Alan Marre, the CMO, all the top brass, to plead with me that it was unwise for the Secretary of State to do this [set up a working party and chair it himself], that it would be dangerous and would upset people on the outside if they were excluded from the working party. I spent twenty minutes explaining that this wasn't a working party, but a brains trust, and that I couldn't work without bringing in people from outside . . . an informal think-tank . . . It is strange how deeply suspicious civil servants are of people being brought in from the outside and of having a mixture of civil servants and outsiders to think out new policies.[2]

[1] See C Ham, *Health Policy in Britain: the politics and organisation of the NHS* (Basingstoke, Palgrave, 1999).

[2] R Crossman, *The Crossman Diaries, Vol. III: Secretary of State for Social Services, 1968–70* (London, Hamish Hamilton, 1977), p. 826. February 1970.

The power of the CMO to progress or hinder the introduction of specific policy initiatives at various points in our history has been palpable. John Charles effectively delayed the introduction of family planning services in the 1950s for very personal reasons. As a devout Roman Catholic, and brother-in-law to Cardinal Basil Hume, he stifled any progress in this area throughout his time as CMO. Godber also was hesitant on the subject of putting family planning advice into hospitals, but opposed Crossman's proposals for different reasons:

> George Godber was a tremendous problem on this, holding back on it, saying it was terribly difficult and that there would be major trouble. Eventually when Bea Serota [Minister of Health] saw the President of the Royal College of Obstetricians and Gynaecologists, she found that he was urging us to do more. The fact is that George has been unduly sensitive. He regards Family Planning and the pill and all these things as not pukkah doctoring of the sort that the Ministry deals with.[3]

At the other end of the spectrum from the individual interventions of senior civil servants were the Royal Commissions. They became a favourite legitimisation technique used by governments to pursue particular policy agendas. CMOs have been closely involved in many of the health-related ones, either through steering the choice of chairman and members, or through more direct participation. A Royal Commission was often an ideal opportunity to involve senior members of the medical profession in decisions which related to their field of expertise or interest. This is more subtle than outright rigging, but has at times cast Ministers in a less than favourable light.[4]

While Royal Commissions are formed specifically to address timely issues, a further mechanism has been developed to secure external advice for Ministers – advisory committees. These are not only vehicles for professional interests such as salaries and working conditions, but groups of carefully selected senior doctors or scientists who can provide expert advice on their area of specialism. Although an advisory body was initially created to serve the new Ministry of Health in 1919, the function was not fully exploited. A rare example of inter-war expert advisory committees was the Nutrition Committee established in 1931 to analyse nutrition surveys and advise on policies to tackle perceived 'malnutrition' in some parts of Britain.[5] We will return later to the role of advisory committees in the post-war period.

The Ministry of Health and the Medical Research Council

The development of nutrition research and policy in the 1930s illustrates the problems of prioritising research within government, and the tension between

---

[3] Ibid., p. 749. December 1969.

[4] See, for example, Barbara Castle and David Owen's pleasure at appointing Alec Merrison in 1975 as Chair of the Royal Commission on the National Health Service (1976–79), recounted in P Hennessy, *Whitehall* (London, Pimlico, 2001), p. 549. Merrison (1924–1989), who was Vice Chancellor of Bristol University (1969–84) had already chaired the Committee of Inquiry into the Regulation of the Medical Profession, 1972–75.

[5] C Petty, 'Primary research and public health: the prioritisation of nutrition research in inter-war Britain', in J Austoker and L Bryder (eds), *Historical Perspectives on the MRC* (Oxford, Oxford University Press, 1989), pp. 83–108.

the Ministry of Health and the Medical Research Council (MRC). The relationships between Newman, the seventh CMO, and the Secretaries of the MRC, Walter Fletcher and his successor Edward Mellanby, exemplify this. Although a concordat had been agreed between the Ministry and the MRC in 1923, which defined their respective research responsibilities, there was a considerable grey area in the middle.[6] There were problems on both sides. Fletcher was irritated by the refusal of Newman at the Ministry of Health to acknowledge the usefulness of biochemical experiments in determining causes of malnutrition. Thus in 1931 Fletcher wrote to Dawson, an influential health adviser, who had recently become a member of the MRC:

> The medical administrators have delayed inexcusably to use the abundant new knowledge that has been pouring out of the laboratories in the last fifteen years . . . Physiology teaches us that faulty nutrition is far worse for our populations than faulty housing [one of Newman's favoured projects]. We waste millions a year by not using the new knowledge we have.[7]

The relationship was almost completely severed when Newman used his 1931 Annual Report to claim that the diet of the pregnant woman was 'a matter of common sense'. Fletcher's irate reply highlighted the potential damage to future MRC bids for Treasury funding for nutritional research.[8] When Mellanby replaced Fletcher as the MRC's Secretary in 1934, he attempted to use the Ministry's Expert Advisory Committee to refocus attention on the development of nutritional standards and supplements. In fact the membership of the Ministry's panel of experts was almost identical to that on the MRC's Nutrition Committee.[9] For the first time, the political parameters of expert advice were being defined partly by external agencies.

Nutrition was only one area of potential collaboration. Various attempts to improve working relations between the Ministry of Health and the MRC in the period 1920–1939 had been wrecked by similar territorial disputes. A joint Vaccination Committee never really got off the ground: the MRC was criticised for not supporting experimental work on infectious diseases such as diphtheria, whilst the Ministry of Health would not be a conduit to local Medical Officers of Health who had responsibility for vaccination services. Both organisations were castigated for their reluctance to consider merging their respective laboratory services.[10]

There was very little interchange of personnel or ideas until the development of plans in 1938 for a wartime Emergency Public Health Laboratory Service, which was to be jointly managed by the Ministry of Health and the MRC. A further sign

---

[6] L Bryder 'Public health research and the MRC', in Austoker and Bryder (eds), *Historical Perspectives*, pp. 59–81. This is a very good account of the failed experiment of a joint MH/MRC committee on vaccination which was formed in 1926. Bryder also discusses the research output of the Ministry of Health, which included some 90 reports published between 1920 and 1939.

[7] MRC 2100/1. Fletcher to Dawson, 15.04.1931.

[8] MRC 1190. Fletcher to Newman, 22.10.1931.

[9] Petty, *Primary Research*, p. 99.

[10] Ibid.

of improved relations was the formation of a Preventive Committee by the MRC in 1939 with Wilson Jameson as its Chair. His appointment the following year as CMO did go some way to bridging the chasm between these two organisations. Six specialist subcommittees were very quickly formed to deal with mass immunisation against diphtheria, whooping cough vaccination, cross-infection on hospital wards, measles, infant mortality due to enteritis and the control of school infections. All of the resultant policies were later supported by the newly created Emergency Public Health Laboratory Service.[11]

In the post-war period, there was renewed impetus to foster in-house medical research, as well as forging stronger links with external agencies like the MRC. However, by the early 1960s it was increasingly clear that the MRC was firmly fixed on clinical research, and that it gave little priority to social and epidemiological research. Godber sought to remedy this in 1962 when he created a new research organisation for the Department of Health and Social Security (DHSS). He turned to his long-standing associate Dick Cohen (1907–1998), Second Secretary at the MRC, with whom he had had considerable contact through the MRC's Clinical Research Board (on which the CMOs of the Health Departments sat as assessors). Godber invited Cohen to join him at the DHSS as Deputy CMO to lead the new research programme.

Cohen proved enormously influential through his connections with other MRC colleagues, including Archie Cochrane (1909–1988), Director of the MRC's Epidemiology Research Unit. With the approval of Godber as CMO, he supported a range of innovative research projects which exploited expertise in a number of institutions, including Alan Williams' Health Economics Unit at York University and Walter Holland's Social Medicine and Health Services Research Unit at St Thomas's Medical School. Beginning in 1962, Godber managed to secure £5,000 annual funding for Cohen's programme from the 'CMO's Fund'. By 1972–73 Departmental research funding had risen to nearly £3.5 million annually and questions were already being asked about the political role of a government department in health services research. The Rothschild Green Paper had been published in 1971, which was translated into the White Paper, *A Framework for Government Research and Development*, in 1972.[12] An outcome of this analysis was the creation in 1972 of a new committee structure and the post of Chief Scientist, which Cohen held for a year until his retirement, when he was succeeded by Douglas Black (1913–2002). By retaining a research organisation within the Department of Health and Social Security, Godber had succeeded in keeping some control over the prioritisation of projects to address health service and public health research needs.

External influences on policy

In parallel with the development of 'internal' research expertise, and serving a different purpose, the 1946 National Health Service Act rejuvenated the culture of external advice through the creation of nine Standing Medical Advisory Committees. Their remit was to advise Ministers through the Central Health Services Council, but they also had the freedom to investigate and report on other

[11] Bryder, *Public Health Research*, p. 74.

[12] *A Framework for Government Research and Development*, Cmd. 4814 (London, HMSO, 1971); *A Framework for Government Research and Development*, Cmd. 5046 (London, HMSO, 1972).

topics as they deemed appropriate. As with the composition of the Central Health Services Council, there was a delay in agreeing their membership. The CMO (Jameson) was a permanent member of the Medical, Maternity and Midwifery and the Tuberculosis Standing Advisory Committees; the Deputy CMO (Charles) was on the Medical, Ophthalmic and Mental Health Standing Advisory Committees. Interestingly Godber, although a relatively junior member of staff in 1948, was also on the Ophthalmic Standing Advisory Committee.[13]

The Standing Medical Advisory Committees presented their advice directly to the Minister of Health. However, this advice was usually interpreted for the Minister by the CMO. The CMO also had a group of external consultant advisers – one to represent each medical specialty. In 1976, when Yellowlees was CMO, there were 49 advisers; by the time Acheson left office in 1991 this number had increased to over 100, reflecting the proliferation in medical specialties in that short period of time. The consultant advisers held this position over several years, and interacted not only with the CMO but also with the senior policy officials, providing an immediate and reliable source of information on developments within clinical medicine and medical research.

The Nuffield Trust and the King's Fund

Two significant independent organisations have developed as influential 'think-tanks' on health policy: the Nuffield Provincial Hospitals Trust (now the Nuffield Trust) and the King's Fund, which began life as The Prince of Wales' Fund for the Hospitals of London. At various times CMOs have had strong links with both organisations and have used them for independent advice or as a source of ideas on health policy.

The Nuffield Provincial Hospitals Trust was founded by Lord Nuffield, a motor industry magnate, in 1939. Its remit was to facilitate the co-ordination of regional hospital services, which in the pre-NHS period involved a confusing array of municipal, old Poor Law and voluntary hospitals which had no regional logistics. As discussed in Chapter 5, the Trust embarked on a national survey of hospitals with the support of the Minister of Health, Walter Elliot (only the second Minister of Health to be medically qualified). Its report, published in 1941 as *A National Hospital Service*, was well-received by the Ministry of Health, and added pressure to consolidate the initial progress towards a unified hospital service made under the 1929 Local Government Act.[14]

George Godber provides an excellent example of how CMOs have involved such organisations in policy formation 'by stealth'. His suggestion to Gordon MacLachlan, Secretary of the Nuffield Provincial Hospitals Trust, for a series of policy seminars on 'Future Trends in Medicine' resulted in an historic workshop at Christ Church, Oxford in 1957, which paved the way for significant developments, including postgraduate medical education and general practitioner standards.[15]

[13] MH 133/492. Standing Medical Advisory Committee constitution.
[14] Nuffield Provincial Hospitals Trust, *A National Hospital Service: a memorandum on the coordination of hospital service* (Oxford, The Trust, 1941).
[15] See I Craft *et al.* (eds), *Specialised Futures: essays in honour of Sir George Godber* (London, Oxford University Press for the Nuffield Provincial Hospitals Trust, 1975) for a review of some of Godber's policy interests.

This was Godber's preferred *modus operandi* – to listen to young doctors, sow the seeds of ideas with a group of influential people and then to watch them flourish into firm policy proposals later. His advice to a junior civil servant in his department was that you must have 'total willingness to be humble. You can achieve anything in this place if you insist that it is somebody else's idea'.[16]

The King's Fund was founded in 1897 to raise funds for the voluntary (charity) hospitals. Although its initial *raison d'être* was the efficient provision of medical services for London, it later widened its area of interest to include national health services. Jameson was the first CMO to have sustained contact with the King's Fund, and many subsequent CMOs have been members of its General Council. In 1943 Jameson was appointed to a King's Fund Committee on Hospital Diet, chaired by Sir Jack Drummond, Scientific Adviser to the Ministry of Food. He continued to maintain his interest and contact in the Fund, and in 1948 was appointed to the Fund's Management Committee. He was the first serving CMO to have held such a significant post within an independent advisory organisation. After his retirement as CMO in 1950, he resigned from the Management Committee in order to be employed by the Fund as a medical adviser and Chairman of the Managing Committees for the Staff Colleges for Hospital Administration and Ward Sisters, positions he held until 1960.[17]

This employment was a financial necessity for Jameson as much as a welcome opportunity to continue his work; although his salary on retirement had been £3,000, his pension was £500 per annum with a lump sum of £4,828.[18] His post-CMO contribution through the King's Fund was perhaps as important to the development of health policy as his time in Whitehall. To Jameson, it was a pleasanter environment. He had commented to a colleague that 'the atmosphere [at the Ministry] was heavily charged with politics and I could never get accustomed to the annoyances caused me by the obstructive tactics of much of the civil service, not the fault of individuals but rather of the machine'.[19] At the King's Fund Jameson's qualities were fully exploited and he was valued for his insight into Whitehall and for his sound judgement.[20]

George Godber also saw the value of the King's Fund both to him as CMO and to the wider formation of health policy. He used the Fund extensively as a sounding board and to further specific research interests. He was appointed to the Fund's General Council in 1961, the year after he became CMO, and was enthusiastic about the creation of a 'hospital centre' at the Fund which would

[16] Senior medical civil servant interview, 28.08.2002.
[17] F Prochaska, *Philanthropy and the Hospitals of London: The King's Fund, 1897–1990* (Oxford, Clarendon Press, 1992), pp. 144, 187, 199. Four Staff Colleges had been formed by the King's Fund: for Ward Sisters (1949), for Matrons (1953), for Hospital Administrators (1951) and a School for Hospital Caterers (1951). Jameson also gave lectures on public health and the NHS.
[18] N Goodman, *Wilson Jameson, Architect of National Health* (London, George Allen and Unwin, 1970), p. 149.
[19] Ibid., pp. 148–66.
[20] Goodman's biography includes some rather odd information on Jameson's personality which must be taken with a pinch of salt, but, if true, illustrates how attitudes to support staff have changed since the 1950s. It is claimed that he kept a bottle of nail varnish remover and cotton wool in his desk drawer in case any secretary dared to wear red nail varnish in his presence.

analyse the operations of the NHS. He also persuaded the Fund to provide training courses for Ministry and NHS staff from 1960. Most significant were the management courses for doctors in 1964, which 'was a notable departure, for it brought together consultants and senior administrators in a neutral setting'.[21]

The King's Fund was, however, more than just a 'think-tank'. Through its Emergency Beds Service it provided a clearing-house for admissions to London hospitals, which Godber, who became the chair of the Emergency Beds Service Committee in 1972, described as 'a barometer of the health of London'. Godber, like Jameson, enjoyed close relations with the King's Fund even after his retirement. In 1976 he served (with Sir Francis Avery Jones and Professor Ian McColl) on a Fund subcommittee, which submitted evidence to the Royal Commission on the Health Service. Its critical stance on the NHS's administrative complexity, poor industrial relations and 'infusion of party political dogma' was seen by many in the medical profession and Whitehall as Godber's personal comment on the service he had helped to found. He was later instrumental in the establishment of the King's Fund Institute in 1986, having visited the American Institute of Medicine which had greatly impressed him.[22]

Standing Medical Advisory Committees, think-tanks and external consultant advisers are, however, only as good as the system within which they operate. The CMO's role in ensuring their continued co-operation and goodwill, for what is an unpaid and sometimes onerous duty, has been critical. It required the CMO to remain abreast of significant developments across the spectrum of medical and scientific specialties, and to have a personal and effective network of contacts to be called upon at short notice. Two of the best recent examples of how the CMO had exploited this resource are AIDS and BSE.

AIDS: a plague for the twentieth century

Acquired immune deficiency syndrome – AIDS – generated public and governmental fear in Britain in the 1980s. It was initially identified among gay communities in the United States, appearing as a mix of symptoms which were subsequently understood as resulting from infection with the human immunodeficiency virus (HIV). As the number of cases increased, historical parallels were sought, most usually with other socially stigmatised diseases such as syphilis. But this 'new' disease also generated some refreshing commentary on the wider perspectives of health and medicine.[23] It required an integration of previously discrete biomedical and cultural models of transmission, variously incorporating epidemiology, screening and education programmes. In the process, AIDS exposed the tensions between 'expertise' and the integration of pressure groups into the policy-making process.

Although significant numbers of HIV cases were seen in the USA, the disease was initially well-contained in Britain, mainly due to the pre-emptive planning of the Conservative Government. This history concentrates on events in Britain at

[21] Prochaska, *Philanthropy*, p. 212.

[22] G Godber, 'Does Britain need an Academy of Medicine?' *Times Health Supplement*, 19.02.1982, p. 9; *British Medical Journal*, 1979, (II), 1611.

[23] E Fee and D Fox (eds), *AIDS: the burdens of history* (Berkeley, University of California Press, 1988).

the time that AIDS first emerged and not with the subsequent and devastating impact of the disease globally and in Africa in particular. As with the nineteenth century epidemics of cholera, initially the resultant public fear was almost as bad as the disease itself. The public response precipitated the development of a hard-hitting health education campaign, and, as with sexually transmitted diseases in the Second World War, brought the CMO into the media spotlight.

It has been claimed that AIDS was seen primarily as a public health issue in the UK because of the leading role played by the Chief Medical Officer.[24] This suggests a far greater degree of authority for the post than perhaps even its recent holders would assert. Yet it is clear that the American and British responses to the epidemic were markedly different, to a degree which cannot be explained by their historically divergent healthcare systems, or the fact that such public health issues in the USA are handled at the state rather than the national level. The AIDS epidemic in Britain provided a rare opportunity to engage in a debate on exactly what public health means to government and the public at the end of the twentieth century, and one positive outcome was a reaffirmation of the import-ance of the CMO post.

AIDS also exposed some of the weaknesses of an uncritical engagement with history. Much analysis of the recent past has been in what could be broadly termed 'heroes and villains' style. A common theme of the narratives of AIDS has been of delays to policy caused by homophobic politicians and civil servants. This perspective is exacerbated when the leading actors attempt to tell the story 'their way'. Norman Fowler, Secretary of State for Health and Social Services between 1981 and 1987, devoted a chapter of his memoirs to AIDS, predictably per-sonalising the progression of a health education campaign from his first govern-ment AIDS press briefing on the steps of 10 Downing Street on 11 November 1986.[25]

Fowler's history of AIDS is invariably Whiggish, moving smoothly from recognition of the problem in Britain and establishment of a government Cabinet Committee, to his fact-finding trips in 1987 to the USA and Europe. His auto-biographical positioning of himself ('I had the time to devote to the issue which no new Secretary of State could have managed. A crisis of this kind justifies long-serving ministers.') does not do justice to the practical realities of managing this new health threat. In this 'history', Acheson, Fowler's CMO, is relegated to the position of passive supplier of statistics. Yet without the expert briefings of Department of Health and Social Security officials, there would have been little impetus at the Ministerial level to target AIDS. The Prime Minister, Margaret Thatcher, was not moved to action (and expenditure) unless a watertight case could be made. It is testimony to the persuasive powers of Acheson as the Government's chief health adviser that she authorised the establishment of a Cabinet Committee under the chairmanship of the Deputy Prime Minister, William Whitelaw.

---

[24] J Lewis, 'Public health doctors and AIDS as a public health issue', in V Berridge and P Strong (eds), *AIDS and Contemporary History* (Cambridge, Cambridge University Press, 1993), pp. 37–54; V Berridge, 'History in public health; who needs it?', *Lancet*, 2000, 356, 1923–5.

[25] N Fowler, *Ministers Decide: a personal memoir of the Thatcher years* (London, Chapmans, 1991).

When Fowler made his explicit press statement in November 1986, there were already over 500 cases of AIDS in Britain, and an estimated 25,000 people who were HIV positive. With no effective treatment nor any prospect of a vaccine, the British authorities had decided that a frank health education campaign was required to alert the public about how the disease was transmitted. The opposite approach was taken by the American administration under President Ronald Reagan, which maintained a stoical silence in the face of high prevalence rates in the traditionally gay communities of California and drug-using neighbourhoods of New York City. The 'gay' element to the disease has usually been interpreted as a handicap to the development of an effective AIDS policy, allowing various authorities to justify their narrow interpretation of risk and moral blame. In the UK, churches refused to support a health education campaign which seemed to condone sexual promiscuity. The government's response was to use a leaflet, poster and television campaign to explode the myths on how the disease was transmitted. The leaflet, entitled '*AIDS – don't die of ignorance*', was delivered to over 23 million homes. It was stark in its warning:

> Any man or woman can get the AIDS virus depending on their behaviour. It is not just a homosexual disease. There is no cure. And it kills . . . Because the virus can be present in semen and vaginal fluid, this means for most people the only real danger comes through having sexual intercourse with an infected person. This means vaginal or anal sex. (It could also be that oral sex can be risky, particularly if semen is taken into the mouth.) So the virus can be passed from man to man, man to woman and woman to man.

The television campaign, which variously featured a tombstone and an iceberg, was one of the most memorable ever mounted. The government also considered (but rejected) a Ministerial broadcast – an unprecedented step which not even the recent Falklands War had merited. Follow-up polling showed impressive and immediate results: by February 1987, 98 per cent of the public were aware that AIDS could be transmitted by sexual intercourse and needle sharing. The television campaign had been seen by 95 per cent of the British population. Fowler was keen to push home this intensive media onslaught and persuaded the authorities at the British Broadcasting Corporation (BBC) and the Independent Broadcasting Authority to integrate AIDS themes into programming, including influential 'soap opera' storylines.

In parallel with the awareness-raising campaigns came detailed policy initiatives on how accurately to track the disease in the population and how to reduce transmission. Harm minimisation rather than prohibition was the underlying 'liberal consensus' response to the crisis.[26] The Cabinet Committee quickly dismissed the suggestion that compulsory testing for AIDS should be introduced. Instead innovative pilot schemes such as needle exchanges for drug users were developed, inspired by similar schemes which had been established in Amsterdam and Berlin. Safe sex rather than no sex was the message of the day.

How then did the CMO fit into this Ministerial decision-making machine? Well before Fowler made his Downing Street press statement in November 1986, the

[26] V Berridge, *AIDS in the UK: the making of policy, 1981–1994* (Oxford, Oxford University Press, 1996), p. 7.

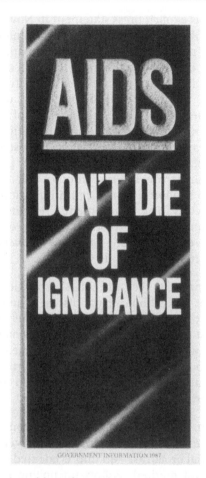

Figure 6.1 Department of Health and Social Security AIDS leaflet, 1987. © Wellcome Library. Reproduced with permission.

Department of Health and Social Security had become aware of the new disease, its progress in the USA and its arrival in the UK. An Expert Advisory Group on AIDS (EAGA) was selected and initially chaired by Acheson in January 1985. Yet, as Virginia Berridge has noted, AIDS was a blank sheet. There was no pre-existing policy or pressure groups. Although gay groups had the initial advantage, they soon appeared marginalised by the government, whilst at the same time the politicians themselves were constantly outmanoeuvred by the civil servants by virtue of the novelty of the disease and the potential for political embarrassment.[27]

In this novel scenario, Acheson became the intermediary. His liaison between the medical profession (who provided the expertise) and the gay groups (who initially provided the majority of the patients) was a powerful riposte to Ministerial authority. It further illustrated the resurgence of the specialty of public health medicine and its essential skills of epidemiology and health education. Acheson had witnessed the emasculation of public health at community level since the abolition of the post of Medical Officer of Health in 1974. The

[27] Ibid, p. 8.

restyled specialty of 'community medicine' lacked leadership and a positive image within the medical profession and suffered from chronic vacancy and career structure problems. Acheson saw part of his CMO role as to reinvigorate the specialty. From 1985 he chaired a committee to investigate the public health function. AIDS provided an opportune moment to return to the older, more trusted nomenclature of 'public health medicine'. The committee report, published in 1988, at the height of public and government attention on AIDS, recommended a rejuvenation of epidemiological expertise and improved career prospects for public health practitioners. It could not have been better for the profession or the disease.

Acheson 'ate and slept AIDS from 1985 onwards'.[28] His skills first and foremost as an epidemiologist made him acutely aware that the cases which had presented in Britain at this stage might well be the tip of a much bigger iceberg. His passionate conviction that this epidemic must be quashed before it could take hold was one of his main strengths in persuading the government and his colleagues to take the disease seriously. This testimony from a Department of Health colleague encapsulates his single-minded commitment:

> It was very, very exciting – to be involved at a high level on a new disease which the CMO regarded as important . . . Donald was difficult, he wanted instant answers from civil service doctors and didn't use the Communicable Disease Surveillance Centre in the way he used us. At the time he was a tartar . . . to expect an erudite article on his desk in half an hour because of a *Sun* article! . . . He would ring up and say he was still at the Medical Research Council and would be back in an hour. This was at 6.30 p.m.! He had a flat near the Department of Health and would hold meetings at 8 p.m. He used to go home on Friday evening for the weekend . . . we all breathed a sigh of relief![29]

Other senior civil service colleagues and journalists interviewed by Berridge for her analysis of the formation of British AIDS policy put a different spin on Acheson's enthusiasm. Some saw it as a 'godsend' for him, a public health project that he 'had been given to play with' and which he naturally found more stimulating than some of the routine NHS management issues.[30] Another senior medical civil servant commented in an interview for this book that Acheson 'did a Senior Medical Officer's job four rungs down the ladder better than anyone else could have done it, but he didn't do his own job. Staff meetings were totally dominated by AIDS debates'.[31]

Shortly after he became CMO in 1983 Acheson invited representatives from the main gay pressure groups, including the Terrence Higgins Trust, to join an informal alliance. He was then able to steer some Departmental funding into gay health services support. This did not endear him to DHSS senior officials, who felt that he had perhaps placed himself in a compromised position:

> He took on the chair of the Expert Advisory Group on AIDS, it was a heavy burden . . . and he was also chairing the Public Health

[28] Ibid, p. 68.
[29] Medical civil servant interview, recounted in Berridge, *AIDS in the UK*, p. 68.
[30] Ibid., p. 69.
[31] Senior medical civil servant interview, 28.08.2002.

Committee at the same time, so he was under strain . . . It over-
burdened him and put him in an awkward position. The Advisory
Group was hijacked by a homosexual group among the doctors . . .
There was a danger of lobbies . . . Acheson was about to meet the
English Collective of Prostitutes![32]

With the formation of the Expert Advisory Group on AIDS in 1985, Acheson
called upon a long-standing mechanism for influencing policy formation. Expert
advisory groups, composed of medical and scientific experts, had long been used
by the CMO to gather advice from which ministers could develop policy. In a new
policy area such as AIDS, independent expert advice became an essential tool
through which politically sensitive recommendations could be 'repackaged' with
the badge of scientific authority and integrity. Thus the initial membership of the
Expert Advisory Group on AIDS, when it was chaired by the Deputy CMO Dr
Michael Abrams, was heavily weighted with haematologists and health service
advisers. There was no representation at first from the gay community. The
formative early years of the Expert Advisory Group on AIDS saw the development of a liberal policy response, which drew substantially on the historical
context of past sexually transmitted disease policies. It also reflected the inherent
professional medical policy values of the confidentiality of doctor–patient relationships, opposition to routine testing and compulsory notification.[33] In this
period, up to the awakening of significant political interest in late 1986, the expert
advisers set the course for the ethos of subsequent policy direction.

Acheson was again instrumental in the escalation of AIDS policy from an
internal Department of Health and Social Security project into a governmental
concern. Throughout the first year of the Expert Advisory Group on AIDS
existence, he pushed for Ministerial involvement. He prepared a briefing paper
for Kenneth Clarke, the then Secretary of State for Health, who delegated the new
Minister for Health, Barney Hayhoe, to attend a meeting of the Expert Advisory
Group on AIDS in October 1985. A direct outcome from this was the formation of
an inter-Ministerial steering group for AIDS in December 1985, through which
Acheson could co-ordinate policy development in appropriate government
departments. When government money became available on a useful scale at
the end of 1985 (£6.3m AIDS package; £2.5m for the national health education
campaign), Acheson was in a pivotal position in prioritising the various services,
including a Department of Health and Social Security AIDS Unit with a telephone
helpline for professionals, and funding for the Public Health Laboratory Service
and regional health authorities to provide screening and counselling services.

It was, however, the health education campaign which best highlighted the
role of the CMO as policy broker. The huge budget meant that a substantial,
sustained campaign could be mounted, which the public would not be able to
avoid. Its accuracy and direction therefore became a critical issue. Despite his
personal sensibilities, Acheson's professional approach to the issue meant that he
immersed himself in briefings on gay sexual habits. He was unsure about the
strategy of explicit advertising, and preferred euphemisms such as 'back passage'
to anal or rectal sex. Yet it was his name and his professional authority which

[32] Senior civil servant interview, recounted in Berridge, *AIDS in the UK*, p. 69.
[33] D Porter and R Porter, 'The enforcement of health: the British debate', in E Fee and D Fox
(eds), *AIDS: the burdens of history* (Berkeley, California University Press, 1988), pp. 97–120.

were used to front the first advertisement which appeared in the press on 16 March 1986, along with his three other UK CMO colleagues. The adverts were subsequently criticised for their vagueness: although safe sex was advocated, the public appeared unsure exactly what this meant. Under pressure from the Health Education Advisory Group, subsequent media campaigns had to be more blatant.

Virginia Berridge sees the AIDS crisis of the late 1980s as a prime example of the 'durability of post-war policy traditions and the power of civil servants to define issues to politicians'.[34] Within this group of civil servants and politicians, Acheson was supreme, shaping expert scientific and media advice in a fluid policy environment, fully supported by the Permanent Secretary, Sir Kenneth Stowe, who was enormously influential throughout Whitehall and Westminster. Stowe, using a Foreign Office document which highlighted the potential scale of the imminent epidemic in Africa, had been instrumental in persuading the Prime Minister to authorise the creation of the Cabinet Committee on AIDS. With this high-level attention, Acheson's role as expert 'gatekeeper' became even more significant.

The dilemma for the Cabinet Committee, which held its first meeting on 11 November 1986 (and met six more times before Christmas), was how to resource and steer AIDS policy without being seen to become too 'hands on'. Although Fowler took a lot of the media attention for his personal AIDS crusade, in reality the detailed development of policy remained in the hands of the civil servants, who were free to pursue a liberal agenda which might have seemed to some to be at odds with the traditional conservative ethos of the then Conservative government. The urgency with which the media and the church approached the subject also put the government under pressure. This facilitated a move to a national rather than party political approach following the House of Commons debate on AIDS on 21 November 1986. The subsequent £20m advertising campaign, including the leaflet drop to 23 million households, refocused attention away from a predominantly gay risk to a health problem for the British population as a whole.

Acheson had obtained Fowler's agreement for this leafleting before the Cabinet Committee had been formed, and because it had already been made public through a newspaper, the government could not renege on its commitment. Thereafter, the AIDS media campaign was to be co-ordinated at arm's length by the government through the new Health Education Authority, which replaced the former Health Education Council. Acheson worked closely with Fowler and a small group of civil servants to brief the TWBA advertising agency on the message to be put across. Throughout the development of the campaign he was cautious in balancing correct information to avoid causing public panic. There were some lighter moments, such as Fowler's reported 'Crikey' when the finer details of oral sex were explained to him, and Acheson's £5 bet with the advertising guru Sami Harari that the word 'condom' would not make it onto television.[35]

The peak of the campaign, an AIDS Week on television in February 1987, owed much to Acheson's vision of broadening the focus away from the initial gay target group. The television week incorporated 19 hours of public service broadcasting across all the four television channels – a blitzkrieg approach, to use a militaristic

[34] Berridge, *AIDS in the UK*, p. 102.
[35] Ibid., p. 112.

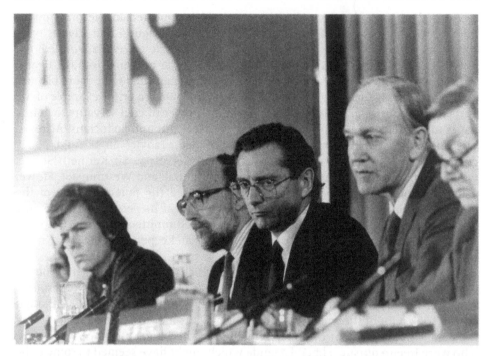

Figure 6.2 An AIDS press conference. From left: Romola Christopherson, Sir Donald Acheson, Norman Fowler, Sir James Gowans and Professor Sir Patrick Forrest. © Topfoto. Reproduced with permission.

metaphor in the spirit of this perceived 'war'. Acheson was also very much aware of the AIDS risk for intravenous drug users. He had visited pioneering needle exchanges in Amsterdam and Berlin, and was also receiving informal briefings from pilot schemes that had quietly been established in some British cities. In 1987 he spearheaded a government policy which combined needle exchanges with youth radio campaigns such as Radio One's *Drug Alert*.[36] Again, his medical authority was critical in obtaining government approval for what was in effect a scheme which condoned illegal drug use.

Yet the continuing uncertainty over the transmission mechanisms for HIV caused ongoing concerns for Acheson. Even the medical profession managed to cause public panic over the safety of blood transfusions, when in January 1987, Dr John Dawson, head of the British Medical Association's professional division, advised that anyone who had had more than one sexual partner in the last four years should not donate blood. The effect on blood donations was instantaneous, and Acheson insisted that a joint British Medical Association and Department of Health and Social Security damage-limitation statement be issued. Later that year, the British Medical Association again angered pressure groups and the government when a conference debate surprisingly upheld the motion that it was acceptable for doctors to perform tests for AIDS without the knowledge or

[36] One of the regional pioneers of needle exchanges, who had briefed Acheson on their success, was piqued to find his ideas passed off by Acheson as his own. Senior medical civil servant interview, 10.03.2000.

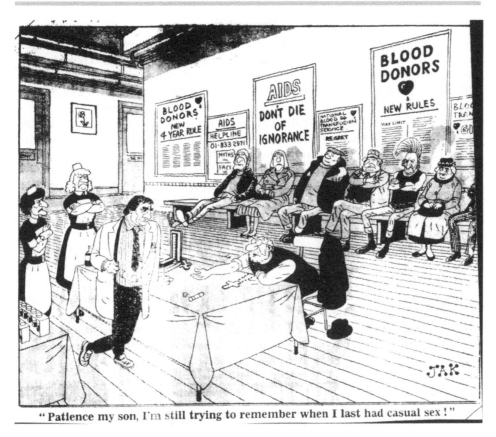

"Patience my son, I'm still **trying** to remember when I last had casual sex!"

Figure 6.3 *Evening Standard*, 7th January 1987. Cartoon by Jak [Raymond Jackson] on the new four-year rule for blood donors. © Solo Syndication. Reproduced with permission.

consent of the patient. Although the British Medical Association retreated from this controversial position at its annual meeting in 1989, serious damage had been done to the increasingly precarious bond between doctor and patient.[37] It was precisely this sort of scaremongering that Acheson sought to avoid, for fear that any element of compulsion in testing would drive the problem underground.

The issue of anonymous screening was one of the few areas in which Acheson's epidemiologically based proposals did not immediately find success. The parliamentary Social Services Select Committee had decided to conduct an investigation into AIDS early in 1987. Its final report was broadly supportive of government policies on AIDS developed so far, but it differed on this crucial issue. Although the Public Health Laboratory Service had engaged in limited anonymous screening of blood in the early years of the AIDS crisis to determine the extent of the infection in the population, it had halted the programme in 1985. There was no consensus within the medical profession on the ethical issues around such testing, but strong claims had been made for its usefulness by such eminent epidemiologists as Sir Richard Doll. Acheson had also tentatively floated the proposal with the Social

[37] Porter and Porter, 'The enforcement of health', p. 115.

Services Select Committee in February 1987, but faced strong opposition for jeopardising public trust in medical confidentiality.[38] It was not until AIDS became 'normalised' as a disease that the issue of anonymous screening as a methodology to track the progress of the 'epidemic' was finally accepted in 1989. This coincided with, and perhaps reflected, the downgrading of AIDS as a political issue since the Cabinet Committee was disbanded in the same year.

Alongside the heightened health education campaign, there was also consider-able investment in research into the disease with the aim of developing a vaccine and a cure. Although Acheson had been accused of bias in favouring early AIDS funding for epidemiology rather than biomedical research, the MRC's subsequent large-scale investment in an AIDS-directed programme in 1987 was beyond his control. Criticism of the MRC's own prioritisation of vaccine development over treatment research attracted its own long-standing criticism from clinicians and gay groups alike.[39]

Acheson's role on the issue within the World Health Organization was also crucial for the development of domestic policy. He acted as a broker in the development of international guidelines on infected healthcare workers, using his position on the Executive Board of the World Health Organization and as a delegate to the World Health Assembly. As the timetable of international AIDS meetings and conferences filled up in the mid-1980s, it was Acheson who ensured that the dominant ideology remained the British liberal consensus approach.[40] It was Acheson again who served as co-chair of the steering committee for the World Summit of Ministers of Health on Programmes for AIDS Prevention, which was held in London in January 1988, drawing together delegates from 148 countries, three-quarters of them government Ministers. This produced the London Declaration on AIDS Prevention, which reflected Acheson's guiding hand in its targets of education, free exchange of information and the need to protect human rights and dignity.[41]

By early 1988 the structure and function of the Expert Advisory Group on AIDS had been considerably altered. From the original small tight-knit team in which the majority of AIDS policy was made 'on the hoof' with Acheson's constant presence, it had matured into a central committee with a flexible number of specialist subcommittees in which external experts were now outnumbered by civil servants. Although Acheson had initially chaired the Expert Advisory Group on AIDS, it was Hilary Pickles, the Medical Head of the Department of Health and Social Security's AIDS Unit, who in later years acted as the main filter between the Expert Advisory Group on AIDS subcommittees and the CMO. Also, the Expert Advisory Group on AIDS soon found that it was no longer the sole governmental advisory committee on the subject: others were developed to tackle related issues such as AIDS and the NHS.

While removing himself from the front line, Acheson was maintaining close control over all AIDS-related policy developments. For example, some members of the Expert Advisory Group on AIDS Monitoring and Surveillance Subcommittee (established in April 1987) were convinced that the CMO was being shown drafts of

[38] Berridge, *Aids in the UK*, p. 149.
[39] Ibid., pp. 117–19.
[40] Senior medical civil servant interview, 10.03.2000.
[41] Berridge, *Aids in the UK*, p. 163.

their reports before they came back to the Committee. He was also influential in persuading the Royal College of Midwives to delay their public criticism of antenatal screening until after the politicians had had a chance to debate all the findings of the Subcommittee. The breakthrough which Acheson had been delicately engineering came with Ken Clarke's decisive support for anonymous testing shortly after he took up his post as Secretary of State for Health in 1988.

By the time that Acheson retired in October 1991, AIDS had already passed through several distinct phases, from the initial shock threat of an epidemic to the managed culture of a chronic condition (although not of course in the global context). It was consciously re-evaluated by the incoming CMO, Kenneth Calman, who decided not to follow Acheson's example of chairing the Expert Advisory Group on AIDS himself, but to delegate initially to the Deputy CMO, Michael Abrams, and then from 1992 to the other Deputy CMO, Jeremy Metters.

In the following year, 1993, the special Department of Health and Social Security AIDS Unit was merged into a general Communicable Disease Unit. This structural 'downgrading' was emphasised by emerging statistics which indicated that AIDS was then not likely to reach epidemic proportions in Britain. Indeed, the 'failure' to observe the predicted cases at the time caused difficulties in maintaining the impetus for the heterosexual health education campaign. The Chief Medical Officer's Annual Report for 1990 was criticised for the way in which it attributed the rise in heterosexual cases to the sexual activity of British people while abroad. It did not clearly state that the heterosexual AIDS cases which were now being seen in Britain were almost all among recently arrived African immigrants.[42]

In an era of continual personnel 'flux' in Whitehall it is interesting to speculate how much the AIDS epidemic in Britain was shaped by the personality, outlook and professional interest of the CMO, Donald Acheson. How differently would the emerging problem have been handled if the disease had appeared as a significant health threat a few years earlier, when Henry Yellowlees was CMO? The personality factor is significant, and also becomes apparent when one examines the impact of the switch to the more assertive Ministerial team of Virginia Bottomley as Secretary of State for Health with Brian Mawhinney and Tim Yeo as junior Ministers in April 1992. Although they pursued harder lines on drugs policies, relations were not so close with the Health Education Council, and civil servants feared that many of Acheson's carefully won media battles of the late 1980s would be undone.

There is a vast amount of literature now available on how AIDS can be used as a metaphor for the condition of society and civil liberties at the end of the twentieth century.[43] The disease has also been used as a lens through which the redefinition of the discipline of public health can be scrutinised. Yet this brief analysis, by shifting the focus onto the CMO, has also illustrated the vulnerability of policy making to personal and professional enthusiasms.

What is clear is the pivotal position of the CMO as intermediary between government, the public and experts. Acheson continually refined this role through his experience of managing the AIDS crisis. His leadership and scientific credibility proved to be vital in a number of significant areas, including his selection of members for the Expert Advisory Group on AIDS, the success of the

[42] Ibid., p. 248.
[43] E Fee and D Fox (eds), *AIDS: the burdens of history* (Berkeley, University of California Press, 1988).

'open door' approach to the gay community in the early years, the development of a liberal 'harm minimisation' policy as well as the subsequent refinement towards a more epidemiologically founded strategy of disease surveillance. Acheson was at the heart of the process of defining risk (groups and/or behaviours) and in the translation of political concerns into scientifically neutral policy, fronted by experts. Even after AIDS policies became embedded into mainstream governmental structures, Acheson was able to influence their development through his wide network of contacts. The CMO's function within other government departments such as the Home Office, the Foreign Office and Education reinforced the centrality of this position. Acheson's very personal commitment to the AIDS cause undoubtedly was fundamental to the successful avoidance of a larger-scale British epidemic.

The BSE crisis

A decade after AIDS received attention in Britain, the recognition of a new human disease, variant Creutzfeldt–Jakob disease (vCJD), in the spring of 1996 plunged the country and the CMO into a new public health crisis. Although the peak of this crisis may not yet be as clear as that for AIDS in Britain, the episode provides an essential component of our portrait of the overloaded role of the CMO at the end of the twentieth century. Crises do not wait their turn until others have moved off the agenda: one of the essential skills of the CMO is the ability to juggle an unpredictable workload, to be able to spot a crisis in the making and to solicit expertise accordingly. This has been a repeated pressure which has engaged all CMOs from John Simon onwards – from the coincidence of cholera threats and smallpox vaccination scares for Richard Thorne Thorne in the 1890s, to the management of an Emergency Medical Service and rising rates of sexually transmitted diseases during the Second World War for Wilson Jameson. Very few CMOs have had a quiet ride.

Although cattle were probably infected by bovine spongiform encephalopathy (BSE) as early as the 1970s, the long incubation period meant that this new disease with its alarming symptoms did not receive government attention until the Central Veterinary Laboratory investigated the death of a cow in September 1985. By the end of 1987 the Ministry of Agriculture, Fisheries and Food officials had become concerned at the increasing number of cases and questioned whether it was acceptable for cattle showing signs of 'mad cow disease' to be slaughtered for human consumption. Because of the similarity of BSE to scrapie, a disease found in sheep, the accepted wisdom throughout the early years was that this was an animal disease, which posed no threat to human health. This was the context within which one of the most potentially serious public health crises of recent years began.

On 20 March 1996, the government confirmed the public's fear – that BSE might be passed on to humans in the form of the new disease, new variant Creutzfeldt–Jakob disease (nvCJD).[44] The seriousness of this issue demanded an official inquiry, which was initiated in 1998 under the chairmanship of Sir Nicholas Phillips (later Lord Phillips of Worth Matravers). By the time the inquiry report was published in

[44] The scientific evidence for this link was not published until 6 April: RG Will, JW Ironside, M Zeilder et. al., 'A new variant of Creutzfeldt–Jakob disease in the UK', *Lancet*, 1996, 347, 921–5.

November 2000, it was estimated that over 80 people, mainly young, had died or were dying from the human form of BSE.[45] It is too early to attempt to write a definitive history of the BSE crisis, but the episode is a very useful illustration of the role of the CMO in assembling and communicating policy advice and how it is used by the government. It also elaborates on issues touched on elsewhere in this study, especially the heavy workload borne by the CMO, and the impact of the cuts made to departmental staff and resources in the 1980s and 1990s.

Acheson was first advised of the BSE cases through a letter from the Ministry of Agriculture, Fisheries and Food Permanent Secretary, Sir Derek Andrews, on 3 March 1988, several months after the disease had been recognised as a potentially serious problem. The letter, requesting the CMO's advice, had been sent after discussion with John MacGregor, the Minister for Agriculture, Fisheries and Food, who for economic reasons was keen to avoid a compulsory slaughter and compensation scheme for diseased cattle.

Acheson's witness statement to the later inquiry makes clear his considerable duties at this time. He was CMO not only to the Department of Health and Social Security (from 1988 the Department of Health), but also to other government departments including the Ministry of Agriculture, Fisheries and Food. As a grade 1 civil servant he also had the right to attend the weekly meeting of Permanent Secretaries, which he used to ensure the co-ordination of health issues throughout Whitehall. The late 1980s also witnessed a number of significant initiatives which he as CMO was closely involved with, including the continuing AIDS campaign, the National Health Service review (which had been announced apparently without the Department of Health and Social Security's prior knowledge by Prime Minister Margaret Thatcher in January 1988), breast cancer screening, and food safety issues.

A report on the review of the Senior Open Structure of the Department of Health and Social Security in 1986, colloquially known after its chairman as the Moseley Report, had commented on the heavy workload of Acheson as CMO: 'The sheer scale of personal responsibility seemed to us to have dimensions which distinguish it even from some of the highest posts of all within Whitehall.'[46] As discussed in Chapter 4, this opinion was confirmed in the 1988 review of the Deputy Chief Medical Officer posts in the Department of Health and Social Security by Patrick Benner and Malcolm Godfrey. They stated that it was 'a matter of urgency and importance that some means should be found of reducing the burden, not merely for the sake of the post-holder [Acheson] but also because it must be dangerous, and therefore against the public interest that the crucially important, sensitive and high-profile functions of the post should have to be performed against a background of such an unremitting degree of overload'.[47]

The Philips Inquiry Report acknowledged that Acheson had been placed in a difficult position in March 1988 by the Ministry of Agriculture, Fisheries and Food's request for a prompt decision on the risk to humans from BSE. His

[45] The full BSE report, including witness statements and transcripts of oral hearings, can be found at www.bse.org.uk. See also TH Pennington, *When Food Kills* (Oxford, Oxford University Press, 2003).

[46] *Report on the Review of the Senior Open Structure, DHSS* (Moseley Report) (April 1986), pp. 29–31.

[47] *Review of the Deputy Chief Medical Officer (DCMO) Posts in DHSS* (August 1988), report by Mr Patrick Benner and Dr Malcolm Godfrey, p. 4.

immediate response was personally to call and chair two interdepartmental meetings on BSE within 25 working days of being informed of the situation by the Ministry. By Whitehall standards this represents an extraordinarily short response time and demonstrates how seriously Acheson perceived the situation, and how he exploited his authority as CMO to convene high-level meetings. He also used the regular Wednesday morning meeting held by the Cabinet Secretary to make a statement about the outbreak of the BSE epidemic to all his Permanent Secretary colleagues, including those from the Welsh and Scottish Offices.

At quickly convened interdepartmental meetings, Acheson brought together the relevant internal advisers: Ed Harris, Deputy CMO with responsibility for advice on microbiological and scientific issues; Spence Galbraith, Director of the Communicable Disease Surveillance Centre; Joan Davies, Deputy Director of the Public Health Laboratory Service; Sylvia Gardner, the virologist at the Public Health Laboratory Service with the relevant interest; Bill Watson, Director of the Central Veterinary Laboratory; and Alistair Cruickshank, Ministry of Agriculture, Fisheries and Food Under-Secretary dealing with policy issues related to food safety. Together they considered three options: (a) that the threat was sufficient to require immediate action (i.e. banning consumption of cattle products); (b) that an expert group should be formed to consider what action should be taken; and (c) that no action need be taken to protect human health. The unanimous view of the meeting was that Acheson should adopt option (b), and that no immediate action was needed.

On 21 March 1988 Acheson briefed John Moore, Secretary of State at the Department of Health and Social Security that this new disease might hold serious implications for human health, and Moore agreed to his recommendation for the formation of an expert advisory group. This was the only possible course of action – the Treasury would not countenance option (a) without independent expert advice, but Acheson had a duty as CMO to advise his Minister on action that would not leave him vulnerable to criticism of inaction from either the public or Parliament. As CMO, Acheson himself had few statutory powers, except for certain duties in respect of diseases such as smallpox, plague and cholera. As Acheson recorded:

> The limitations of my powers had already been demonstrated to me earlier in 1988 when a very large outbreak of paratyphoid fever occurred in Birmingham following a meal consumed in a disused factory at celebrations of the fortieth anniversary of the independence of India. I tried to insist that the officers of the Birmingham Local Authority should call on the expertise of the PHLS [Public Health Laboratory Service] and its Communicable Disease Surveillance Centre to assist them. They declined to seek help. I was advised by the then Permanent Secretary, Sir Kenneth Stowe, that the CMO had no powers to overrule officers of a local authority.[48]

Acheson did not choose to delegate this, initially veterinary, problem to his Deputy CMO, Ed Harris, which he could easily have done. Despite the Moseley and Benner–Godfrey Reviews on staffing within the Department, Acheson had been relieved of virtually none of his workload. In fact, as part of the Whitehall-wide target to reduce staff, he had lost a considerable number of medical staff, including a

---

[48] BSE Inquiry, witness statement of Sir Donald Acheson. No.251A, p. 19.

reduction of Deputy CMOs from three to two. The ongoing Whitehall reviews meant that Acheson estimated he was spending '20 to 25 per cent of my work defending my people from further cuts throughout my years in office . . . it was incessant'.[49] Yet he judged that this new disease was an issue which required the direct input of the CMO's time and authority to ensure its proper progression. It also represented a personal interest for him as an epidemiologist, as evidenced by the inclusion of a discussion on CJD in his Annual Report as CMO in 1985.[50]

Instead of advising an immediate ban on consumption of diseased cattle, Acheson convened an expert working party. This reflected long-standing good practice for CMOs when faced with a new health risk, of which they had insufficient personal knowledge. He therefore advised the Department of Health and Social Security and the Ministry of Agriculture, Fisheries and Food on the appropriate composition for an expert working party to examine the implications of BSE 'in relation both to animal health and any possible human health implications'. There was very little reliable scientific research into transmissible spongiform encephalopathies, of which the bovine form is just one type. The long incubation periods (around five years in cattle, one to three years in laboratory mice) meant that there was a strong possibility that an epidemic was already well-established when the first cases presented in 1985–86.[51] In identifying appropriate members for an expert team, Acheson had little room for manoeuvre.

In 1998 Acheson supplied to the BSE Inquiry a list of 31 committees and nine series of regular meetings which were operational between 1988 and 1991, providing a classic illustration of how the CMO solicits advice from the medical and scientific community.[52] Some of these were well-established 'standing committees', originating in the 1946 National Health Service Act; others, such as the Expert Advisory Group on AIDS, had been formed in response to new health concerns. From his panel of consultant advisers, Acheson selected Sir Richard Southwood to chair the BSE group. Southwood was Chair of the National Radiological Protection Board and a highly respected scientist. Acheson knew him well personally and was aware that he had already successfully chaired a Royal Commission on Environmental Pollution. The other members of the working party were also eminent professionals, personally selected by Acheson for their knowledge of this obscure area of science. They included (Michael) Anthony Epstein, who, according to Acheson, had narrowly missed out on getting a Nobel Prize for his discovery of the Epstein–Barr virus; Sir John (later Lord) Walton, the 'doyen of British neurology'; and William Martin, an academic veterinary scientist and Director of the Edinburgh Institute.[53]

Having established the Southwood Working Party, and arranged for a joint secretariat from the Department of Health and Social Security and Ministry of Agriculture, Fisheries and Food to service it, Acheson presented an initial list of questions for consideration. He then followed established civil service procedure

[49] BSE Inquiry, oral transcript of evidence from Sir Donald Acheson, 06.11.1998, p. 103.
[50] *On the State of the Public Health*, being the Chief Medical Officer's Annual Report for 1985 (London, HMSO, 1985), pp. 49–50.
[51] M Schwartz, *How the Cows Turned Mad*, trans. E Schneider (Berkeley, University of California Press, 2003).
[52] See BSE Inquiry website, www.bse.org.uk.
[53] BSE Inquiry, oral transcript of evidence from Sir Donald Acheson, 06.11.1998, p. 51–2.

and had no further involvement with the work of this advisory group, reflecting the principle that it should be completely independent from government influence and, more importantly, from political pressure from Ministers. He had learnt this lesson during the AIDS crisis, when he had initially chaired the Expert Advisory Group on AIDS, partly because 'it had very special aspects which a lot of people found very difficult to deal with'.[54] He subsequently realised that it was inappropriate to be involved in formulating advice which he would then have to receive and approve in his capacity as CMO. He had therefore found an independent expert to chair the Expert Advisory Group on AIDS.

The composition and performance of the Southwood Working Party was thus crucial to the success of the government in managing the BSE affair. As Acheson explained in his witness statement: 'For a CMO not to accept expert advice properly considered and submitted would have serious implications and had this become more than exceptional, would have led to the collapse of the CMO's and therefore the DH's [Department of Health] scientific advisory machinery.'[55]

The Southwood Working Party, at the request of Acheson, produced immediate interim advisory briefings following each of its meetings in June, November and December 1988. This facilitated an ongoing review of risk within both the Department of Health and the Ministry of Agriculture, Fisheries and Food. All the Working Party's major recommendations were implemented before the final report was published in February 1989. As BSE was essentially a scientific issue, the medical staff within the Department took the lead. Acheson had given careful thought to his nomination for the Department of Health and Social Security member of the Secretariat. His choice of Hilary Pickles reflected her superior medical and research qualifications. She had already served as Scientific Secretary for the Expert Advisory Group on AIDS and had proved very competent at disseminating scientific information within the Department.

Pickles continued to act as the lead person in the Department of Health on BSE after the end of the Southwood Working Party. She officially reported through Jeremy Metters (who was promoted to Deputy CMO in August 1989), but she also updated Acheson directly, usually in person, immediately after significant developments. Acheson then reported direct to Ministers. As Sir Christopher France succinctly put it to the BSE Inquiry: 'It was *not* necessary for administrators to draft advice for medical officials to offer to Ministers. That is one of the points of having medical *civil servants*.'[56]

After the publication of the Southwood Report, Acheson arranged for it to be evaluated by his deputy, Ed Harris, to provide a reassurance that the Working Party had considered all the available evidence and addressed the issues directed to it. Acheson was therefore able to make a submission to the Secretary of State on 9 February 1989, in which he stated that 'On the evidence given in the report I accept that the risk to Man has been extremely small and that . . . every reasonable step has already been taken to minimise any theoretical risk of transmission by destruction of affected cattle'. He endorsed the report as 'a thorough study of the problem with sound and balanced conclusions'.[57] The report was also favourably reviewed in the scientific press.

---

[54] Ibid., p. 65.
[55] BSE Inquiry, witness statement of Sir Donald Acheson. No.251A, p. 9.
[56] BSE Inquiry, witness statement of Sir Christopher France. No.275B, p. 17.
[57] BSE Inquiry evidence. YB89/2.9/9.1.

One of the main recommendations of the Southwood Report was the need to establish a group specifically to look at BSE research. This was subsequently formed in February 1989, chaired by David Tyrrell, who had been a member of the Committee for Dangerous Pathogens and who was already recognised as a distinguished medical virologist and an expert on spongiform encephalopathies. The Tyrrell Committee published its report in January 1990, which highlighted the need for ongoing research into BSE. Arising out of this was the formation in April 1990 of a standing committee, the Spongiform Encephalopathy Advisory Committee, known as SEAC. Sir Richard Southwood declined to continue his involvement because of the pressure of other work, but Tyrrell agreed to serve as Chair and Pickles continued to act as Scientific Secretary.

The advice provided by these various bodies was communicated to Ministers through the CMO, and only after his personal evaluation. Ultimately, however, as with the translation of all advice into policy, it was a Ministerial decision what to adopt and what to refuse. For example, there was a potential conflict of policy interest over the implications of a specified bovine offal ban. The early BSE cases all showed evidence of the disease as confined to the brain and nervous system of cattle. The Southwood Working Party had not recommended a ban on human consumption of these parts of cows, but the Ministry of Agriculture, Fisheries and Food wished to institute one in May 1990. Acheson objected, not to the ban in principle, which would provide a 'belt and braces' security function, but because the review he had requested on the use of bovine material in medicines, especially vaccines, had not yet been completed: 'I had to weigh up what I knew was a very real risk, to the health and lives of those children whose parents might fail to vaccinate as a result of a scare, against what I was advised was a remote risk from ingesting bovine offal.'[58] In the event, the Ministry's announcement of the ban in September 1990 generated minimal media attention, and Acheson's fears were not realised.

As scientific research into BSE progressed, the Spongiform Encephalopathy Advisory Committee advised the Ministry of Agriculture, Fisheries and Food and the Department of Health on required precautionary legislation. The initial ban on specified bovine offal made in 1988 was intended to eliminate the disease being transferred between cattle, especially after the discovery that 'meat and bone-meal' feedstuffs, which incorporated recycled parts of slaughtered cattle, were the major source of new infection. There was an agreement between the Ministry and the Department of Health that departmental responsibility for the implementation of legislation would depend on whether the issues were primarily animal or human. Thus the enforcement of regulations in abattoirs for the full removal of specified bovine offals and their destruction came under the Ministry of Agriculture, Fisheries and Food's control. Its assurance (that the local authority surveillance of abattoirs was satisfactory) was integral to the subsequent assurances given by Acheson as CMO that specified bovine offals were not reaching the human food chain.

But this was not the reality of the situation. A suspected case of BSE in a cat in May 1990 provoked a number of panic reports in newspapers that there might be a possibility of transmission of the disease between species, and also, therefore, to humans. On 15 May 1990, Acheson was advised that the scale of public alarm

---

[58] Ibid., p. 46.

was so great that it justified a statement from him. He attempted to call an emergency meeting of the Spongiform Encephalopathy Advisory Committee to agree the wording of such a statement, but under extreme pressure from Ministers for an immediate statement, had to be content with contacting them individually by telephone. They all agreed that the risk posed to human health by BSE was still remote, and that beef was still safe to eat.

A written statement was issued by Acheson to health authorities and local authorities on 15 May 1990, and also published as a press release with accompanying explanatory notes by the Department of Health Press Office on 16 May 1990. On the same day he made a videotaped interview to be used for television news programmes. However, Acheson's statement was edited down to leave a single sentence: 'There is no risk associated with eating British beef and everyone, children, adults, patients in hospital, can be quite confident that it is safe to eat beef.'[59] As he said in his witness statement to the Phillips Inquiry: 'It is inconceivable that I made a public health pronouncement to be used by the media on this or any other matter which consisted of only a single sentence. Therefore it is self-evident that this sentence has been extracted from a longer interview, removing it completely from its surrounding context.'[60]

The core of Acheson's message to the public was intended to be that beef was 'safe' to eat. He never intended to say 'no risk' – a phrase which an experienced epidemiologist such as Acheson would have been wary of using. The written press statement had used the words 'no scientific justification' instead.

The concept of risk, and the position of CMO as the public's trusted medical expert, is one which we will return to in more detail in Chapter 7, but it illustrates how the government relied on a statement from one person, the acknowledged expert, to allay public fears. Had the same statement been made by Kenneth Clarke, then Secretary of State for Health, it would have lacked the vital 'scientific' credibility which the public had come to demand in health crises. Certainly John Gummer's persuasion tactics as Minister for Agriculture, Fisheries and Food, when he fed a beefburger to his young daughter in front of television cameras at an agricultural show, were met with widespread public derision and have become infamous.

One of Acheson's final actions on BSE before he retired in September 1991 was to call for the appointment of a research supremo – an expert to identify and direct future research priorities for BSE. He had successfully created such a role before. He had appointed Sir James Gowans, Secretary of the Medical Research Council, to oversee the development of research on AIDS. The primary benefit to be gained was that this circumvented the normal delays in bidding and refereeing required to initiate research. Gowans, as AIDS research supremo, would have been able to go straight to key individuals and ask them to put aside their current projects to do directed research for him. However, there was considerable opposition to this idea from both the Ministry of Agriculture, Fisheries and Food and from the Agricultural and Food Research Council. The latter did not wish to be under the control of anyone other than their own immediate directors.[61] As with the issue of the Spongiform Encephalopathy Advisory

[59] BSE Inquiry, oral transcript of evidence from Sir Donald Acheson, 06.11.1998, p. 128.
[60] BSE Inquiry, witness statement of Sir Donald Acheson. No.251B, p. 1.
[61] BSE Inquiry, oral transcript of evidence from Sir Donald Acheson, 06.11.1998, p. 10.

Committee's reporting line, it required intervention from Permanent Secretaries to try to resolve this problem. In this case Acheson's authority as CMO did not prove sufficient.

When Kenneth Calman moved from being CMO for Scotland to the English post in 1991 his guiding principles were very much in line with those of his predecessors – namely that all actions should be based on scientific evidence and where evidence was lacking a precautionary principle should be adopted. Interestingly, he was not simultaneously appointed as CMO to the Ministry of Agriculture, Fisheries and Food. Calman has suggested that the appointment might have been delayed because of the impending report from the Banks Review on the Structure of the Department of Health.[62] However, this did not appear until 1994, and would seem to have been a minor concern in comparison to the accepted need to have stronger communications between the Ministry and the Department of Health, which had been identified at Permanent Secretary level. Calman appeared satisfied that BSE was under control when he came into office in September 1991. Having made investigations to assure himself of the comprehensiveness of current research, he did not see the issue of a BSE research supremo as a 'primary concern', and he solicited an assurance from the Spongiform Encephalopathy Advisory Committee that there were no new discoveries casting doubt upon existing policies.

However, in August 1992, Calman was alerted to the existence of a farmer with suspected CJD. When this farmer died in February 1993, a post-mortem examination confirmed that it was a case of CJD, and Calman responded to heightened media concerns by issuing a press statement on 11 March 1993. On advice from the Spongiform Encephalopathy Advisory Committee, he gave an assurance that there was still no scientific evidence to link BSE in cattle with CJD in humans, and that beef should still be considered safe to eat.

Further suspected cases of the disease were reported to the CJD Surveillance Unit in 1993, but the one which caused most public concern was that of the sixteen-year-old girl, which the press were linking to the consumption of hamburgers. Calman again made a press statement reiterating his view that beef was safe on 26 January 1994. By June 1994, new experiments showed that the BSE agent had been found in cattle tissue outside the brain and spinal cord, and threw into question the presence of the disease in offal from calves under six months old, which was still being sold as 'safe' for human consumption. An emergency meeting of the Spongiform Encephalopathy Advisory Committee was called on 25 June 1994 to decide whether the advice to Ministers and the public needed to be amended. This resulted in a further press statement, this time jointly from Calman and the Chief Veterinary Officer, Keith Meldrum, that the ban on specified bovine offal would be extended to calves as a precaution.

By this stage, the Spongiform Encephalopathy Advisory Committee appears to have been under pressure to provide advice quickly to Ministers. Calman recalled that at their meeting on 25 June 1994, the Committee members were concerned that they 'were expected to produce top-class scientific opinions in a rush' and that this was an 'unrealistic expectation'.[63] The Committee continued to be a concern for Calman into the autumn of 1994, when he suggested to William

[62] BSE Inquiry, witness statement of Sir Kenneth Calman. No.179, section 71.
[63] Ibid., section 65.

Waldegrave, then Minister for Agriculture, Fisheries and Food, that the clinical membership of the Committee needed strengthening and that it required a new Chairman. Professor John Pattison, who was also a Public Health Laboratory Service board member, was subsequently appointed as Chair in 1995.

One of the biggest problems in the BSE crisis emerged on 23 October 1995, when Calman received a letter from Meldrum, the Chief Veterinary Officer, informing him for the first time that four instances of incomplete removal of the spinal cord in abattoirs had been detected through a Ministry of Agriculture, Fisheries and Food programme of unannounced inspections. Meldrum summarised this discovery as 'disappointing'. Calman considered this a massive understatement, especially since he had relied on the Ministry's assurance that this could not happen. That assurance had enabled him to make all his public pronouncements on the safety of beef since he became CMO for England in 1991.

In the next few days, a Cabinet subcommittee deliberated over how this news should broken to Ministers. Calman found the initial draft statement unsatisfactory, in that it did not acknowledge the full potential risk. He asked to have the statement reworded. This was 'a step too far' for the Ministry officials. They were keen that Ministers be told that the Ministry of Agriculture, Fisheries and Food did not know of any specific cases where specified bovine offal material had entered the human food chain. Calman agreed to a slightly reworded statement, which left Ministers in no doubt that there was an issue of public health to be addressed.

Calman then met with Baroness Cumberledge (the Department of Health Minister with responsibility for BSE) and Richard Packer (the Permanent Secretary to the Ministry of Agriculture, Fisheries and Food, 1993–2000). Further investigations revealed the extent of unsatisfactory abattoir and feed mill inspection programmes, which had been under the control of the Ministry through the Meat Hygiene Service. Calman requested a meeting with Douglas Hogg (the Minister for Agriculture, Fisheries and Food). This was held on 7 November 1995, at which Calman stated that he was not prepared to give any further public assurances on the safety of beef, given the possible contamination by specified bovine offals. Douglas Hogg was left to make a statement about his meeting with representatives of abattoir owners and operators which 'created a great deal of media interest'.[64]

In the light of this new information, Calman resolved further to strengthen the 'human' health expertise on the Spongiform Encephalopathy Advisory Committee, a move which was supported by its Chairman Professor John Pattison. The Committee advised that the vertebrae from adult cattle should not be used in 'mechanically recovered meat'. Such meat was obtained by subjecting cattle carcasses to high-pressure water jets to remove remaining scraps, which were usually destined for cheap sausages and pies. This process, more than any other within the abattoir, risked contamination of meat with BSE agents. However, 'mechanically recovered meat' had so far failed to generate sustained interest from either the Ministry of Agriculture, Fisheries and Food or the Department of Health, despite the Welsh CMO Deirdre Hine's requests in 1991 for investigations into production processes and the risk of contamination. The new advice from the Spongiform Encephalopathy Advisory Committee was forwarded to Stephen

---

[64] Ibid., section 101–2.

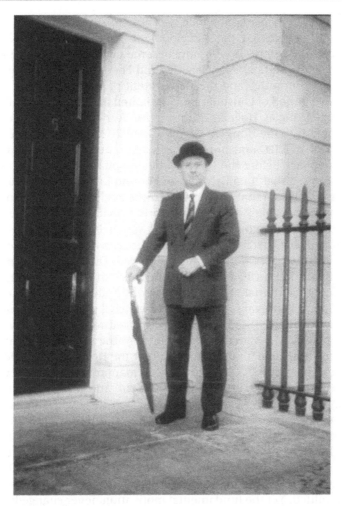

Figure 6.4 'The Classic Civil Servant': Kenneth Calman poking fun at himself. © Kenneth Calman. Reproduced with permission.

Dorrell, then Secretary of State for Health, by Calman. The Prime Minister, John Major, was also briefed in a Cabinet discussion on 7 December 1995, and approved the issue of a Specified Bovine Offal (Amendment) Order on 15 December 1995 to prohibit the use of 'mechanically recovered meat' containing material from the vertebral column.

There had been a number of new suspected cases of CJD during 1995, including a fourth farmer (a statistical unlikelihood which worried the Spongiform Encephalopathy Advisory Committee), and an abattoir worker. However, it was in March 1996 that the CJD Surveillance Centre in Edinburgh submitted to the Committee sufficient reliable evidence of a cluster of cases of the disease in twelve people aged under 40 years, which showed distinct new pathological features. It was clear that this was a 'new variant' of CJD, considered to be almost certainly related to BSE in cattle. Calman, on advice from the Spongiform Encephalopathy Advisory Committee, briefed Stephen Dorrell and wrote to Packer at the Ministry of Agriculture, Fisheries and Food to try to halt the production of publicity material which was now incorrect in the light of the new findings. He also discussed this development with the other UK CMOs and informed the Prime Minister, who now became personally involved in meetings with the Ministry of Agriculture, Fisheries and Food, the Spongiform Encephalopathy Advisory Committee and the Department of Health.

This intensive period of consultation culminated in Stephen Dorrell as Minister for Health and Douglas Hogg as Minister for Agriculture, Fisheries and Food making statements to the House of Commons on 20 March 1996. They confirmed the existence of nvCJD, and provided a reassurance that these infections had probably taken place before the specified bovine offal ban was imposed in 1989. Calman emphasised that 'I had always sought and followed the advice of experts in the field and repeated that any new scientific evidence would be passed to the public as soon as possible'.[65] He subsequently provided a comprehensive action plan for officials and the government on 26 March 1996.

BSE illustrated that there were even some areas where there were insufficient experts within Britain, let alone within Whitehall. One of the recommendations of the 1994 Banks Report had been that the mechanisms and resources open to the CMO to obtain external medical and scientific advice should be examined in detail. Therefore, John Evans, a former medical civil servant, who had retired as Deputy Secretary at the DHSS in 1984, was asked to lead a review. His report, which was published in March 1995, was not music to Calman's ears as he had hoped for some independent confirmation that the Department of Health should bolster rather than cut its expert medical manpower. In the event, Evans acknowledged that it would be more efficient and cost-effective to exploit external experts as the need arose. This reflected the increasing complexity of issues on which the Department needed advice, and BSE was a case in point.

As the crisis deepened, between the discovery of the first bovine cases in 1986, through to the recognition that the specified bovine offal bans were not watertight in 1995, and the confirmation of human nvCJD in March 1996, the CMO played a critical role, alternating between proactivity and reactivity as events and resources permitted. Yet the fundamental motivation never changed: to safeguard the health of the public through the application of three key principles: (a) to solicit independent expert advice to enable the Ministers to make a scientifically rigorous decision on policy, (b) to communicate that advice and appropriate scenario planning throughout Whitehall, government and the health service, and, most importantly, (c) to inform the public.

This last item sounds deceptively easy. Yet it requires a degree of sophistication on both sides: the CMO has to consider when a public statement is necessary, and the public must have the ability to comprehend the information supplied. At the heart of this dialogue lie differing conceptions of risk. Calman had taken a personal interest in 'risk theory' over many years, publishing papers and books on the subject.[66] He sought to develop this further by creating a Risk Communication Group within the Department of Health in 1995.[67] The Phillips Report

---

[65] Ibid., section 121.

[66] P Bennett and K Calman (eds), *Risk Communication and Public Health* (Oxford, Oxford University Press, 1999).

[67] For more details, see *Annual Report on the State of the Public Health for 1995* (London, HMSO, 1996).

commented on the assumptions of Acheson and Calman about how the public would interpret their statements, in terms of both risk and the state of scientific information on BSE. Along with Robert Kendell, the Scottish CMO, they had not explicitly stated that their opinions on the 'safety' of beef were dependent on the strict compliance with the precautionary measures for animal feeds and abattoir processes. The government's overriding aim was to prevent an 'alarmist over-reaction' from the public, given that it considered the risk to human health from BSE was remote. Thus, the Phillips Report concluded, when the government did make the admission of a causal relationship between BSE and nvCJD in March 1996, the public felt betrayed: 'Confidence in government pronouncements about risk was a further casualty of BSE.'[68]

Conclusion

The AIDS and BSE crises are examples which expose the vital role of the CMO in the interpretation and management of significant new health risks. In much the same way as the late nineteenth century CMOs had to cope with diseases where the aetiology was unknown, such as smallpox and scarlatina, late twentieth century CMOs also had to take personal responsibility for understanding the latest scientific research and judging the quality of the findings and the direction of future research. It would have been equally appropriate here to discuss the role of Yellowlees and the Ebola virus in the 1970s. All these examples illuminate how governments have too often generally reacted to risk problems with an essentially 'paternalistic' form of policy making.[69] There are lessons to be learnt here on how the CMO has been positioned within Whitehall, how he has managed the 'gatekeeper' function for both internal and external advice, and, crucially, how he has guided government and the public on the understanding of risk.

[68] BSE Inquiry, vol. 1, Executive Summary of the Report of the Inquiry, p. xviii.
[69] R Klein, 'The politics of risk: the case of BSE', *British Medical Journal*, 2000, 321, 1091–2.

Conclusion

Chapter 7

The nation's doctor

A glance through the official portraits of the fourteen CMOs reveals no one who would feature in a popular history in the way that many politicians would. Of course, the public of the day may sometimes have heard of their CMO. Godber was even the subject of newspaper cartoons. It is only in the era of television that the CMO has been a publicly recognisable figure. This really applies to CMOs who have held office during the recent past – Acheson and Calman – who appeared on television in response to major public health crises such as AIDS. For example, one 'urban myth' circulated in the Department of Health following Acheson's visit to Moscow with Kenneth Clarke (the Secretary of State for Health) in 1990 was based on an encounter with British tourists in Red Square:

Tourist to Mr Clarke:	'It is Mr Clarke, isn't it?'
Mr Clarke:	'Yes.'
Tourist to companion:	'I told you so when I saw him standing next to the Chief Medical Officer.'

Many earlier CMOs, with the possible exceptions of Simon, Jameson and Godber, were probably known only to the medical profession and Whitehall.

One of the earliest and most important functions which the office of CMO acquired was to report on the state of the public health – its current condition, predicted risks to it and strategies for improvement. Since John Simon took up the post of Medical Officer to the Privy Council in 1855, the CMO has communicated with a widening group. The modern CMO is recognised as the public face of state medicine. Although Simon's primary contact was with Parliament and the small band of Medical Officers of Health in local authorities, the public increasingly desired, and subsequently expected, to be informed of significant health problems.

There are subtle indications of this, from the more frequent reporting of health issues in national newspapers to the increased print runs for the CMO's Annual Reports. The intermittent coverage triggered by the epidemics of cholera, typhus fever and other infectious diseases, prominent in the nineteenth century, were gradually replaced by a more sustained interest in personal as well as public health, especially after the introduction of National Insurance in 1911. By the time the Ministry of Health was created in 1919, one of George Newman's primary strategies was to target the individual in his campaign for preventive medicine. This required, above all, a public which was educated in health matters. It also reflected, for the first time in Britain, increasing access to modern healthcare and the resurgence in self-medication, which was facilitated by the expansion of pharmacist companies such as Boots. The introduction of radio as a means of mass communication in the 1920s also had a significant impact on the CMO's media strategies.[1]

By the end of the twentieth century, the CMO had the capacity to communicate direct with the majority of the British public and, through the National Health Service, with all members of the medical profession. The techniques may have changed and the issues have broadened since John Simon's time, but the underlying principles remained the same: risk assessment and considered advice, delivered with care and based on scientific evidence from the best available intelligence systems.

John Simon and freedom of speech

Through his involvement with the construction of the 1858 and 1859 Public Health Acts, Simon secured one of the most vital functions of the CMO – the right to report independently on *any* matters concerning public health. It was his confident assertion of this function that gave him authority with Parliament and the public soon after his appointment. For example, he constructed the documentation required to convince Parliament of the need to legislate for compulsory smallpox vaccination. He solicited information on historical and contemporary vaccination procedures from ten foreign governments. In all, 542 European doctors completed his questionnaire on vaccination practices. In Parliament, Mr HA Bruce proclaimed that 'this inquiry was as exhaustive and complete as ingenuity could devise'.[2] Simon not only provided the theory behind vaccination, he also prepared detailed instructions on how to put such a national system into practice.

Like so many of his Victorian contemporaries, Simon had an unshakeable faith in the power of information and perhaps naïvely believed that an accumulation of facts should be sufficient to induce change. He urged that:

> The local public and the general public and the government and the legislature ought to have before them the precise facts of each case where a preventable or partly preventable disease prevails to great excess in any particular district.[3]

The way in which these facts were interpreted was crucial – the brute force of sanitarian dogmatism had to be replaced by sensitive scientific pragmatism. The publication of Simon's *Sanitary Papers* in 1858 had aroused the antagonism of his two keenest enemies, Edwin Chadwick and Florence Nightingale, and, to a lesser extent, of William Farr at the General Register Office. Chadwick and Nightingale bitterly opposed the novel methods of statistical analysis which Simon encouraged his protégé, Dr Edward Headlam Greenhow, to develop, calling it a 'shallow and erroneous system of statistics' which put 'contagion on the same footing as witchcraft and superstition'.[4] They could not countenance any theory which

---

[1] See A Karpf, *Doctoring the Media* (London, Routledge, 1988) for details of George Newman's handling of the media.

[2] Hansard, clxxxii, 11.04.1866, col.1096. Debate on the Vaccination Bill.

[3] Simon, *Sanitary Papers*, PP 1857–8, xxiii, p. 310.

[4] Nightingale Papers, British Library, MS 43,398, 19.08.1858, Nightingale to Chadwick; 43,399, draft note by Nightingale, April 1861.

threatened the Chadwickian philosophy of 'sanitary reform', and used every opportunity to disparage the *Sanitary Papers* through the press and at meetings of the Sanitary Science Association. To Chadwick and Nightingale's dismay, the extensive press coverage of the *Sanitary Papers* worked in Simon's favour, consolidating his already significant public persona, and strengthening his hand with government in the drafting of public health legislation in 1858. The main lesson from this is Simon's demonstration of the necessity for objectivity in determining public health policy. His own rejection within only ten years of some of the miasmatic principles which had underpinned his earlier *Sanitary Papers* is testimony to this new philosophy of relying on the best evidence.

The tradition of the Chief Medical Officer's Annual Reports

Section five of the 1859 Public Health Act was one of the most momentous legislative developments in the history of public health. This short section reads:

> The Medical Officer shall from time to time report to the Privy Council
> in relation to any matters concerning the public health or such matters
> as may be referred to him for that purpose.[5]

The Times immediately acknowledged the significance of Simon's achievement: 'What will be obtained will be publicity and only that moral compulsion to do something . . . which publicity may impose.'[6] The Act also required the submission from the CMO of an Annual Report to Parliament on the state of the public health, containing his personal professional assessment of the public's health, with complete freedom from government sanction. He was thereafter free to select matters for investigation and report, gaining in the process, as Mr Lowe said during the parliamentary debate on the Bill, 'quasi-judicial' authority for his post.[7] Simon had no need to disseminate his views through anonymous reports or through rigged committees. He revelled in the freedom to claim authorship for his ideas, and, as *The Times* noted, his authorship meant that these ideas were 'universally regarded as conclusive on the questions with which they deal'.[8] Simon enjoyed the full and considerable support of the British national and medical press during his time as CMO. This was undoubtedly a relief to him as he remembered the part the press had played in Chadwick's downfall. His Annual Reports were covered in *The Times* and other leading newspapers. They consistently praised him for his 'most shrewd practicality with the most penetrating scientific acumen', and as a public servant who 'deserves the public gratitude'.[9]

The pithy reports which Simon personally wrote between 1858 and 1876 ignored mundane and routine business and cut straight to the heart of contemporary health issues. Once past the perfunctory obsequiousness to his Whitehall masters, Simon's reports provided him with a unique opportunity to castigate government for its failure to implement policies to improve public health. They

---

[5] Public Health Act, 1859. 22 & 23 Vict. c.iii.
[6] *The Times*, 19.07.1859.
[7] Hansard, clv, 19.07.1859, col.15. Third reading of the Public Health Bill.
[8] *The Times*, 01.02.1864; 04.10.1864; 23.11.1872.
[9] *The Times*, 10.08.1866; 27.08.1868; 04.04.1874; 12.08.1874.

seem amazing documents even now. One cannot begin to assess the reaction such uncensored criticism must have provoked at the time. Simon cultivated a style of report which was guaranteed to appeal to his public supporters. He wrote introductory essays which brought together the main findings from the voluminous statistical appendices. Even Chadwick was forced to admit that Simon had a talent as a writer and that his reports 'invariably attract the attention they merit'.[10] *The Times* later praised them as 'terse, forcible and graphic', powerful through their 'real eloquence, intense and fervid, reaching a climax of a deep and almost terrible earnestness'.[11]

Simon also used his reports to publicise the research which he had been able to commission through his department. There were wide-ranging reports on industrial health, housing for the poor, the impact of maternal employment on infant mortality, the proposed regulation of druggists, a systematic study of hospital provision in Britain with European comparisons, to name but a few of the many topics. Simon engaged the most eminent scientists to undertake these researches. Thus the young pathologist JLW Thudichum and John Gamgee, Principal of the Edinburgh Veterinary College, were personally selected by Simon to investigate the problem of parasitic diseases in meat destined for human consumption.[12] He was all too aware of the impact that his style of report could have. He continued the habit he had started in his years as Medical Officer of Health for the City of London of sending out copies of his reports to individuals whom he knew to be influential. His enemies were later to castigate him, considering the abuse of public money on unnecessary quantities of official publications.[13]

Simon's relationship with the press was close – some would now perhaps say it was unprofessionally intimate. He took a keen interest in how his work was reported. His office subscribed to all the main newspapers and periodicals, and these were often delivered first to his home in Kensington Square so that he and his wife could read them over breakfast, before being taken later on to Richmond Terrace.[14] He was in frequent contact with JT Delane, the editor of *The Times*, who had been a close personal friend to Simon and his wife since the late 1840s. He also knew the manager and proprietor of *The Times*, and several of the leader writers, who were all useful connections. Florence Nightingale accused him of writing supposedly anonymous editorials on sanitary matters. He almost certainly was the author of anonymous letters to *The Times* in 1856 in support of the proposed Medical Education Bill, and again in 1862 when St Thomas's hospital was threatened with relocation out of the city centre.[15] Other articles contained so much 'inside' information about his office that his hand was obviously behind them. If he did not personally write for the press, he had close colleagues who did:

[10] Nightingale Papers, MSS 45,770, 21.08.1858, Chadwick to Nightingale. *Lancet*, 1867, (II), 167; 1868, (I), 201; 1869, (II), 352–3.
[11] *The Times*, 25.07.1904. *British Medical Journal*, 17.09.1887, (II), 628.
[12] *Fifth Report of the Medical Officer of the Privy Council*, PP.1863.
[13] MH 19/210. Lambert minute, 06.03.1875; T.9/12, 24.06.1864, 22.06.1866; PC 7/11, 13.06.1861; PC7/19, 16.07.1870.
[14] R Lambert, *Sir John Simon and English Social Administration* (London, MacGibbon & Kee, 1963), p. 298.
[15] Ibid., p. 462. Lambert notes that the letters, which are kept in the Simon archive at the Royal College of Surgeons, are signed STH – Surgeon to St Thomas's Hospital.

Robert Lowe, Vice President of the Local Government Board, wrote editorials for *The Times*, and Simon's clerk, Herbert Preston-Thomas, wrote articles on public health for the *Morning Post*.[16]

Simon was fully aware of how to achieve influence through the media. For example, he accepted the Presidency of the Medical Teachers Association in 1867, which was little more than a pressure group for reform of the General Medical Council (GMC). Simon had opposed the GMC since its formation in 1858 because it had not adopted his favoured 'one-portal' entry system for aspiring medical practitioners. He knew that his speech to the Medical Teachers Association in January 1868 would receive widespread attention and he used the occasion to launch a bitter attack on the GMC – its 'utter corruption', low examination standards and general incompetence in regulating the medical profession. He did not have to mention the GMC by name – the press knew only too well that this was the object of his wrath.[17] His speech generated coverage and support from the medical press and ultimately contributed to the reform of the GMC (1886). Simon used similar tactics with the Royal College of Surgeons. He began with outspoken public criticism, and when elected to the Council of the College, cajoled its members into accepting reform.

Simon's outspokenness was tolerated by his superiors in government through-out the 1850s and 1860s, but with the arrival of Gladstone's Government in 1871, and Simon's move into the newly created Local Government Board, the mood was less indulgent. Both Stansfeld as President of the Board and Lambert as Permanent Secretary decided that Simon's revised (more junior) position at the Board did not give him the right to issue his own Annual Reports. Thus in 1872 and 1873 he was reduced to publishing only a small and authorised section within the main report of the Local Government Board.[18] Simon had been gagged. The *Lancet* hoped that despite this setback, the Medical Department (of the Board) would prove 'too tough and big a morsel for the insensitive and anaconda-like swallow of the Poor Law organisation'.[19] The journal maintained a watch over the fate of medicine at the Board in the early 1870s, noting gloomily the 'suicidal policy . . . and practical suppression of Mr Simon and his staff'.[20] In 1875 it concluded that 'Mr Simon has been relegated to some departmental limbo'.[21] Simon's plight was also covered by the *Pall Mall Gazette* and *The Times*. However, even his loyal supporters in the press could not achieve Simon's goal of becoming reintegrated to policy-making circles within Whitehall.

Simon resumed writing his own, independent Annual Reports in 1874,

---

[16] H Preston-Thomas, *The Work and Play of a Government Inspector* (William Blackwood and Sons, Edinburgh, 1909), p. 34.

[17] *Lancet*, 25.01.1868, (I), 115–18, 134, 575, 831. *British Medical Journal*, 25.01.1868, (I), 65, 75; 22.02.1868, (I), 169.

[18] MH 19/211. Lambert to Treasury, 23.03.1876; Lambert to Treasury, 06.04.1876.

[19] *Lancet*, 07.12.1872, (II), 822.

[20] *Lancet*, 13.04.1872, (I), 363; 13.04.1872, (I), 514; 15.06.1872, (I), 837; 12.10.1872, (II), 532; 02.11.1872, (II), 642; 30.11.1872, (II), 786; 26.07.1873, (II), 124; 02.08.1873, (II), 158; 27.12.1873, (II), 913; 03.01.1874, (I), 21; 17.01.1874, (I), 95; 31.01.1874, (I), 169; 18.04.1874, (I), 562; 31.10.1874, (II), 630. See also coverage in the *British Medical Journal*, 30.11.1872, (II), 607; 28.06.1873, (I), 722; 16.08.1873, (II), 78; 28.02.1874, (I), 279; 07.02.1874, (I), 178. *Practitioner*, 1874, (XII), 233, 386; 1875, (XIV), 153, 232.

[21] *Lancet*, 1875, (I), 582.

following Disraeli's Conservative victory in the general election. Lambert remained as Secretary, but Stansfeld was replaced by the more amenable Sclater Booth and Simon was then able to re-establish his freedom of speech. His last three Annual Reports, between 1874 and his resignation in 1876, were pure Simon. He relished the renewed opportunity to speak his mind and push the tolerance of government to the limit with his public opposition to its plans. In the 1874 report, he openly criticised the system of employment for local Medical Officers of Health and claimed that he was the man to remedy this fault. He used his 1875 report to point out that shortage of resources was costing lives:

> I have thought it essential to put before you, as a matter of proportion, how slight, except in regards of smallpox, is the cognizance which the Board hitherto takes, and how far apart are its exertions of skilled influence, in regard of those local defaults of disease prevention which annually cost many tens of thousands of lives . . . The quantity of medical inspecting-force available to the Department for this branch of service is about equal to the employment of three Inspectors . . . the sanitary jurisdictions of England are . . . 1,558 and the mortality as due to causes more or less under control of the law . . . amounts, in the common estimate of informed persons, to at least 12,000 deaths per annum.[22]

Simon's last reports were hailed in *The Times* as 'a manifesto of considerable importance'. The *Practitioner* viewed his outspokenness as a 'dignified protest' against the Board's policy and the 'formal enumeration' of a better one.[23] The impact was less than Simon hoped for and was counter-productive in his relationships at the Board and his longer-term security in the post. At the very least, though, he kept sanitary reform at the forefront of the opposition and the public's mind.

The value of the CMO's Annual Report was evident again when restrictions were placed on Simon's successor in 1877. As part of the Whitehall-wide rationalisation exercises, the Treasury demanded that expensive lithographs and illustrations be discontinued. This was despite complaints that this would detract from the usefulness of the Report. The print run was also limited to 1,000 (400 for Parliament, 400 for the Local Government Board and 200 for sale to the public). The public copies sold out within a fortnight of issue.[24] Yet the Annual Reports contained much more than general demographic and epidemiological information. They also included reports on special investigations by the CMO's medical staff, which provided vital information and guidance for local Medical Officers. However, because of limited circulation, these useful Reports (e.g. Thorne Thorne's on isolation hospitals in 1882) failed to reach the target audience. There were only 775 copies printed of Thorne Thorne's Report, most of which were sent to Parliament and Local Government Board officials, and 225 put on sale. Thorne Thorne campaigned to have free copies sent to all the 1,600

---

[22] *Report of the Medical Officer of the Privy Council and Local Government Board*, NS.4, PP.1875, xl, pp. 11–12.
[23] Lambert, *Simon*, p. 551. *The Times*, 12.08.1874; *Practitioner*, 1874, (XIII), 144–5.
[24] MH 19/212. Seaton to Lambert, 22.07.1878.

local Medical Officers of Health, but the Treasury compromised with an additional print run of 50 copies.[25]

Again in 1883 Buchanan petitioned the Treasury to increase the print run for the Principal (Chief) Medical Officer's Annual Report, stimulated by a request from a local Medical Officer of Health to be put on the annual mailing list. Buchanan wrote pessimistically:

> Do you think this application from an intelligent Medical Officer of Health might well raise the larger question whether health officers who have occasion for these volumes ought not to receive them on application? The more we trust and expect people to do what they ought to do, the more reason there is for showing them what their duty is, and the way of doing it; and a health officer to whom shillings are of consequence and whose S.A. [sanitary authority] would not think of purchasing a book for him, wants aids and models and instruction which as our reports afford . . . Such a man, when our inspectors visit his district, puts time and brains at our disposal, and is at all times prepared to give time and trouble to answer all questions put to him for the sake of knowledge beyond mere sanitary administration.
>
> Of course we shall hear that the reports cannot thus be given away except at some great cost, but their value would be more amply returned in the form of increased efficiency of Medical Officers of Health.[26]

During the years at the Local Government Board the Annual Report continued to suffer from cutbacks, and, more seriously, from substantial delays in publication, mainly caused by the huge workload of the CMO. The 1889 Report was not issued until mid-1891, and Dr Parson's Report on the influenza epidemic of 1889–90 was not available until 1892.

> It is unfortunate for Dr Buchanan that the larger portion of his annual report is invariably out of date by the time that the blue book which contains it is given to the world. We have before commented on the extraordinary delay in the publication of a report which is, we understand, due on March 31st, is dated August, and is not out until the following February. It is impossible to expect much interest to be excited by the chronicle of events some of which happened two years ago . . .[27]

However, part of the Medical Department's workload entailed the preparation of circulars, memoranda and reminders which were sent out by the Medical Department to sanitary authorities, Medical Officers of Health and Boards of Guardians. This aspect of health communication had increased dramatically since the early 1860s, reaching an output of some 119 items in the 29 months between October 1878 and February 1881.[28]

---

[25] MH 19/214. Thorne Thorne for Medical Officer to Rotton, 19.09.1882.

[26] MH 19/215. Buchanan to JT Hibbert, 07.06.1883.

[27] *British Medical Journal*, 19.02.1887, (I), 409.

[28] RM McLeod, 'The frustration of state medicine', *Medical History*, 1967, XI, 19. MacLeod calculates that in the period 1866–71 there were 62 circulars and memoranda issued.

On the state of the public health

Simon's annual reports had been published as part of the 'blue books' series of the Local Government Board, although sometimes designated as an 'appendix' to the main report. When the Ministry of Health was formed in 1919, the CMO's Report took on a more prominent role, printed separately from the first part of the Ministry's Annual Report. The new title, *On the State of the Public Health*, reflected Newman's optimism for the preventive medicine ethos of the Ministry. He dedicated a substantial amount of his personal time to the preparation of his Annual Report, perhaps at the expense of more useful projects. By the end of his time in office, they had become voluminous publications, requiring the assistance of several civil servants to prepare.

His successor, MacNalty, had a very different perspective on official reports. Although he enjoyed writing and published an enormous number of historical books, including the official medical history of the Second World War, after he retired, during his time in office he produced the statutory reports with reluctance. One reviewer of a MacNalty Annual Report on the health of the school child submitted a postcard reading:

> This Report is the work of MacNalty and Glover,
> Glover the text and MacNalty the cover.[29]

The individual literary style of the CMOs has always been secondary to the traditional structure and content of the Annual Reports. The weather has been a persistent opening theme, although this owes more to the ancient Hippocratic principle of the association between climate and health than to the British obsession with observing the minutiae of weather conditions.[30] This extract from Jameson's Annual Report of 1947 is typical (although the degree of climatic detail did decline in later reports):

> The eighth year of austerity, 1947, was a testing year. Its first three months formed a winter of exceptional severity . . . these three months of bitter snow and bitter cold were followed by the heaviest floods for 53 years, which did great damage, killed thousands of sheep and lambs, delayed spring sowing . . .[31]

George Godber, who became CMO in 1960, ensured that his first Annual Report received coverage in national and local newspapers. *The Financial Times*, the *New Daily*, *The Guardian* and large regional papers like the *Liverpool Echo* all discussed the main contents of the Report.[32] The *Daily Mail* reprinted in detail the discussion on lung cancer and the *British Medical Journal*'s suggestions for government action on smoking:

[29] N Goodman, *Wilson Jameson, Architect of National Health* (London, George Allen and Unwin, 1970), p. 138.
[30] I am grateful to Geoffrey Rivett for reminding me of this tradition within the Annual Reports. G Rivett, *From Cradle to Grave: fifty years of the NHS* (London, King's Fund, 1998), p. 48.
[31] *On the State of the Public Health. Report of the CMO for 1947* (London, HMSO, 1949).
[32] *Financial Times*, 14.12.1961; *New Daily*, 14.12.1961. *The Guardian* gave the Report two columns, 15.12.1961. MH 55/2226. Press cuttings in the Ministry of Health files.

- reduce smoking in public places
- forbid smoking in theatres and cinemas
- stop the issue of cheap cigarettes to young servicemen
- enforce the law prohibiting the sale of cigarettes to children under 16
- 'There is a strong case for curtailing tobacco advertisements. In Sweden, they are forbidden.'[33]

The public's increased interest in health matters in part stimulated the expansion of editorial and publication staff within Whitehall. By the mid-1970s, when Henry Yellowlees was CMO, there was a substantial team working on the production of the Annual Report of the Department of Health and Social Security and its companion volume, *On the State of the Public Health*. This team also prepared the series *Reports on Health and Social Subjects*, which had begun in 1920 shortly after the establishment of the Ministry of Health, and by 1976 had published 139 booklets on such subjects as the *Reports on Confidential Inquiries into Maternal Deaths in England and Wales*. All these were Stationery Office (formerly HMSO) documents, and available for purchase by the public as well as being provided free to doctors.

With the expansion of the Department of Health and Social Security responsibilities, the all-inclusive format of the CMO's Annual Report with the statistical summaries made for cumbersome reading. They remained useful reference tools, but apart from the limited personal introduction they lacked vitality and vision for the 'health of the public'. There had been a perceptible decline in size: from the 1968 report of 276 pages to around 100 pages for the reports of the late 1970s and early 1980s. These bore little resemblance to the passionate reports written personally by John Simon between 1858 and 1876.

Guidance for the medical profession

While the CMO's Annual Report is ostensibly for the primary benefit of Parliament and the public, additional mechanisms were developed to communicate with doctors. By the 1980s the amount of information issued by the Department of Health, which the CMO had to approve, was substantial. The channels used varied according to the target audience but the output was enormous: by 1985 there were 918 health circulars in force (some dating back to 1948), numerous advice notices were issued on medical products and 'Dear Doctor' letters went out each year from the CMO to all medical practitioners.[34]

In 2001 the Report of the Select Committee on Health noted that the number of CMO letters had fallen to between three and five per year, which reflected the increase in other forms of CMO communication with the medical profession. For those CMOs who had relied heavily on communication through 'letters', it is interesting to see how their personal style and sense of authority was conveyed. The approach of Godber and Yellowlees, for example, could not be more different: Godber's enormous respect for clinical practitioners is evident in his tone. He usually made the supporting facts and figures behind the topic the key component, with the message of required action almost a throwaway comment at the

---

[33] *Daily Mail*, 15.12.1961.
[34] *Report on the Review of the Senior Open Structure, DHSS* (Moseley Report) (April 1986), pp. 107–8.

end. He preferred the doctor to evaluate the evidence presented and agree with his suggestion. Yellowlees, on the other hand, favoured straightforward delivery of the instruction and did not give such weight to providing the rationale and evidence behind his pronouncements. In 1994 a quarterly bulletin, the *CMO's Update*, was introduced. This was designed to communicate non-urgent information to all doctors in England as well as being read by other health professionals, including nurses and pharmacists.

New communications technology was being exploited by the end of the twentieth century. The Public Health Link System was introduced in 1994 as an electronic urgent message system. The CMO's office sent alerts and other information to health authorities for distribution through a 'cascade' to nominated professionals (including general practitioners, practice nurses, community services pharmacists, medical directors in hospitals). A pager alert mechanism was used so that health authorities were aware that a message had been sent and they were classified for distribution within either six hours (*immediate*) or 24 hours (*urgent*).[35]

In 2001 it was estimated that urgent and immediate communications were sent on average 15 times a year, containing information on drugs, infections, vaccines and other public health measures. More recently, email alerts have superseded the telephone/pager cascade system, and, in 1997, the first CMO's website was established for Kenneth Calman.

Jameson: the fireside CMO

Newman had actively sought a public role for the CMO, partly, one suspects, to bolster his personal status. He was also aware of the potential of radio to take health education into British homes. He did not personally make broadcasts, but maintained control over the health content of all BBC programmes. In the interwar period, its relationship with the government was such that the BBC bowed to pressure on programme content and its invited speakers were vetted. In 1928, the minutes of the BBC's Controversy Committee noted that:

> Sir George Newman [Chief Medical Officer at the Ministry of Health] took great interest in talks by medical men and on medical subjects, and . . . in addition to supervising all questions of broadcasts by medical men he often asked to see the manuscripts of talks on medical or semi-medical subjects to be given by non-medical men. In spite of this the Ministry . . . refused to admit that it acted in an advisory capacity to the BBC or had any say in the question of what talks were suitable or unsuitable. This attitude puts the BBC in a very difficult position.[36]

Newman had further strengthened his control over the BBC by also acting as the General Medical Council's nominee for the approval of any medicine-related scripts. Gradually, however, the relationship improved, and the Ministry of Health began to make suggestions for radio programmes rather than merely

---

[35] Select Committee on Health, Second Report 2001, Annex G, The Chief Medical Officer's Communications.
[36] Cited in Karpf, *Doctoring the Media*, p. 38.

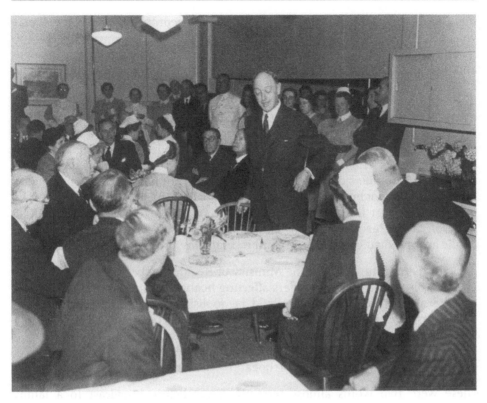

Figure 7.1 Jameson giving a speech at the opening of new kitchens at the London Hospital in Whitechapel, London, after they were damaged during the Blitz. 8th August 1945. © Getty Images. Reproduced with permission.

monitoring BBC output. In MacNalty's era (1935–1940) the Ministry also began to employ Press Officers and to issue press notices.

It was the arrival of Jameson, and the advent of the Second World War, which had the biggest impact on how the CMO engaged the media and the public on the nation's health. Within a few months of coming into the Ministry of Health, Jameson held monthly press conferences to give details of the current health situation and to launch health promotion campaigns. Jameson was a natural presenter – relaxed, often talking without notes, and willing to answer questions from journalists.

On 5 May 1941 Jameson made his first radio broadcast. The theme was diphtheria, and the purpose was to persuade parents to have their children immunised. This was a golden opportunity. The blackout had forced people to remain at home in the evenings, where the radio became the prime source of entertainment and, of course, of news about the war. Jameson had a huge potential audience and his measured Scottish delivery proved enormously popular. His carefully worded broadcast described the distressing features of the disease: 'Have you ever seen a child suffering from a severe attack of diphtheria – the dirty, evil-smelling throat, the swollen neck glands, the horrible forms of paralysis . . . .' He moved on to explain how the Canadians had successfully tackled the disease, and ended with: 'In my view it's nothing short of a disgrace that there's still so much diphtheria about. There needn't be if only you will play your part.'[37]

Jameson's broadcast was augmented with national media publicity campaigns and the diphtheria immunisation rate improved from eight per cent of children in 1940 to 50 per cent in 1942.[38] This was probably the first time that a civil servant had made a radio broadcast. It was a novel event, but not as amazing as the subject for his second one: venereal disease. In October 1942, following a similar broadcast by the American Surgeon General, Thomas Parran, Jameson arranged a slot just after the nine o'clock evening news on the BBC's Home Service. This was peak time for listener numbers. The BBC, when told of the sensitive subject for his speech, was alarmed and another slot was offered which would not have such a big audience. Jameson would not budge. He had the support of his Minister, Ernest Brown, who was also a Baptist lay preacher, but the latter's backing was somewhat timid. Jameson talked his way into this embarrassing topic slowly, first reminding the public how tuberculosis had been until recently an unmentionable disease:

> It is part of the policy of the Ministry of Health to take the public into its confidence over all matters affecting health . . . there is nothing to be alarmed about, but it would be foolish of me to pretend that everything is just as it should be, when in fact it is not. The two black spots are tuberculosis and venereal disease . . .
>
> And now a few words about venereal disease, the two chief forms of which are syphilis and gonorrhoea.[39]

These were two words almost certainly never before broadcast to a family audience, definitely not the stuff of post-dinner conversation. Jameson explained the symptoms of the diseases and the appalling lack of awareness about the free treatment which could be obtained for them:

> How are we going to deal with this situation? I will tell you how we shall never be able to deal with it – or with any other situation – and that is by running away from it, shutting our eyes to its existence, by refusing to discuss it, or by withholding from young people information regarding its dangers . . . So let us decide here and now that we shall no longer tolerate this hush-hush attitude regarding venereal disease. With the help of an enlightened public opinion we could easily reduce these diseases to insignificant proportions, and I hope you will lend your support to our efforts to rid this country of yet another of its social plagues.[40]

His talk was reprinted in full in *The Listener* magazine, along with an editorial which concluded that Jameson had done the nation a great service in broaching

---

[37] Full text of this broadcast is reprinted in Goodman, *Wilson Jameson*, pp. 188–9.

[38] Jameson, of course, did not choose to enlighten the public that Britain had lagged behind Canada in diphtheria immunisation because it did not have the funds or the staffing to mount such a large-scale campaign. For an analysis of this scandalous delay, which cost some 6,000 infant deaths per year, see J Lewis, 'The prevention of diphtheria in Canada and Britain, 1914–1945', *Journal of Social History*, 1986, 20, 163–76.

[39] Goodman, *Wilson Jameson*, pp. 190–4.

[40] Ibid.

this difficult subject: 'He treated sex-hygiene with the deftness and assurance of a bomb-disposal expert.' The public responded amazingly well to Jameson's frankness and his 'sympathetic, common-sensible Scottish voice', *Social Survey* carried out a poll which showed that 90 per cent of the public approved of breaking this taboo. The broadcast was followed up by a Central Council for Health Education conference on venereal disease (chaired by the Archbishop of Canterbury), and a poster and film campaign: 'ten plain facts about venereal disease'.

Communication was central to Jameson's passion for public health. After the successes of the diphtheria and venereal disease campaigns he worked closely with the Ministry of Health Public Relations Officer, Thomas Fife Clark, to design posters and commission a number of health education campaigns. He championed the cause of health information in his public speeches and lectures, including the Harveian Oration at the Royal College of Physicians in October 1942 and at the Royal Sanitary Institute in 1946, telling his audience that he put measures for 'telling the public the truth' second only to new medical breakthroughs such as penicillin and DDT.[41] He also travelled to the USA and Canada during the war to lecture on how Britain was ensuring the health of its population in wartime conditions. He was aware of the power of the mainstream media and particularly of films. Cinema going, already popular, took on a new urgency during the war, as the newsreels shown before the film were the only way of 'seeing' the progress of the war, in contrast to the radio coverage. The Ministry of Health, concerned about a dramatic rise in infestations of head lice during the war, asked film stars to change their hairstyles so that shorter hair (which would be easier to disinfect) would become more fashionable.

One introduction to a broadcast from 1945 sums up Jameson as the archetypal 'public' CMO – the nation's own family doctor:

> I present to you the gentleman who feels the national pulse, inspects the national tongue, and then assures us in the blandest and most comforting manner in the world that, on the whole, we are keeping rather better than we feel.[42]

Like his mentor Jameson, Godber worked hard at maintaining good relations with the press, in particular the medical press, notably the *British Medical Journal* and the *Lancet*. Occasionally his consideration was not appreciated within the Department of Health and Social Security. Crossman (Secretary of State) noted in his diary in April 1970, in the run-up to the publication of the controversial report on the contraceptive pill:

> 'Oh,' said the officials, 'the daily press will get a copy of the *BMJ* the day before publication and they can print what they like.' Peter [Brown – Director of Information at DHSS] said it was essential to brief the press beforehand, so that the newspapers would have a

---

[41] DDT (dichlorodiphenyltrichloroethane) was introduced in 1942 as a very effective insecticide, particularly used against malaria-carrying mosquitoes. Penicillin was the first successful antibiotic to be developed in 1943, following the work of Alexander Fleming, Howard Florey and Ernst Chain.

[42] Goodman, *Wilson Jameson*, p. 143.

proper statement on the morning when the *BMJ* is published. We have had great trouble co-ordinating all this, because the CMO has the strange idea that the editor of the *BMJ* must be allowed his tantrums, which means that we are deciding our timing solely at his dictation. But it's a good example of Godber's total concern with the doctors. He was apparently much less concerned with the effects on the women. I have to keep both in mind.[43]

Godber presided over a period in which the public really woke up to a medicalised society for the first time, aware of the potential of new miracle drugs like penicillin. There was also intense public interest in (and affection for) the new National Health Service. On its tenth anniversary in 1958 there were several newspaper stories in which the triumphant tones of British success were accompanied by criticism of the state of the nation's hospitals.[44] Despite receiving an annual 50–60 per cent of the NHS budget, and considerable investment in nearly all hospitals, if not that many new buildings, there was mounting media dissatisfaction with the failure to modernise at a faster pace.[45] The public was increasingly exposed to the hospital as the pre-eminent site of medical expertise through a number of seminal television programmes, including documentary series such as *Your Life in Their Hands*, which was presented by Dr Charles Fletcher, who came to rival the 'Radio Doctor' Charles Hill as a national media 'medical personality'.

The more powerful influence of television compared to radio was soon recognised by the Ministry of Health. The CMO's Annual Report for 1958 reported that the Ministry would be using a new television serial based on a hospital emergency ward to promote blood donations.[46] The medical profession was not always so eager for uncontrolled television coverage: the BBC's series *Your Life in Their Hands* was criticised by the British Medical Association because it could give the public the wrong impression on health and medicine, especially as eight of the ten programmes were filmed in hospitals and showed such eye-catching items as surgery.[47]

The public's love affair with hospitals also had an impact on the relative image of the general practitioner. It proved very difficult in the first decade of the National Health Service to provide funding for practice modernisation or the development of group practices, and even Godber, while Deputy CMO, resorted to an unusual degree of public criticism of the skewed investment in hospitals.[48] With this intense media focus on an image of health as the white-coated professional in the high-technology hospital, it was an uphill battle for public health professionals, including the CMO, to present a more balanced picture of health determinants.

---

[43] R Crossman, *The Crossman Diaries, Vol. III* (London, Hamish Hamilton, 1977), p. 878.
[44] *Daily Mail*, 'How Sick is the Health Service', 01.07.1958; *News Chronicle*, 'Our Hospitals are Out of Date – That's the Hard Truth', 09.05.1958.
[45] D Fox, *Health Policies, Health Politics: the British and American experience, 1911–1965* (New Jersey, Princeton University Press, 1986), p. 170.
[46] *On the State of the Public Health in 1958* (London, HMSO, Cmd. 871), p. 40.
[47] See D Fox, *Health Policies*, for a full discussion on the media's love affair with medicine in this period. Also the commentary in the *British Medical Journal*, beginning with 'Disease education by the BBC', 15.02.1958, (I), 388–9, and continuing on pages 449–50, 456, 510, 592, 899.
[48] G Godber, 'Health services, past, present and future', *Lancet*, 1958, (II), 3.

Don't die of ignorance

By the 1980s there had been a sea change in public expectation of information on health issues. A 1986 Department of Health and Social Security report calculated that the Department received around 1,000 calls a week from the press and broadcasting media, and over 2,000 from the public to the Health Inquiry Office. It also noted the enormous range and quantity of information issued: in 1985 there were 400 press notices, 250 different leaflets (with a total print run of over 100 million), 100 different posters, 800 pages of information on Prestel and £5 million worth of advertising (television, newspapers, magazines).[49]

Yet one significant impetus to the public's new expectations was the deliberate change in the speed and format of dissemination of information adopted for the AIDS crisis in 1986. The usual secrecy which until that time surrounded Cabinet committees was laid aside, and the new *ad hoc* Committee on AIDS, chaired by Lord Whitelaw, Lord President of the Council, was initially publicised in *The Independent* newspaper.[50] This was followed within a fortnight by the remarkable media briefing which Norman Fowler, Secretary of State for Social Services, gave in Downing Street on the outcome of the AIDS Committee. This was done with such haste, in order to convey the government's sense of urgency and action on the subject, that it took place before the Cabinet Secretariat had even had time to type up the Committee minutes.[51]

The emergence of this frightening disease was responsible for a dramatic transformation in the public's perception of the CMO. It was not sufficient to have Norman Fowler expounding the benefits of condoms on the steps of 10 Downing Street (supposedly with Margaret Thatcher watching from behind the net curtains). The public now increasingly demanded the reassurance which only a medical practitioner could offer. The CMO had to talk directly to the public, through television, radio and newspaper interviews. Donald Acheson, the thirteenth CMO, became the recognisable face of state medicine, and his persona as an authoritative yet benevolent expert was just what was required. Since then the trend for the CMO to make more frequent public statements on current health crises appears to have been irreversible. This was no doubt media driven rather than department led, but it also reflects both a commitment to a more open style of government and a conscious revision of the communications strategy.

The role of the CMO, and his press statements in the BSE crisis, have already been discussed in detail in Chapter 6. However, one direct observation which his role prompted came out through the House of Commons Agriculture Select Committee's report in July 1990, which advised that instead of relying on the CMO in a 'fire-fighting' role, the Department of Health should have a more systematic way of dealing with media scares.[52] Acheson also commented in 1998 that the pressure on him to appear in the media was sometimes intense: 'In an extreme case there might be anything up to ten different "bids" from TV/radio channels on a single day. If Ministers did not wish to appear there was usually no

[49] *Report on the Review of the Senior Open Structure, DHSS* (Moseley Report) (April 1986), p. 108.
[50] C Hughes, 'Cabinet takes up the battle against AIDS', *The Independent*, 03.11.1986.
[51] C Brown, 'AIDS warning will go to every home', *The Independent*, 12.11.1986.
[52] Report of the Agriculture Select Committee, 1990, para. 75.

alternative to my agreeing to do it myself.'[53] He also noted: 'When one becomes a civil servant one very quickly has to take into account Ministers' relationships with the public and public relations and how things will look.'[54]

Other examples of the CMO being used to make public warnings on behalf of Ministers include those on salmonella in powdered milk and botulism linked to hazelnut yoghurt.[55] One food scare which has been singled out for sustained public recognition is that of salmonella in eggs. In this scare, it was the junior Health Minister, Edwina Currie, who made an 'off the cuff' statement during a radio interview in December 1988 in which she said that 'most of the egg production in this country is sadly infected with salmonella'. The rest of the media immediately interpreted this as meaning that most British eggs were infected and within days sales of eggs had plummeted, causing a crisis in the farming industry.

Acheson, as CMO, quickly drafted full-page newspaper advertisements and issued public statements which sought to accurately convey the facts, and to reassure the public that although there were some limited risks for vulnerable people (pregnant women, the elderly) from raw or lightly cooked eggs, that the rest of the population had nothing to fear. This was robust advice supported by scientific evidence, but, as Acheson noted, for some interested parties it did not appear to go far enough:

> However, a junior Minister in MAFF [Ministry of Agriculture, Fisheries and Food] sent for me and put intense pressure on me to make a less carefully qualified statement about the safety of eggs. Bearing in mind that there were several thousand cases of food poisoning annually due to infected eggs and some deaths, I was not prepared to do this. I sought the support of my Secretary of State, Mr Kenneth Clarke, and the pressure from MAFF stopped.[56]

It was within this context of an increasing number of health scares in the 1980s and early 1990s that the public had to decipher subsequent crises, such as those on the 'safety' of beef in 1990. The zenith of public hysteria was reached in May 1990, prompting the Ministry of Agriculture, Fisheries and Food to issue a press briefing entitled 'British Beef is Safe. Gummer'. This was followed by statements to the public from Lady Wilcox, Chair of the National Consumer Council and statements to the National Health Service (jointly from Acheson and the Parliamentary Under Secretary). For the first time in the episode, the media statements explicitly invoked the personal medical authority of Acheson:

> British beef can be eaten safely by everyone, both adults and children, the Chief Medical Officer, Sir Donald Acheson, confirmed today. This advice has been given to the National Health Service. Sir Donald said: 'I have taken advice from the leading scientific and medical experts in this field. I have checked with them again today. They have consist-

---

[53] BSE Inquiry, witness statement of Sir Donald Acheson. No.251, section 33.

[54] BSE Inquiry, transcript of evidence from Sir Donald Acheson (T79), p. 57.

[55] M O'Mahony, E Mitchell, RJ Gilbert, 'An outbreak of food-borne botulism associated with contaminated hazelnut yoghurt', *Epidemiology and Infection*, 1990, 104, 389–95.

[56] BSE Inquiry, transcript of evidence from Sir Donald Acheson (T79), section 35.

ently advised in the past that there is no scientific justification for not eating British beef and this continues to be their advice. I therefore have no hesitation in saying that beef can be eaten safely by everyone, both adults and children, including patients in hospital.'[57]

However, as we discussed in detail in Chapter 6, issuing a statement is one thing; but there is no assurance that the media will use it in its entirety or in appropriate context.

Conclusion

By the end of the twentieth century there was a wide range of mechanisms through which the CMO could communicate with the medical profession, Parliament and the public. The Annual Report continued to retain a real and symbolic importance, especially as a statement of the freedom which the CMO enjoys from governmental control. The Annual Reports, when used efficiently, raised awareness of the risks faced not only by the public but also the risk faced by government if they failed to heed this public expression of measured medical advice. The reports were often used as 'early warning systems' of impending health issues. The later ones no longer provide a bland, straight-to-archive chronicle of the Department's annual activities. Time alone will tell if this newer, risk-awareness format is effective in influencing the behaviour of the general public.

The freedom of speech which the CMO has enjoyed at various times under-pinned the confidence which was placed in him to undertake risk analysis for both the public and the state. This trust was also dependent on the public's perception of the CMO as impartial and unbiased – beyond the reach of drug companies and similar vested interests. In an increasingly unintelligible scientific era there is a greater need than ever for experts who can guide the public through the moral maze of responsibility for their individual health and that of the wider community. Whether this advice is adopted or ignored is another matter, but it has been the CMO's business to ensure that it is there, easily accessible and understandable, for all those who wish to have it.

[57] Ibid., section 86.

Chapter 8

Reflections: a job is what you make it

Aside from producing their Annual Reports, many of the CMOs published books or papers during and after their time in office. Looking back over this body of work, sometimes written in reflective terms on the challenges for the future, sometimes tightly focused on intractable contemporary problems, sometimes searching the past to draw inspiration from the public health titans of yesteryear, the words seem to be imbued with a common restlessness of spirit.

When Newsholme, in his 1932 book *Medicine and the State*, pointed to two ideals at the heart of all civilised communities – that the health of every individual is a social concern and responsibility and that medical care for every individual is an essential condition – he was unconsciously revealing the breadth of his own vision for the job he found himself in.[1] He was also close to encapsulating in words a goal for any government of modern times.

The essential qualities

Most of the fourteen CMOs, when the baton was passed to them, saw before them challenges on a major scale which they were hungry to tackle. Their appointment as CMO gave them a unique opportunity to change things for the better and they remained restless in pursuit of such ideals. Some of the fourteen looked away from this grand vision, perhaps dazzled and intimidated by its breadth. They were content to hold the office and the prestige that went with it. Others were defeated by the internal politics of government or by external events. Those who left the most successful legacies of achievement had at least one of three important qualities.

First, they were able to master the art of getting things done within Whitehall. This was a culture which was by turns stultifying, driven by petty jealousies, deeply conservative and highly resistant to change. The ability to navigate these dark waters with subtlety and ingenuity whilst avoiding a reputation for deviousness and intrigue required great skill.

The second quality that the successful CMOs possessed was their ability to become indispensable to Ministers. Someone who reliably and consistently gives the right advice, with a full assessment of the context and likely consequences, accrues enormous power and influence within the Whitehall machine. It is clear that there were several periods in the history of the post, at times of crisis or doubt, when a frequently issued instruction on the Ministerial corridor was 'Get me the CMO'.

Simon, the first CMO, exemplifies this ideal. With consummate skill he

[1] A Newsholme, *Medicine and the State: the relation between the private and the official practice of medicine, with special reference to public health* (London, George Allen & Unwin for the Milbank Memorial Fund, 1932).

developed a wide range of influential political contacts and allies. At the peak of his power and influence he was not just shaping government policy through his advice, he was identifying the problems and championing and leading the reforms necessary to address them. He became indispensable to the government, although they perhaps did not realise nor even want it. It is sad to reflect on the waning of his influence and his eventual departure as a broken man. Perhaps he had just been there too long in a situation where too many parts of the Whitehall machine resented his influence and pioneering zeal.

Wilson Jameson, the second of the truly great CMOs, was firmly and unquestionably relied upon by Health Ministers to do what they could not do alone: deliver the medical profession's support for that post-war ideal of a comprehensive national health service, free to all, and based entirely on need, not the ability to pay. Jameson's legacy is formidable for this achievement alone.

Godber, a medical giant of his day, was equally talented in operating the Whitehall machine. Often using his extensive external network of colleagues and experts to stimulate action, he would play down his own views until the moment was right to advocate a new policy or initiative which, by that time, had gained a powerful coalition of external support which Ministers would find difficult to resist. He also showed great courage and integrity in pushing forward action on smoking after years of government neglect and procrastination.

The best of the CMOs also had the ability to communicate well, to be able to espouse a clear vision, to inspire and motivate others to want to deliver it, to be able to explain complex subjects simply, to be able to persuade and to be able to reassure. Too few people in leadership positions have these communication skills in depth but they were characteristic of some of the men whose histories we have explored. A very few of the fourteen combined all three qualities – they understood the Whitehall machine and how to harness its power, they had the unreserved respect of Ministers and they were gifted communicators. Some of these men were selected precisely because they had already demonstrated these aptitudes in other posts, and because the CMO post needed a strong character to balance a more powerful medical profession or difficult political climate.

Seizing the day

The post of CMO has perfectly fitted the old adage 'a job is what you make it'. The job description has always been pretty broad and general. It offered the individual the chance to create opportunities within boundaries that are not clearly drawn. Throughout its history, the post has been significant within the public service. From the outset, in 1855, it has had a national overview of health and increasingly from the early twentieth century it has had a direct responsibility for the development of health services. It has been part of the government of the day but not a political appointment. It holds high civil service ranking but with a degree of independence and autonomy which has no parallel in other Permanent Secretary posts. It sits in the centre of a complex, triangular relationship between the government, the medical profession and the public. Many of the fourteen CMOs used this unique positioning of the post together with their personal qualities to achieve a great deal. The job was indeed what they made it.

The CMO role in modern times has many similarities with the job done by the earliest holders of the post. The need to analyse, understand and contextualise the main health problems of the day was as relevant to Godber and Calman as it was to Simon and Newman. The importance of a CMO who championed a cause and galvanised commitment to addressing it is as evident in Acheson's response to the earliest cases of AIDS as it was in Newsholme's response to tuberculosis. When Aneurin Bevan rose to his feet, at the end of an intimate dinner to thank those who had worked most closely with him in the planning of the new National Health Service, and proposed the toast, 'To the new National Health Service, coupled with the name of Wilson Jameson', he was acknowledging the power potentially invested in the post of CMO when held by someone who has gained the trust and respect of those at the highest levels of government.

Redefining the health agenda

Leading, championing, investigating, influencing, planning and driving change – these are the common threads which run through the role of CMO from 1855 to 1998. Yet there was a clear discontinuity in 1919 with the creation of a Ministry of Health, combined with the appointment of Newman, which gave health a centre-stage position in government for the first time. Perhaps, though, the traditional role of the CMO really began to change in the second half of the twentieth century as the country itself changed after the end of the Second World War. The CMO role (and that of government and public services as a whole) began to be shaped by the needs and expectations of a modern consumer society. The impact was not immediate but the seeds of change sown in the late 1940s were those which have created the climate and context in which the modern CMO has had to operate.

A number of issues stand out. Firstly, the relationship of the CMO with the public through the print and broadcast media. When Wilson Jameson made his bold and imaginative decision in 1942 to give a radio talk at peak listening hours on the BBC on (what was then called) venereal disease, the post of CMO entered a new era. It became the voice, if not yet the face, of the nation's health. The epithet most commonly applied to the CMO by journalists and profile writers is 'the nation's doctor'. Wilson Jameson that night was indeed the epitome of the family's doctor, joining listeners by the fireside with a stern message yet delivered with warmth, kindness and humanity.

Looking back at it today the broadcast is a landmark: the CMO building a bridge of communication to the public that he serves and cares for through the medium that had sustained them during the dark days of war. Considering that seminal broadcast in the context of how the relationship with the media has subsequently developed, the contrast between the CMO in the 1940s and his counterparts in the late twentieth century could not be more stark.

Although earlier CMOs had had extensive dealings with the print and broadcast media, the relationship was essentially one between authoritative spokesman and passive recipient. It was during the 1980s and early 1990s, when Acheson and Calman held office, that the attitude of mass media towards government and managers of public services changed most, and the media climate became turbulent. Journalists began to ask increasingly awkward and provoking questions of the government and its spokespeople. The skills of investigative journalism, symbolised by the *Washington Post's* Woodward and Bernstein and their role in uncovering the Watergate scandal in 1972, were being honed. The tradition of governments in withholding information and only releasing what was thought good for people to hear was challenged as it came to be regarded by news editors as paternalistic and anachronistic.

At the beginning of the 1960s, a decade of social upheaval which ushered in the age of consumerism, John F Kennedy sent a message to Congress. He included 'the right to be informed' amongst the four rights of a consumer. Today, this appears even more prescient for voters and taxpayers when electing their governments. Although America had already moved towards more open governance in the second half of the twentieth century, it has not been such an issue in Britain. Given the independence, professional integrity and freedom from politics traditionally associated with the British CMO role, it was ironic that when the hurricane hit it was the last of the two CMOs in our historical account who were in the eye of the storm.

The epidemic of bovine spongiform encephalopathy (BSE) or 'mad cow disease' and the subsequent emergence of its human form, variant Creutzfeldt–Jakob disease (vCJD), was the point of meltdown in public confidence in health information and health advice coming from the government. The two CMOs covering this period (Acheson and Calman) continued, however, to fulfil the (by then) established role of the holder of the office – to be the main government spokesman in giving the public information about a problem, setting out the context and providing advice on what action people should take to reduce the risk to themselves and their families.

The media and the subsequent Judicial Enquiry Report criticised the government for failing to take effective action quickly enough, for complacency in the face of an unknown but potentially serious risk to human health, and for being unduly reassuring to the public. The enduring media image of the BSE crisis was of a Cabinet Minister feeding a beefburger to his daughter in a misguided attempt to reassure the public that British beef was safe. Symbolic perhaps of this particular crisis was the way in which the balance was struck between politics and public health, with the latter becoming subordinate to other considerations, and potentially damaging to the public confidence in the CMO.

The warning signs were perhaps already there in another smaller crisis in 1988 when politics once again marginalised public health. On that occasion, Health Minister Edwina Currie's off-the-cuff remark about the risks of salmonella infection from British eggs generated a public furore in which the focus of media attention was on the viability and commercial interest of the egg industry. That particular crisis cost Currie her place in government. In retrospect, it also established a precedent that, because a major issue involving risk and population health would inevitably become controversial and political, then political handling would be a necessity. Moreover, after witnessing the fate of Edwina Currie, it would be a brave politician who, when faced with a similar situation in the future, would take pre-emptive, precautionary action to protect the public health when doing so would threaten a major industry with dire economic consequences.

It was unfortunate that the BSE crisis broke when there had been no acknowledgement nor any debate on the genuine dilemmas at the heart of decision making involving risk to the public health from food, agriculture or other environmental hazards. The fundamentals had not been sorted out. The methodologies for objective, scientific assessment of risk in such situations were not well-developed. The ground rules for taking precautionary action to protect the public when no definite risk had been established had not been written or even properly discussed. There was no precedent for the communication of public health advice in situations where there was scientific uncertainty and that uncertainty needed to be conveyed to the public. Phrases such as 'no evidence that . . .' conveyed a measure of reassurance that may have misled the public. The whole language of risk communication was unclear: what did 'safe' actually mean?

The BSE crisis engendered a breakdown of trust in health and scientific advice provided by the government. There are some who appear still to believe that on public health matters governments tend to cover up risks, protect vested interests, and reassure rather than truly inform. It was unfortunate that the CMOs of the day were caught up in this catastrophic affair.[2] They had even agreed that they would resign *en masse* if the government refused to accept their specific advice to ban specified bovine offal from entering the food chain. Four CMO resignations would have sent a stark message to the public on government competence – it was therefore a message which the Ministers took very seriously.[3] However, the reality was that credibility in public health advice needed to be restored once the crisis was over. Calman, the fourteenth CMO, addressed the issues of risk and risk communication, writing and speaking widely on the subject and producing guidance for government officials and practitioners.[4] However, it is difficult to say to what extent this has secured public confidence in expert health advice.

A National Medical Service?

The second issue that stands out in the working life of the modern CMO compared to his predecessors is the predominance of healthcare issues in comparison to public health concerns. When the National Health Service was established in 1948, its architects believed that it would become largely a health maintenance service. Infectious diseases, the big killers of the past, were regarded as being on the way to being conquered thanks to vaccines and the potential of antibiotics. There were high hopes for preventive medicine.

These predictions proved spectacularly wrong. The NHS became the major focus of public, media and political attention from the late 1960s onwards. As the population aged, as medical technology rapidly advanced, as therapeutic opportunities widened, the costs of the service rocketed. Need and demand outstripped supply and available resources. The NHS became a political football. Its real and perceived problems continue to fill acres of newsprint each year.

As the focus of the government, and Health Ministers in particular, remained firmly on the NHS, the CMO of the day became heavily involved in helping to shape policy, finding solutions to seemingly intractable healthcare problems and

[2] There are currently four Chief Medical Officer posts: England (from 1855), Scotland (from 1929), Wales (from 1969), Northern Ireland (from 1922). The latter three posts have traditionally been seen as subordinate to the English Chief Medical Officer, but from 1991 the group has strengthened its communications and team approach to health policy.
[3] Senior medical civil servant interview, 16.05.2000.
[4] P Bennett and K Calman (eds), *Risk Communication and Public Health* (Oxford, Oxford University Press, 1999).

trying to keep the medical profession engaged, particularly at times of major change. Thus Godber was intimately involved in producing the 1962 Hospital Building Programme, developing specialist services and rejuvenating general practice. Other CMOs have chosen to devote their energies to different areas of concern, but all have had to operate within the parameters set by the NHS ethos.

Neither the 1946 National Health Service Act nor its successors actually defined the nature of health, illness and care. More recently, Calman has also drawn attention to the need to educate the public in realistic expectations of what medical science can deliver. Matching public demand with health service potential has never been easy, it creates tension and stress on both sides.[5] However, the CMO is often the individual best placed to progress innovative approaches to such problems. The 'effectiveness and efficiency' principles of Cochrane, for example, were translated by Calman and Hine into both organisationally and clinically effective systems for cancer services in the 1990s.[6] Deirdre Hine, the former CMO for Wales, in her Jephcott lecture in April 1999 at the Royal Society of Medicine, raised (but perhaps not fully supported) a more provocative stance: educate the public that 'Death is inevitable: most major diseases cannot be cured; antibiotics are no use for 'flu; artificial hips wear out; hospitals are dangerous places; drugs all have side effects; most medical treatments achieve only marginal benefits; many don't work at all; screening tests produce false negative results and there are better ways of spending money than on healthcare technology.'[7] In the light of such brutal 'facts' the historian must confront public expectations and government or commercial inconsistencies in effective strategies for achieving health.

Political dogma has been a constant presence in healthcare discussions throughout our period. The modern CMO has therefore had an important part to play in ensuring that government health policy does not become too health service-centred, squeezing out longer-term health improvement as a priority. Some CMOs have been more sympathetic to the political ethos of their Ministers than others. How else can one reconcile Newman's silence at the Ministry of Health in the 1930s, at a time when Medical Officers of Health around Britain were reporting widespread evidence of malnutrition?[8] A stronger CMO might have felt that such evidence demanded his support, or his resignation. It was left to local Medical Officers of Health, like GCM McGonigle, to act as spokesmen for public health.

A change of government can also have a huge impact on the development of healthcare research and its translation into policy. The best example of this was the deliberate attempt in 1980 to suffocate the seminal *Black Report on Inequalities in Health*, produced by a working party initiated by David Ennals, the former

[5] KC Calman, *The Potential for Health* (Oxford, Oxford Medical Publishers, 1998).

[6] AL Cochrane, *Effectiveness and Efficiency: random reflections on health services* (London, Nuffield Provincial Hospitals Trust, 1971); Department of Health, *Report of an Expert Advisory Group on Cancer Services* (London, Department of Health/Welsh Office, 1995).

[7] D Hine, 'For the good that it will do: issues confronting healthcare in the UK', *Journal of the Royal Society of Medicine*, 1999, 92, 332–8.

[8] For a full account of the refusal of Newman and the Ministry to accept such evidence from Medical Officers of Health and pressure groups, see C Webster, 'Healthy or hungry thirties?', *History Workshop Journal*, 1982, 13, 114.

Labour Secretary of State for Health and Social Security in 1977.[9] It was the most unwelcome kind of report for the new Conservative Government to receive a year into its administration. The new Secretary of State, Patrick Jenkin, chose to issue only 260 duplicated copies rather than a proper Department of Health and Social Security publication, and to issue it on the Friday before the August Bank Holiday. The content, however, when efficiently publicised through a press conference at the Royal College of Physicians, provided some unpalatable truths about the inequalities in health and access to health services. The ensuing media attention made it into a (relative) bestseller on the state of the nation's health.[10] The role of the English CMO of the day, Yellowlees, in the production of the Report (it was led by the Chief Scientist, not the CMO) or its dissemination, was never consciously questioned at the time or subsequently. Yet the Scottish CMO, John Brotherston, was actively involved in the inequalities debate.[11]

Acheson, as CMO between 1983 and 1991, made repeated attempts to regenerate public health both within his own post and also as a government priority. The 1987 Inquiry into the Public Health Function, which he chaired at the request of Norman Fowler, the Secretary of State for Health, was a welcome opportunity to balance the managerialism of the earlier Griffiths Report on the National Health Service. Acheson was adamant that if National Health Service Boards were to have allocated places for management, finance and estates representatives, that there should also be a reserved space for a public health specialist at that level, rather than tucked in two or three rungs down the National Health Service management hierarchy. Acheson's subsequent success in initiating a public health White Paper, *The Health of the Nation*, which set targets for population health gain, was also a significant achievement given the ethos of the current Conservative Government, which was so wary of any discussion which acknowledged 'variations' in health (even to use the word 'inequalities' was considered a step too far). He was supported by a vibrant research community which had maintained this theme since the work of Simon and other pioneer public health activists in the mid-nineteenth century.[12]

---

[9] The members of the working party were Sir Douglas Black (Chairman), Professor Jerry Morris, Dr Cyril Smith and Professor Peter Townsend. The Black Report was the subject of a 'witness seminar' held at the London School of Hygiene and Tropical Medicine in 1999. A transcript and supplementary papers were published as a special issue of *Contemporary British History*, 2002, 16 (3): 'Poor health: social inequality before and after the Black Report', edited by Virginia Berridge and Stuart Blume.

[10] P Townsend and N Davidson, *The Black Report* (London, Pelican Books, 1982). See also Berridge and Blume, ibid., for David Player's first-hand account of how the Conservative Government attempted to stymie the follow-up report, Margaret Whitehead's *The Health Divide*, by disbanding the Health Education Council immediately before its publication date in 1987.

[11] Sir John Brotherston (1915–1985), Chief Medical Officer to the Scottish Home and Health Department, 1964–1977. J Brotherston, 'Inequality: is it inevitable?', in CO Carter and J Peel (eds), *Equalities and Inequalities in Health: Proceedings of the Twelfth Annual Symposium of the Eugenics Society, London, 1975* (London, Academic Press, 1976).

[12] See S Macintyre, 'The Black Report and beyond: what are the issues?', *Social Science and Medicine*, 1997, 44 (6), 723–45. This gives an excellent overview of the research before and after the Black Report.

The wider arena

The CMOs have been active too, in the international health arena, with many of them playing leading roles in the development of policies. As John Simon witnessed, diseases do not respect international boundaries. Communication with foreign health experts and participation in the formation of agreed disease prevention strategies quickly became an essential part of the CMO's task. Several CMOs consciously sought to develop their overseas roles. Seaton represented the government at the International Sanitary Conference in Vienna in 1874, Thorne Thorne was seconded several times at the request of the Colonial and Foreign Offices to international conferences, where his fluent French gave him an advantage in steering quarantine agreements. He was appointed as Her Majesty's Plenipotentiary to sign the Convention of Dresden in 1893, Paris in 1894 and Venice in 1897. In recognition of his outstanding international contributions, he was awarded a special increase in salary in 1898. His name was probably more well-known throughout Europe than John Simon's. Arthur Newsholme's most influential international period occurred after his retirement as CMO, when he made a lecture tour in the USA and also travelled to Russia to investigate Soviet health systems.

In the post Second World War era, CMOs have also been closely involved with the development of the World Health Organization, the successor to the League of Nation's Health Assembly which had operated in the inter-war period. John Charles, in particular, devoted a considerable amount of time to his various international roles. He was Chairman of the World Health Organization Executive Board in 1957–58, President of the Twelfth World Health Assembly in 1959 and Chairman of the Fourth Expert Committee on Public Health Administration of the World Health Organization in 1960. After his retirement as CMO he was appointed as a World Health Organization senior adviser in Geneva. Subsequent CMOs have maintained an active participation in the World Health Organization, both to promote British health interests and to develop effective international health policies. Godber led thirteen successive delegations to the World Health Assembly and was a member of the World Health Organization Executive for ten years. The Scottish CMO John Brotherston's significant contribution to international health was marked by the award of a Foreign Office knighthood in 1972.

World Health Assemblies became key events in the diaries of CMOs. Although some complained that the fortnight-long 'jamborees' took up too much time, they have often been key players in developing policies, such as Henry Yellowlees' involvement with the smallpox eradication campaigns in the 1970s and Donald Acheson's work on AIDS in the 1980s. Although there have been periods when the British political climate has not favoured close ties with international organisations (for example in the 1980s when Britain suspended its membership of the United Nations Education, Scientific and Cultural Organization – UNESCO), the CMO's primary interest has been in maintaining relations in the interests of national and international public health. Occasionally more politically sensitive international health developments have been led by the 'territorial' CMOs, for example during the Conservative Government (1979–1997) when the English CMO found it difficult to fund the development of World Health Organization health targets projects, and the lead was taken instead by the Welsh Office.

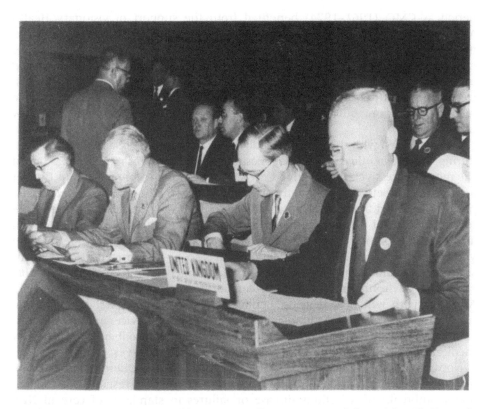

Figure 8.1 World Health Assembly in New Delhi, 1961. From left to right: Sir Kenneth Cowan (CMO Scotland), Sir John Buchanan (Medical Officer of the Commonwealth Department), Norman Roffey (Ministry of Health) and George Godber (CMO England). © Republic News Pictures.

CMOs have also fostered close relationships with their American counterparts, the Surgeon Generals. Wilson Jameson established regular meetings between British, American and Canadian health teams and these events have often proved useful occasions to informally discuss potential policy developments, thus avoiding the issues of strict American freedom of information legislation on written correspondence.

Crisis management

The third area in which the modern CMO has had to do a different job from his predecessors is the management of crises. This is not to ignore the very considerable crises which Simon and his nineteenth century contemporaries encountered – particularly sudden outbreaks of infectious diseases which they could neither predict nor control. However, as we suggested in our introduction, in the twentieth century there were increasing periods of relative calm, when the CMO could manage his priorities and adopt a more proactive stance on public health. Equally, there have been periods when the political climate has been more favourable to the CMO's initiatives. Godber, for example, during his long period as CMO (1961–1974) benefited from the support of visionary Health Ministers such as Enoch Powell. But as one health commentator favourably put it: 'He was a devious manipulator – you have to be.'[13] See, for example, how he chose not to adopt authorship of the three seminal 'cogwheel' reports published by the Ministry of Health between 1967 and 1974 on hospital medical administration. Godber thus distanced himself from any direct potential criticism from the medical profession, but remained in control of the development of this new initiative.[14]

When coupled with the fact that Godber also encountered relatively few 'crises' during his time in office, it is perhaps easier to understand his reputation as one of the most progressive and effective CMOs. The negative comments about Godber are few and far between, and many of them could be read as part of his success: he has been deemed 'incapable and unwilling to delegate' – yet perhaps this desire for overall control was appropriate to the size of team that Godber worked with and their capabilities.[15] Likewise the observation that 'he was wonderful with young people but prickly with peers' could also be interpreted as part of his strategy for maintaining his authority.[16] He worked within a relatively stable economic environment, and had a supportive group of civil servants and Ministers with which to develop significant changes in hospital planning and organisation, specialist consultants, general practitioner services and the progression of issues such as postgraduate medical education. For Godber, there were few medical crises which diverted him from his planned objectives.

Notwithstanding the BSE crisis, the last two CMOs, Acheson and Calman, appeared in the media on a regular basis, for example in response to concern about outbreaks of infectious disease or failures in standards of care in NHS hospitals. This more extensive role was perhaps inevitable given the growth of modern media outlets, the advent of 24-hour news coverage, and the need for a face and a voice to explain complex issues and what was being done about them.

This troubleshooting role in health or health service crises, and the consequent involvement with the media in explaining the background and the action being taken, is far from straightforward. It brings a requirement to speak on behalf of government. In theory this should not be problematic since the CMO is helping the government to develop and implement health policy. In practice, the CMO can easily be drawn into areas of political argument, inappropriate for the impartiality of the post. Few other civil servants speak regularly to the media. Most government policy is explained and defended by Ministers and other elected politicians. It is important that the CMO himself, and particularly government press officers, recognise the dangers of being sucked into a political argument on the back of a seemingly innocuous interview.

The CMO's reputation for integrity has been hard won since 1855 and it is important that it continues to be preserved. In a modern era this requires careful management of the CMO's dealings with a media which is ever hungry for his views and opinions. There have, for example, been suggestions that CMOs should be directly accountable to Parliament – that in the interests of public health and

---

[13] Interview, 22.05.2002.
[14] The reports gained their nickname from the pattern of cogwheels on their covers.
[15] Senior medical civil servant interview, 22.07.2002.
[16] Health commentator interview, 08.06.2000.

open government they should be allowed to give their expert opinion in answer to parliamentary questions.[17]

There have been relatively few periods in the history of the CMO post when the incumbent has had a large cadre of staff accountable to him. Indeed, at many times in the past the size of the CMO's team has been a major bone of contention. Within the senior civil service, the number of people a person is responsible for, and the size of his or her departmental budget, equates to the power of the post. Indeed, the grading and remuneration of civil service posts is determined by such issues.

During the late 1980s and early 1990s, Whitehall became more managerial in its orientation. Within the Department of Health, the National Health Service Executive (which was established to run the NHS) required the Department's senior officials to have a corporate role within the new structure. Both Acheson and Calman had seats on the National Health Service Executive Board. This too brought its tensions. If the CMO was to be involved in the management of the NHS, even at a very strategic level, he was no longer a mere adviser but someone who carried a share of accountability for decisions made, whether good or bad. If the CMO was to accept this role then he needed staff to support him. Neither Acheson (latterly) nor Calman had this support although this was remedied when Calman's post was filled.

Life after CMO?

Even the activities and comments of retired CMOs can hold considerable authority with government, the medical profession and, to a lesser extent, the public. Several have developed substantial post-CMO careers. Both Newman and Newsholme were in demand internationally as visiting speakers and lecturers; Jameson accepted a number of significant roles, including positions at the King's Fund and Chair of the Medical Research Council's Social and Environmental Health Committee. Like other CMOs he also served on Royal Commissions and played an active role in Royal Colleges and medical institutions such as the General Medical Council. He was influential as a member of the steering committee for the establishment of the College of General Practitioners. Charles went on to a further career as an international health adviser at the World Health Organization in Geneva.

Godber perhaps did not develop a retirement role to the extent that he could have, had he wished to. However, when he did make statements they were taken seriously. His speech at the Annual General Meeting of the British Medical Association on 9 July 1980, seven years after his retirement as CMO, still generated discussion and comment.[18] His astute observations on the importance of engaging external expertise and the value of non-political medical leadership were well-received. His plainly worded demand for a system of professional performance review, which the Americans had instituted some five years earlier, was a pointed wake-up call to the government and the medical profession which could not go unheeded. Even in retirement, his influence has been considerable.

[17] 'Labour targets the Chief Medical Officer', *British Medical Journal*, 1996, 312, 998.
[18] GE Godber, 'Doctors in government', *Health Trends*, 1981, 1 (13), 1–4.

As one of his successors put it: 'The Mount Godber volcano is still far from extinct.'[19]

What broad issues arise from this 143-year analysis? It is clear that some elements of the post have remained much the same, and that there are some factors which predicted the success of the CMO in meeting his objectives. There were certainly periods when it was relatively harder to be a CMO. Periods of economic crisis and political uncertainty, in which senior teams changed frequently or the CMO was not part of the 'inner circle', hindered the development of health policies or damaged relations with the medical profession. Outbreaks of diseases were usually beyond human control, but responses to them were very much within the capacity of a well-structured government system.

One factor which we have returned to repeatedly during this study has been that of individual personality and authority. It has underpinned most of the key issues discussed, especially those which have required the CMO to foster White-hall expertise or to be able to obtain it from external sources. Building a national and international reputation was critical to the ability to integrate knowledge and to facilitate the central relationship between the government and the medical profession. The Whitehall and medical communities are remarkably small, in which pedigree, image and the ability to 'network' may often overshadow more substantive qualities. What emerges from the case studies is that both parties have a very clear, almost identical idea of what constitutes a successful CMO, but both sides expect those essential attributes to work in their favour. However, not all CMOs have been conscious of the importance of these issues, and it appears to have been an intermittent concern for their selection panels.

Today's CMO inherits a portfolio which has accrued over a long period. Increasingly, over the last fifteen years it has been shaped by external events, crises and scrutinies of the role of government in relation to public health and the NHS. The portfolio falls into three broad strands: the promotion of the health of the population, the protection of the public health and the enhancement of the quality of clinical care in the NHS. A fourth strand involves a wide range of work in policy making, the review of major health issues and projects, and crisis management. Such work is allocated to the CMO in varying amounts, depending on the degree of confidence which the government has in him. Today's CMO holds this portfolio not as a detached adviser but with accountability for the quality of this work and for the results achieved.

The unique position of the CMO in England is unparalleled throughout the world. Today's CMO inherits the mantle of his fourteen predecessors. His aim must be to pursue a set of health ideals without fear or favour and to preserve for the future the integrity, dignity and influence of the office and its power to do good.

[19] D Acheson, 'Eighty-five not out: essays to honour Sir George Godber', *British Medical Journal*, 1994, 309, 1174–5.

CMO profiles

John Simon

DoB 10.10.1816
DoD 23.07.1904

CMO 1855–1876 (21 years)
Resigned

Simon is probably the one person most associated with Victorian sanitary reform. He was the last of fourteen children in an Anglo-French family, educated partly in Germany before being apprenticed to the first Professor of Surgery at King's College, London in 1833. In 1838 Simon took the MRCS and was appointed as Assistant Surgeon at King's College. After a meteoric rise, he was appointed Lecturer in Surgery at St Thomas's Hospital in 1847, having already published widely on scientific, social and philosophical issues. In 1848, through the efforts of Edwin Chadwick, the first national Public Health Act was passed, which established a General Board of Health (initially without medical representation). Under a local Act in 1848 London established a Public Health Department and Simon was appointed as Medical Officer of Health – the second in the country after Dr William Henry Duncan in Liverpool in 1847. Simon developed the role to collect and interpret mortality and morbidity information on a weekly basis, and to advise on sanitary improvements which were essential – clean water supplies, a sewerage system, less overcrowding, removal of 'nuisances'. All his strategies were made at a time when the exact nature of disease transmission was not understood, but he established for himself a national reputation and his annual reports were widely read. He strongly and publicly advocated the creation of a Ministry of Health, with a constituted parliamentary head and access to impartial expert medical advice. This was not an option compatible with the mid-nineteenth century *laissez-faire* attitude to personal and public health.

In 1855 Simon moved from his London post to be Medical Officer to the General Board of Health, and on that body's dissolution in 1858 he moved to the new Medical Department at the Privy Council. For the first time the country now had a nominated medical adviser. The post at the Privy Council was made permanent (it had been renewed yearly at the General Board of Health). He used his position to publish a series of reviews of health policies, including the effectiveness of smallpox vaccination. One of his most valuable reports came in 1858, *Report on the Sanitary State of the People of England*, which for the first time demonstrated the wide national variations in various disease rates and emphasised the need for impartial, skilled inquiry and publication of such facts.

Simon's conception of public health was as a broad and wide-reaching science. His ambitions for the discipline were constrained by his position within the

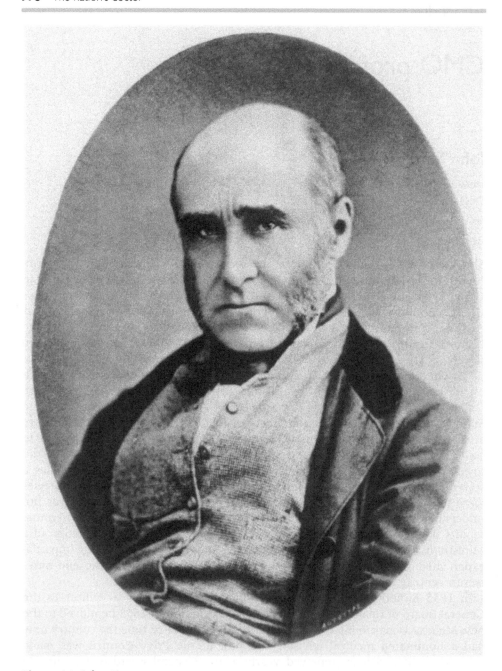

Figure A1 John Simon.

government system, first at the Privy Council, where he had limited statutory duties for vaccination, epidemic disease regulations, quarantine and the Medical Acts. However, he managed to bring together a group of dedicated and enthusiastic medical experts, including his successors – Seaton, Buchanan, Thorne Thorne and Power – who provided him with statistical evidence to substantiate his public health policies. This was evidence-based policy making well before Cochrane. He administered the reformed vaccination system following the 1867 Vaccination Act, and investigated and reported on industrial health, housing conditions and hospital provision. He also advised the Registrar General on how vital statistics could best be collated for health policy purposes and was instrumental in the development of decennial and quarterly supplements for the Registrar General's annual reports. Simon also revised the British government's approach to quarantine measures, and from 1871 a new system of Port Sanitary Authorities was created. His most successful activity during the Privy Council years was to advise the Royal Sanitary Commission in 1868 on the creation of local sanitary authorities.

In 1871 his department was inconsiderately grouped with the Poor Law at the new Local Government Board – an arrangement Simon openly and fiercely criticised, although the new structure included the statutory sanitary authorities which he had advocated. The new Board was little more than the old Poor Law Board, with Simon's Medical Department subordinated to the Poor Law secretariat. It perpetuated all the old traditions of petty interference and over-centralisation. Simon was powerless in the discussions about the creation of the new sanitary districts and the medical investigations were reduced, with some inspections being carried out by non-medical Poor Law inspectors. Simon found the regime and culture at the Local Government Board intolerable and resigned in 1876, disillusioned with his role and the lost opportunities for improving the health of the nation. After his resignation he wrote: 'I believe we had the credit of earnestly endeavouring to learn the truth, and to tell the truth, as to matters which our inquiries regarded.'

During his retirement he continued to write, and published *English Sanitary Institutions* in 1890. Throughout his long life he found inspiration in his close intellectual friendships, most notably with John Ruskin and Sir Edward Burne-Jones.

Obituary: *Lancet*, 1904, (II), 320–5; C Hamlin, 'Simon, Sir John (1816–1904)', *Oxford Dictionary of National Biography* (Oxford, Oxford University Press, 2004); R Lambert, *Sir John Simon 1816–1904 and English Social Administration* (London, McGibbon & Kee, 1963).

Edward Cator Seaton

DoB 1815
DoD 21.01.1880

CMO 1876–1879 (3 years)
Died before officially retiring

Born into a Scottish family and son of a naval surgeon, Seaton studied Medicine at Edinburgh, gaining his MD there in 1837. He moved to London in 1841 and

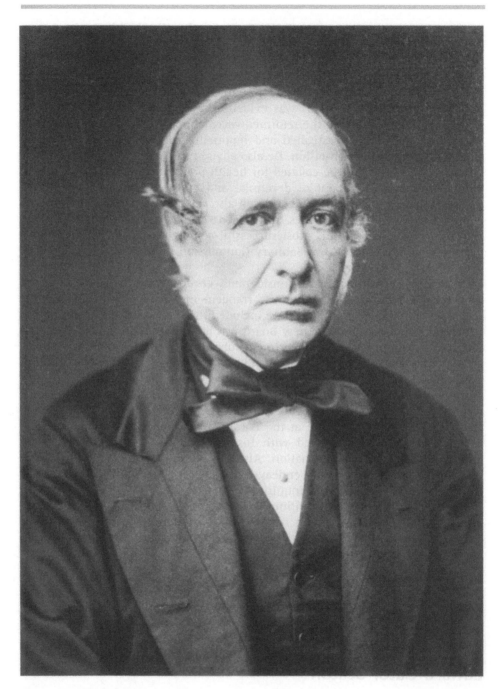

Figure A2 Edward Cator Seaton.

established a practice in Sloane Street, also serving as surgeon to the Chelsea Dispensary. One of his main interests was vaccination. He was appointed as Honorary Secretary to a committee of the Epidemiological Society of London which was formed in 1850 to investigate smallpox vaccination (he also served as President of the Society). The committee's report, which was largely the work of Seaton, was presented to Parliament in 1852 and provided a definitive model for vaccination procedures. Seaton made his professional reputation with this research and John Simon selected Seaton as his vaccination inspector under the 1853 Vaccination Act.

Seaton remained in private practice, although he was increasingly called upon by John Simon for advice on vaccination issues. From 1858 he worked as an Inspector for the Medical Department at the Privy Council under the leadership of Simon, where his investigations illuminated the patchy vaccination arrangements in some parts of the country. His reports provided the evidence for an amendment to the vaccination law. His position at the Privy Council was not made permanent until 1865, when he was appointed as Superintending Inspector of the National Vaccine Establishment, becoming Director there in 1871.

In 1871 Seaton moved with Simon to the new Local Government Board as Senior Assistant Medical Officer. He continued to develop his expertise in vaccination, publishing a *Handbook of Vaccination* in 1867. He also represented the government at the International Sanitary Conference in Vienna in 1874. When John Simon resigned in 1876, Seaton took over the position, although he was paid a smaller salary and suffered from diminished authority. The stresses and low morale at the Medical Department at the Local Government Board un-doubtedly exacerbated his ill-health. He was unable to work fully during his last year, 1879, taking six months' leave to recuperate abroad.

His family was well-connected in the late nineteenth century public health arena with his son serving as Medical Officer of Health for Nottingham, and one of his daughters married to Dr George Buchanan, his successor as CMO. His obituaries commented on his honesty and his reputation as a good disciplinarian. He was also praised for his great power of organisation combined with rare tact and judgement.

Obituary: *British Medical Journal*, 1880, (I), 188–9; D Brunton, 'Seaton, Edward Cator (1815–1880)', *Oxford Dictionary of National Biography* (Oxford, Oxford University Press, 2004).

George Buchanan

DoB 05.11.1831
DoD 05.05.1895

CMO 1880–1892 (12 years)
Retired

George Buchanan was born into a medical family in Clerkenwell, London and graduated MD from University College, London in 1855. He suffered from typhus fever while completing his MD, and he wrote this up later as a case study in Reynolds' *Medicine*. His first post was as Health Officer for the London district of St Giles, where he developed his experience in public health. His particular areas of

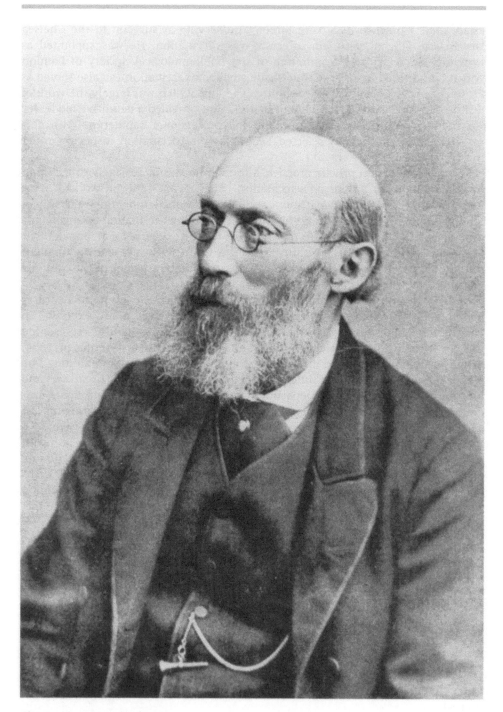

Figure A3 George Buchanan.

interest included the relationship between overcrowding and ill-health and developing anti-smallpox and cholera strategies. He also served as a Medical Officer at the London Fever Hospital and then as Physician at Great Ormond Street Hospital for Sick Children. During his time there he was elected a Fellow of the Royal College of Physicians in 1866 and he delivered the Lettsonian lectures on lung diseases of children in 1867. Between 1861 and 1869 he acted as a temporary inspector for John Simon at the Privy Council, while also making a living as a consultant in children's diseases. He reported and advised on improvements to vaccination policy, resulting in the Amending Act of 1867. He also investigated the typhus outbreaks associated with the 1862 cotton famine, living in affected communities so that he could observe the epidemic more closely. In 1869 he became a permanent Inspector under John Simon at the Privy Council. After the death of Seaton he became Principal Medical Officer in 1880.

His twelve years as CMO witnessed enormous changes to public health policy and practice, informed by new and more accurate theories on how diseases were transmitted, based on the work of Robert Koch and Louis Pasteur. Buchanan had the ability to incorporate this new information into the planning of the Medical Department at the Local Government Board, although his plans were continuously thwarted by the tight financial restrictions imposed by the Treasury. He actively promoted new scientific research. The government of health became increasingly professionalised by the end of the nineteenth century, with the rise of the medical expert balanced by the emergence of the professional civil servant. Buchanan was recognised by his contemporaries as having the necessary 'charm of manner, generosity of spirit and ability to win the confidence, respect and affection of all with whom he came into contact'. He was well-connected in medical circles and recognised the importance of close contact with the Royal Colleges and the General Medical Council (formed in 1858). He was married to his predecessor's daughter, Alice Seaton, who he had met while assisting Seaton with his vaccination studies. His son, George Seaton Buchanan, secured a high-ranking position in his father's department as a Senior Medical Officer.

He retired prematurely in 1892 because of ill-health but was persuaded almost immediately to become Chairman of the Royal Commission on Tuberculosis. His substantial contribution to public health was recognised through his knighthood on his retirement and the creation of the Buchanan gold medal at the Royal Society (the first award of the medal was to John Simon in 1897 as 'Founder of Modern Sanitary Science').

Obituary: *British Medical Journal*, 1895, (I), 1066–7; *Lancet*, 1895, (I), 1224–5; A Hardy, 'Buchanan, Sir George (1831–1895)', *Oxford Dictionary of National Biography* (Oxford, Oxford University Press, 2004).

Richard Thorne Thorne

DoB 13.10.1841
DoD 18.12.1899

CMO 1892–1899 (7 years)
Died in office

Thorne Thorne was educated partly in Europe before returning to England and graduating from London University in 1866. He did his medical training at St Bartholomew's Hospital and held his first post there, before moving as Physician to the Royal Hospital for Diseases of the Chest and the London Fever Hospital. During this time, he occasionally worked as an Inspector for John Simon, investigating and reporting on outbreaks of typhoid fever (substantiating theories that it was a water-borne disease) and the effects of foot and mouth disease on the value of milk supplies. His ability persuaded Simon to offer him a permanent position as Inspector in 1870 and he produced significant reports, including a comprehensive survey of isolation hospital provision in England and continental comparisons.

When he succeeded Buchanan as CMO in 1892, Thorne Thorne inherited a Medical Department with a wide range of statutory duties, but a relatively small staff (two Assistant Medical Officers and 11 permanent Inspectors). His primary duty was to advise the Local Government Board on all matters involving medicine and public health. He thus developed contacts nationally and internationally, particularly during the 1880s cholera pandemic. From 1884 he was seconded several times at the request of the Colonial and Foreign Offices to international conferences, where his fluent French gave him an advantage in steering quarantine agreements. He was appointed as Her Majesty's Plenipotentiary to sign the Convention of Dresden in 1893, Paris in 1894 and Venice in 1897, and in recognition of his outstanding contributions he was awarded a special increase in salary in 1898. His name was probably more well-known throughout Europe than John Simon's.

In addition to developing the role of the CMO in international health affairs, Thorne Thorne also put effort into consolidating the relationship between the government and the medical profession. He replaced John Simon as a Crown Nominee at the General Medical Council in 1895 having previously served on several of its committees and contributed to the drafting of its regulations. As Chairman of its Public Health Committee he helped to frame the regulations for the Diploma in Public Health, and he also directed the negotiations on the Midwives Bill. He also had close relations with the Royal Colleges (he gave the Milroy lecture in 1891). He continued to maintain contact with St Bartholomew's Hospital, lecturing there on hygiene from 1879, and he was appointed to the new Lectureship in Public Health in 1891.

His obituary in the *British Medical Journal* provides a good insight into how he had developed his role as CMO:

> Accurate and painstaking, yet free from pedantry; firm in his own opinion, but courteous in word and manner, he belonged to the very best type of British government official – a body of men who it has been said are the real rulers of the country. But it would be the very

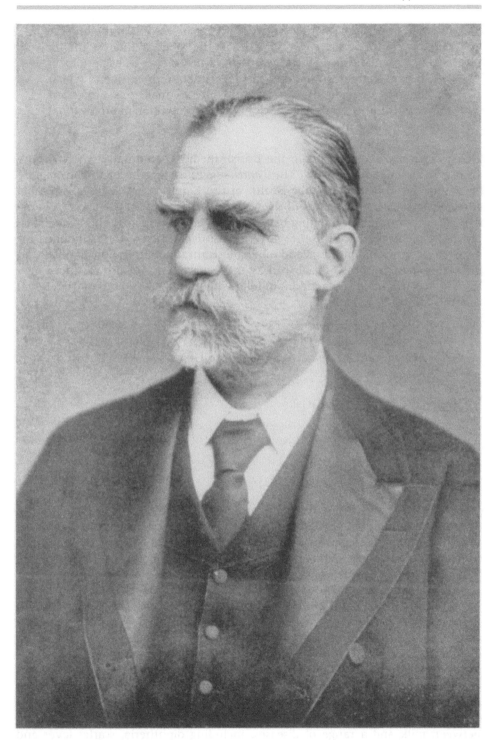

Figure A4 Richard Thorne Thorne.

opposite of truth to say that he ever sank his profession in the official. On the contrary, his eager mind took the keenest interest in the advance of medicine and in the growth of the science of bacteriology, which has so largely influenced the department of medicine to which his life was devoted. He knew, too, how to make his profession respected, and was rightly a stickler for due recognition of professional services by the Government.

There was a real sense of loss in the British medical community when Thorne Thorne died suddenly in 1899. The *Lancet* suggested that he had been 'rapidly becoming the Minister of Public Health of the Empire'. He made considerable advances in securing the status of the Medical Department of the Local Government Board, through negotiating better salaries and contracts for his staff and in providing medical advice to other government departments. He maintained his research interests in diphtheria and tuberculosis throughout his time in office and integrated them into the official work of the Department. He also produced new legislation on smallpox vaccination following the 1898 report of the Royal Commission on Vaccination.

Obituary: *British Medical Journal*, 1899, (II), 1771–3; *Lancet*, 1899, (II), 1762–6; D'A Power, rev. P Wallis, 'Thorne, Sir Richard Thorne (1841–1899)', *Oxford Dictionary of National Biography* (Oxford, Oxford University Press, 2004).

William Henry Power

DoB 15.12.1842
DoD 28.07.1916

CMO 1900–1908 (8 years)
Retired

William Power was of the same generation as his predecessors Richard Thorne Thorne and George Buchanan, and he was also mentored by John Simon for his role in the Medical Department at the Local Government Board. He graduated from University College, London and trained at St Bartholomew's Hospital before working as Resident Medical Officer at the Victoria Park Hospital for Diseases of the Chest. He held several posts in clinical medicine and surgery, having obtained his MRCS in 1864. From 1871 he worked as a temporary Inspector for John Simon and the position was made permanent in 1875. He shared with Simon an active interest in smallpox. During and after the 1871 and 1884 epidemics he conducted a series of investigations which he thought proved that smallpox was an airborne disease, based mainly on his observation that there were more cases around smallpox isolation hospitals. He thus pushed for the relocation of isolation hospitals in less populated areas.

Power also used his epidemiological skills to try to understand the relationship between milk and a range of diseases, including diphtheria, scarlet fever and enteric fever. His meticulous surveys came at a time of scientific debate on whether diseases could be passed between animals and humans, in the absence of any bacteriological proof. In 1887 he directed the Medical Department of the Local Government Board in studying outbreaks of lead poisoning in water

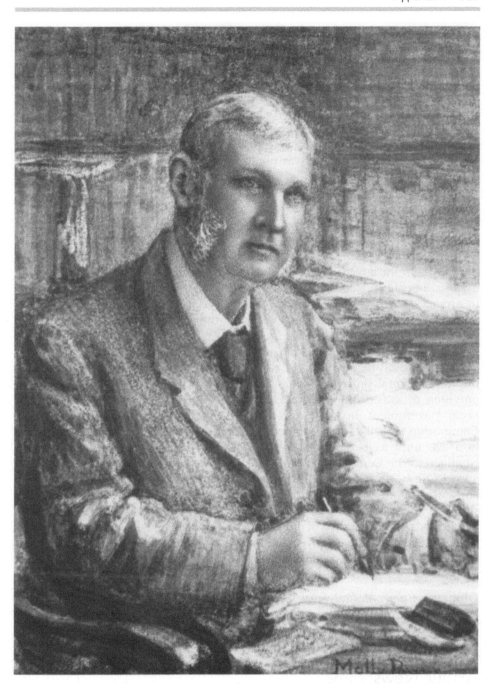

Figure A5 William Henry Power.

supplies. Power hypothesised that the lead pipes were being dissolved by soft moorland waters and he successfully directed the introduction of techniques to reduce the acidity of these waters. He is also renowned for using his extensive natural history knowledge to solve the riddle of how eels got into the water pipes in certain parts of London in the 1880s (he was able to show that eels could move a long distance over land, and that they had been moving from a small stream and then falling through gaps in the cover of a reservoir).

Between 1887 and 1900 he worked as an Assistant Medical Inspector at the Local Government Board. He was not a prominent figure during this time, and apparently was responsible for the training of junior staff in the Medical Department, placing emphasis on their ability to produce high-quality reports based on sound scientific research. This period of public health history is characterised by increasingly frequent local inspections, identifying insanitary areas and forcing local authorities to take action. In 1900, on the sudden death of Richard Thorne Thorne, he was appointed as CMO. His time in this office is significant for the advances made in food safety – with a special subdepartment of the Board being created by Power for this purpose in 1905. Power went so far as to arrange for his Inspectors to travel to meat-processing plants in North and South America to regulate the quality of the meat destined for the British consumer.

Power continued the work of Thorne Thorne on the Royal Commission on Sewage Disposal. He also worked closely with the commissioners appointed for the Royal Commission on Tuberculosis from 1901, particularly investigating the provision of sanatorium accommodation, which was the responsibility of the Local Government Board. He took over as Chairman of the Tuberculosis Commission in 1907 and continued to serve, even after his retirement as CMO in 1908, until its close in 1911. Like his predecessors, he served as Crown Nominee to the General Medical Council and received a range of honours and awards. He was notable for his dedication to his hobbies, including ornithology and duck shooting. According to his obituary in the *British Medical Journal*, 'He shunned any occasion which would bring him prominently before an audience, and he had a physical dread of notoriety. It is impossible to do such a man justice.' His wife died after only four years of marriage, leaving him with two daughters. He was buried at Brookwood Cemetery in Surrey, a few feet away from his close friend, and former CMO, George Buchanan.

Obituary: *British Medical Journal*, 1916, (I), 203–7; *Lancet*, 1916, (I), 244–6; A Hardy, 'Power, Sir William Henry (1842–1916)', *Oxford Dictionary of National Biography* (Oxford, Oxford University Press, 2004).

Arthur Newsholme

DoB 10.02.1857
DoD 17.05.1943

CMO 1908–1919 (11 years)
Retired

In contrast to his predecessor, Power, Arthur Newsholme was a prominent and internationally acclaimed champion of British public health. His time in office

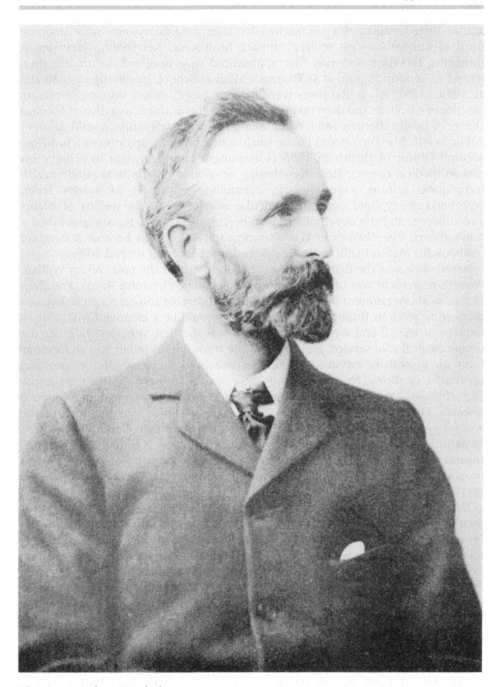

Figure A6 Arthur Newsholme.

spanned the creation of a comprehensive state medical system, only stopping short of universal access to free primary healthcare. Newsholme grew up in Haworth, Yorkshire and was first apprenticed to a Bradford doctor. He then moved to London to train at St Thomas's Medical School, qualifying in 1880 and as MD in 1881. His initial posts were hospital based, before moving to private practice in Clapham and then taking a part-time appointment as a district Medical Officer of Health there in 1884. After taking the new professional qualification in public health (the Diploma in Public Health) he moved to Brighton as a full-time Medical Officer of Health in 1888 (sustaining a loss of income to achieve his chosen medical career). Here Newsholme developed his practical public health techniques, gaining experience in controlling outbreaks of scarlet fever, diphtheria and typhoid fever. His particular interest was in the welfare of infants and children, and the development of tuberculosis services. He also published a seminal text, *The Elements of Vital Statistics*, in 1889, which became a standard textbook for Medical Officers of Health and went through several editions.

Newsholme was the first CMO to be 'headhunted' for the post. When William Power's retirement was imminent, he was approached by John Burns, President of the Local Government Board. Burns had considerable respect for Newsholme's pioneering work in Brighton and thought he would be a creative CMO, able to implement the Liberal welfare reforms. He was the first 'outsider' to enter the senior medical civil service, and oversaw the transition in public health ideology from an essentially environmentalist approach to an emphasis on personal preventive medicine. Newsholme thus developed three new services – maternity and child welfare, tuberculosis medical services and a service for venereal diseases. During his time as CMO much wider reforms were planned to the welfare system, following a Royal Commission on the Poor Law. Newsholme's Department also had to administer the consequences of the new National Insurance Act of 1911, although he had opposed some parts of Lloyd George's proposals because he feared they would compromise the valuable disease prevention work of local authorities.

The First World War stifled some of Newsholme's plans at the Local Government Board and his last year in office was marked by the influenza pandemic. He resigned on the eve of the creation of the Ministry of Health and immediately travelled to the USA where he completed a large lecture tour to promote infant and child welfare. He spent some time lecturing on public health administration at Johns Hopkins University in Baltimore. During his time in America, in his sixties, he also learnt how to drive. He travelled widely in Europe on behalf of the Milbank Fund to make a major study of healthcare systems, which resulted in the publication of *International Studies on the Relation between Private and Official Practice of Medicine* (1931) and *Medicine and the State* (1932). On his return from Russia in 1933 he co-authored a book entitled *Red Medicine* with John Kingsbury, Secretary of the Milbank Fund. Newsholme was a prolific writer, rivalling John Simon in the quality and quantity of his publications, with 25 books and over 160 articles and book chapters to his name, as well as many reports and pamphlets.

Obituary: *British Medical Journal*, 1943, (I), 680–1; *Lancet*, 1943, (I), 696; JM Eyler, 'Newsholme, Sir Arthur (1857–1943)', *Oxford Dictionary of National Biography* (Oxford, Oxford University Press, 2004); JM Eyler, *Sir Arthur Newsholme and State Medicine, 1885–1935* (Cambridge, Cambridge University Press, 1997).

George Newman

DoB 23.10.1870
DoD 26.05.1948

CMO 1919–1935 (16 years)
Retired

Newman inherited a very different role as CMO from that developed by John Simon in the 1850s. He came into a new administrative structure, the Ministry of Health, which for the first time gave health direct government representation. The establishment of the Ministry tested the *status quo* within the civil service between the medical and administrative staff, with Newman battling to have equal access to the Minister alongside the Permanent Secretary. This period also witnessed the development of the CMO's role as arbitrator between the medical profession and the government, as the state began to encroach significantly into the areas of medicine previously respected as the domain of the private practitioner.

Newman was born into a Quaker family in Shropshire. He studied medicine at Edinburgh University, qualifying in 1892 before moving as Assistant Physician to the London Medical Mission. He pursued his interest in public health, lecturing and working part-time for the Medical Officer of Health of the Strand Board of Works on research into local living conditions. In 1894 he registered at King's College, London to study for the Cambridge University Diploma in Public Health, which he passed in 1895. He was then appointed part-time Demonstrator at King's College, teaching practical classes in bacteriology, which allowed him to undertake research for a book, *Bacteria*, published in 1899.

In 1896 he was offered a position as a Medical Inspector at the Local Government Board, but turned it down as he wished for a local authority Medical Officer of Health position. He was appointed part-time Medical Officer of Health to the Holborn Board of Guardians in 1897, while continuing to devote some of his time to Quaker societies (he edited *The Friend's Quarterly Examiner* anonymously from 1899 until his death). His reputation in public health was growing, and he was offered the post of Government Bacteriologist to the India Office, which he declined. His first full-time position as Medical Officer of Health came in 1900 when he was appointed to the new metropolitan borough of Finsbury – a poor, overcrowded area with a high level of infant mortality. Newman spent the next six years instituting strict public health surveillance regimes, health education programmes and an infant milk depot. He developed his academic interest in public health, published several key papers and books, and from 1905 lectured in public health at St Bartholomew's Medical School.

Through his association with Beatrice Webb, Newman presented evidence to the Royal Commission on the Poor Laws, stressing the relatively new idea that the state should provide preventive as well as curative medical services. Through Webb he came into contact with Sir Robert Morant, Permanent Secretary to the Board of Education, and through him he was appointed to the new post of Chief Medical Officer to the Board of Education in 1907, the year in which a system of medical inspection and medical care of school children was established. His appointment was greeted with hostility from some in the medical profession, who took this as a sign of the state's restriction of private practice. Newman

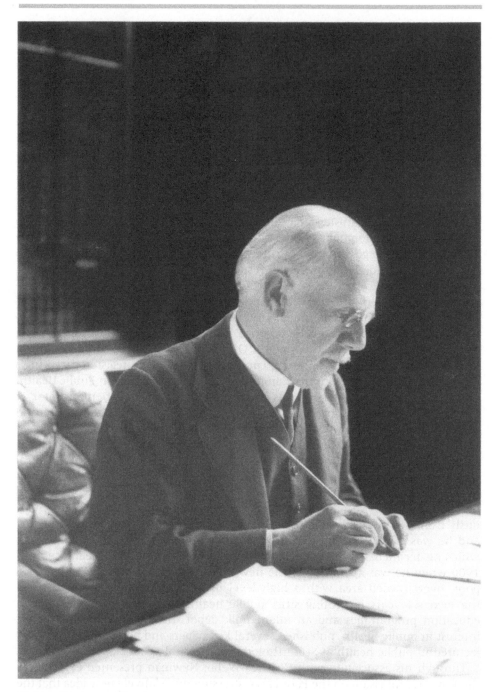

Figure A7 George Newman.

helped to create a comprehensive tuberculosis service out of the National Health Insurance legislation of 1911, and to found the Medical Research Committee (later Medical Research Council) in 1913. His plans for the School Medical Service were delayed due to the outbreak of the First World War in 1914 and he found himself with additional wartime duties, including Medical Officer to the Central Control Board for Liquor Traffic – which he used to express his Quaker temperance beliefs.

From 1916 Newman worked closely with Morant and Addison (Minister for Reconstruction) to develop a plan for a Ministry of Health. On 1 April 1919, Newman was appointed as CMO to the Local Government Board, transferring two months later to the new Ministry alongside Morant as Permanent Secretary and Addison as the first Minister of Health. They had hoped to create an administration in which the medical staff would have equal status and pay with the lay officials. In reality, Newman was not given the official civil service rank of Permanent Secretary which he had wished for. Although he did secure the right to direct access to the Minister (i.e. not through the Permanent Secretary), this was an *ad hominem* concession and did not attach to the post of CMO. His influence in the Ministry was further reduced when Morant died suddenly from influenza in 1920 and when Addison was forced to resign as Minister in 1921.

Having secured the post of CMO within the new Ministry, Newman appeared to lack further creative energy, and his time in office did not produce significant policy developments. He spent his time summarising the state of the nation's health in a series of monumental Annual Reports and in public lectures on his personal vision of preventive medicine. He did, however, work hard at developing a good relationship with the leading members of the medical profession and by continuing as CMO to the Board of Education he ensured co-ordination between medical services. Newman also used his position at the Board of Education in the inter-war years to pursue reforms in medical education, in particular urging that control of clinical training should be taken away from the élite private practitioners and placed with university-based academic teachers.

Obituary: *British Medical Journal*, 1948, (I), 1112–13; *Lancet*, 1948, (I), 888–9; S Sturdy, 'Newman, Sir George (1870–1948)', *Oxford Dictionary of National Biography* (Oxford, Oxford University Press, 2004).

Arthur MacNalty

DoB 20.10.1880
DoD 17.04.1969

CMO 1935–1940 (5 years)
Retired

MacNalty, like so many of the CMOs before him, was born into a medical family. His father was a practitioner in Winchester. MacNalty was educated in Southampton and Oxford and graduated in Physiology in 1904. He completed his medical training at University College, London, qualifying in 1907 at the relatively late age of 27. He then held posts at the Brompton Hospital, specialising in tuberculosis, simultaneously doing research at University College with Sir Victor Horsely on the cerebellum and later with Sir Thomas Lewis on the first use

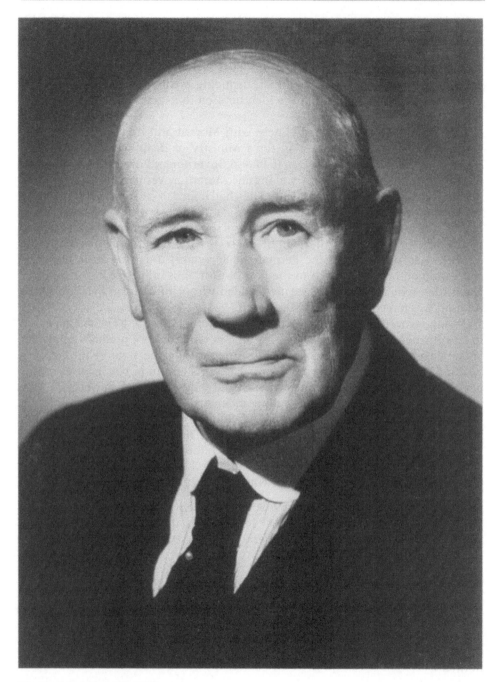

Figure A8 Arthur MacNalty.

of the electrocardiograph for the diagnosis of heart disease. His interest in preventive medicine was encouraged when Sir John Burns, President of the Local Government Board, offered him a medical inspectorship on the advice of Arthur Newsholme in 1913. To prepare for this post, MacNalty worked as an Assistant Medical Officer of Health at Essex County Council. At the Local Government Board he was involved with administering tuberculosis services and served as Secretary to the Medical Research Council's Tuberculosis Committees. He was seconded in 1914 to inspect military camps and hospitals, but continued his research programmes during the war and in 1918 he gave the first clinical review of a 'new' disease – encephalitis lethargica.

From 1919 to 1932 MacNalty was a deputy Senior Medical Officer at the Ministry of Health, working under Newman researching and reporting on tuberculosis treatments, poliomyelitis and the development of the intradermal tuberculin test for bovine tuberculosis. He continued to develop his professional skills, and gained the Diploma in Public Health in 1927, but did not move around the medical divisions within the Ministry as most of the medical staff were expected to do. In 1932 he was promoted to Deputy CMO, the first time an official Deputy had been appointed, possibly because Newman was so often away on CMO duties. His special functions were 'particularly in regard to the better co-ordination and organisation of the work of the medical staff'. He was seen within the Ministry as Newman's heir apparent, although he was not well-known among the public health staff in the country. He succeeded Newman as CMO in 1935 at the age of 55 years. His tenure as CMO was short and overshadowed by the threat of another war in Europe. His time was taken up with planning the Emergency Medical Service (which subsequently formed the basis for the Public Health Laboratory Service) and nursing services for the war (including medical administration of evacuation schemes). He was, however, also responsible for advising the Minister of Health to set up the Athlone Committee to advise on conditions and pay for nursing staff, the implementation of the 1936 Midwives Act and the creation of a cancer service. He also, somewhat belatedly, advised the Minister to make free supplies of diphtheria vaccine available to local authorities in 1940. This was nearly twenty years after the Canadians had introduced a successful national vaccination system. Britain endured an estimated excess 40,000 diphtheria deaths in the 1920s and 1930s because of the reluctance of the government to follow the Canadian example.

MacNalty retired aged 60 years in 1940, ostensibly to coincide with a reorganisation by Malcolm MacDonald, who had been appointed as Minister of Health in May 1940. He was almost immediately appointed by Winston Churchill as Editor-in-Chief of the *Official Medical History of the Second World War*, which he continued to direct from the Ministry of Health headquarters at 23 Saville Row for nearly 30 years until his death (officially as a part-time employee of the Ministry). He contributed several sections to this twenty-volume work, and published a large number of histories and historical novels. He was also commissioned by the Nuffield College Reconstruction Survey in 1941 to contribute to its investigations into the reform of local government and he published *Reform of the Public Health Services* in 1943. He continued to participate very actively in public life after his retirement as CMO, giving a series of lectures to medical institutions, continuing as Crown Nominee to the General Medical Council until 1943, and as an honorary physician to King George VI.

When MacNalty died aged 88 years in 1969, George Godber wrote in the *Lancet*:

> He was essentially a scholar and a physician, and his shyness made him less well-known to his staff than his predecessor had been. But he was a kindly man with an enduring interest, long after his retirement, in the progress of those he had introduced to the Medical Civil Service. To have continued, as he did, working under each of his three successors in turn was a remarkable thing for a senior man to have done in any service. He will be remembered for his erudition and for his kindliness by all with whom he worked.

Obituary: *British Medical Journal*, 1969, (I), 252–3; *Lancet*, 1969, (I), 896–7; GE Godber, rev. M Bevan, 'MacNalty, Sir Arthur Salusbury (1880–1969)', *Oxford Dictionary of National Biography* (Oxford, Oxford University Press, 2004).

(William) Wilson Jameson

DoB 12.05.1885
DoD 18.10.1962

CMO 1940–1950 (10 years)
Retired

Jameson's ten years as CMO witnessed the most dramatic shake-up of healthcare which Britain has ever seen. On 5 July 1948 the National Health Service came to life, delivering free healthcare for all. Jameson had played a vital role in the creation of the NHS, at the same time changing the role of the CMO.

Jameson was born in Perth and educated in Aberdeen. He qualified there in medicine in 1909 before moving to London to a series of hospital posts. After a brief spell in general practice he returned to hospital medicine and gained the Diploma in Public Health at University College, London in 1914. During the First World War he worked at the Royal Army Medical Corps Hygiene Laboratory at Aldershot and was then posted to a hygiene laboratory in Italy. After the war he resumed his teaching at University College and took up a post as Medical Officer of Health in Finchley and St Marylebone in 1920. His first public health publication, *Synopsis of Hygiene*, appeared in the same year.

While pursuing his medical career, Jameson also trained in law and was called to the Bar in 1922. His primary interest, however, was public health, and he obtained a promotion to be Medical Officer of Health for Hornsey in 1925. Four years later he abandoned this practical career and devoted himself to academic medicine, becoming the first Professor of Public Health at London University in 1929, coinciding with the opening of the London School of Hygiene and Tropical Medicine (LSHTM). Jameson's appointment was welcomed by the then CMO George Newman, who saw him as an ally in the development of the discipline of public health. In 1931 he became Dean of the LSHTM, a post he held until his departure for Whitehall in 1940. Jameson made several lengthy trips to Europe, Africa, Asia and North America to develop his interest in industrial health, maternity and child welfare, and tuberculosis. He also constructed a state-of-the-art Diploma in Public Health at the LSHTM, calling upon a wide range of eminent experts to provide guest lectures, which attracted students from all over

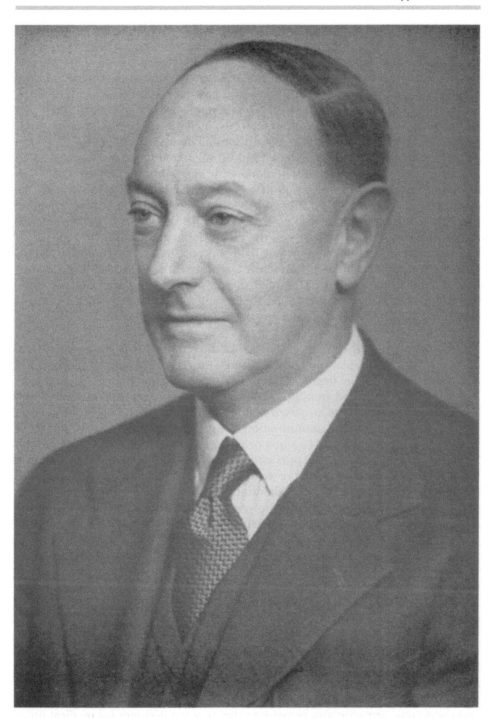

Figure A9 Wilson Jameson.

the world. He proved a valuable link between academic, practical and government health circles, integrating members of the Ministry of Health and the Medical Research Council into the Board of Management at the LSHTM, and serving himself on numerous government advisory committees. He was also a member of the Preposterous Club (pre- and post-parturition), which had seven obstetricians, seven paediatricians and seven public health specialists. They met five times a year to discuss common interests, including a special set of meetings before the 1936 Midwives Bill to assist informally with its production.

When George Newman retired in 1935 he suggested that Jameson should be the next CMO. He was short-listed along with MacNalty, the Deputy CMO, but did not have the necessary range of experience or reputation to succeed. He apparently also expressed a dislike of the Ministry culture at that time, claiming that 'the whole atmosphere is like a badly run girls' school'. This was a reference to the continued bickering between the medical and administrative staff, which had persisted since John Simon first held the post in 1855. When MacNalty's retirement drew near in 1940, Jameson was now considered ideal for the post, having proved his worth in a number of areas, including serving as part-time medical adviser to the Colonial Office. He was still reluctant to consider the post of CMO and required some persuading from the Minister of Health, Malcolm MacDonald.

Jameson became the ninth CMO on 12 November 1940 and immediately became involved in planning the wartime Emergency Medical Services. He advocated a much higher degree of public health information than his predecessors had used, and instituted monthly press conferences at the Ministry of Health shortly after his arrival. He also used radio broadcasts to reach large audiences on subjects such as diphtheria immunisation (May 1941) and the sensitive subject of venereal disease (October 1942 – in a peak-time slot after the 9 p.m. BBC news). Widespread press and Ministry publicity for sexual health followed after Jameson broke this taboo. He advised on the medical aspects of food rationing, and pressed for the Emergency Public Health Laboratory Service to be continued after the end of the war. His most influential role, however, was in the detailed planning for the National Health Service. His position as the government's medical spokesperson brought him into conflict with the profession, in particular the British Medical Association. Jameson was used by the Ministry to 'fly kites' of tentative proposals to test the reaction of the medical profession. His ability to do this while retaining the confidence of both sides is testament to his tact and skill. In July 1945 Aneurin Bevan became Minister of Health and found Jameson a useful ally and supporter in progressing his NHS plans.

Jameson was 63 years old when the National Health Service finally came into operation in 1948, and he retired at the civil service limit of 65 years in 1950. He had reinvented the role of the CMO as the main bridge between the government and the medical profession – a critical position now that doctors were salaried within the National Health Service and required sensitive handling of their pay and conditions. Jameson also recognised the new requirement for medical input into the development of hospital and primary care services. Healthcare services came to dominate the role of the CMO, at the expense of the preventive model favoured by earlier CMOs. The attachment to public health was becoming more tenuous. Jameson recognised the importance of this side of his role, but found it difficult to prioritise when faced with a huge increase in international health meetings and domestic health service planning. He had a reputation within the Ministry for being a more approachable CMO than some of his predecessors. He frequently dropped into his staff's rooms unannounced for advice, rather than summoning them to his office. Jameson also achieved a long-needed restructuring of the Ministry's hierarchy, ensuring that the medical and administrative sides were ranked equally, although the medical side did not have executive powers and the Permanent Secretary was officially head of the office. Jameson as CMO retained his direct access right to the Minister, at the same time resolving some of the chronic antagonisms within the Ministry. He also instituted regular 'Thursday morning' meetings with his senior medical staff and encouraged collaboration with medical staff in other government departments.

In addition to his role in the development of the National Health Service, Jameson should also be remembered for the parts he played in prioritising the nutrition of children and expectant mothers through his chairmanship of a committee at the Ministry of Food, and for his work as a member of the Goodenough Committee (1942–44) through which he steered the post-war reorganisation of medical education. He also continued to be active in health policy formation after his retirement in 1950 through his ten-year role as medical adviser to the King Edward's Hospital Fund for London.

Obituary: *British Medical Journal*, 1962, (II), 1131–3; *Lancet*, 1962, (II), 889–91; GE Godber, 'Jameson, Sir (William) Wilson (1885–1962)', *Oxford Dictionary of National Biography* (Oxford, Oxford University Press, 2004); N Goodman, *Wilson Jameson: architect of national health* (London, George Allen and Unwin Ltd, 1970).

John Charles

DoB 26.07.1893
DoD 06.04.1971

CMO 1950–1960 (10 years)
Retired

John Charles was a complete contrast to Wilson Jameson. He was a quiet, reserved man who disliked public speaking and did little to actively develop the role of the CMO. He was educated in the North East, qualifying in medicine at Durham University College of Medicine in 1916. He served with the Royal Army Medical Corps during the First World War, staying on with the Army of Occupation in Germany from 1919 to 1924. He took the Diploma in Public Health at Cambridge in 1925 and returned to Newcastle-upon-Tyne as a tuberculosis officer at the City Infectious Diseases Hospital. He was appointed as Assistant Medical Officer of Health for Newcastle upon Tyne in 1928 and promoted to Medical Officer of Health in 1932, lecturing at the same time in public health at Durham University. Charles was an excellent practical public health doctor, who could unite academics and general practitioners in the development of innovative services. His reputation gained him an invitation from Jameson to work in Whitehall and he moved to the Ministry of Health in 1944 as a Deputy CMO, where he assisted with planning the National Health Service. He joined Sir Weldon Champneys-Dalrymple, the other Deputy CMO, an

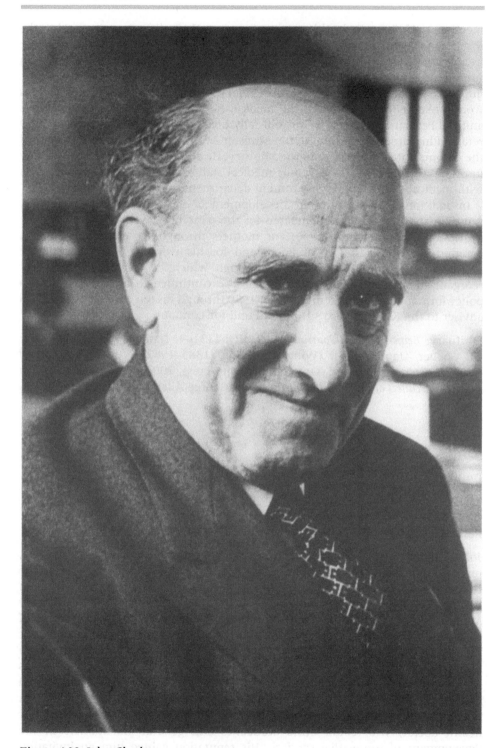

Figure A10 John Charles.

old-style medical civil servant who was not viewed as a serious contender for the 'top job'.

When Charles succeeded Jameson in 1950 he became the first CMO to be appointed to the Home Office as well as the Ministry of Health and the Ministry of Education. He encountered a greater range and intensity of medical work than his predecessors had experienced, and a much more rapid integration of scientific and medical research. It has been suggested that Charles was kept in post as CMO longer than he should have been because he was content with the Ministry's weak stance on the smoking issue. He should have retired at 65 years in 1958 under civil service rules.

Charles preferred to devote his attention to his role at the World Health Organization. He was Chairman of its Executive Board in 1957–58, President of the Twelfth World Health Assembly in 1959 and Chairman of the Fourth Expert Committee on Public Health Administration in 1960. After his retirement as CMO he was appointed as a World Health Organization senior adviser in Geneva, and used his considerable expertise in international health issues to great advantage. At home, he was respected for his 'consolidation' of the NHS and the quiet unassuming way in which he exercised his authority.

Obituary: *British Medical Journal*, 1971, (I), 173; *Lancet*, 1971, (I), 812–13.

George Godber

DoB 04.08.1908

CMO 1960–1973 (13 years)
Retired

George Godber is widely acclaimed as one of the country's greatest Chief Medical Officers. He brought to the post a degree of professional integrity which has not been surpassed. He was educated at Bedford School before moving to a scholar-ship place at New College, Oxford. He completed his medical training in London, qualifying in 1933. Because he lost one eye in an accident, the medical specialties which were open to him were more limited. He was House Physician at the London Hospital under Arthur Ellis (later Regius Professor at Oxford) and the only career he wanted was to be involved from the outset with the anticipated new National Health Service. Godber therefore took the Diploma in Public Health (in addition to the MRCP) at the London School of Hygiene and Tropical Medicine. He was taught there by Jameson, before he became CMO in 1940, beginning what was to become a lasting association. Jameson, while Dean at the LSHTM, was scathing about the Ministry of Health. This did not deter Godber, who found himself a public health position to pass the couple of years until he was five years' qualified – an entrance requirement imposed by the medical civil service.

Godber's entrance into civil service life was unconventional. After the outbreak of the Second World War he was posted to the Birmingham region as an Assistant Medical Officer. From there he was delegated to work single-handedly in Nottingham administering the Emergency Medical Services, liaising between the local Medical Officers of Health and the Ministry in London. When Jameson became CMO in 1940 he delegated to Godber the task of compiling the Midlands

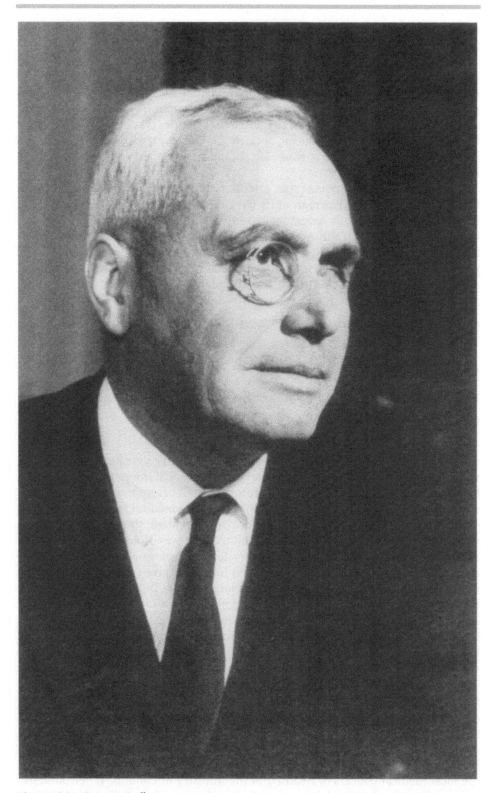

Figure A11 George Godber.

section of the Nuffield Hospitals Survey. Godber accomplished this while carrying out his routine regional duties in Nottingham, and, having impressed his former tutor, he was summoned by Jameson to Whitehall to act as his personal assistant (although still nominally running the Nottingham office).

Godber was intimately involved with the planning of the National Health Service. He frequently took John Charles' place at meetings between Bevan and the medical profession. His major contribution was to advise on the nationalisation of the hospitals, using his expert knowledge from having worked in a region. He also served as secretary to the group formed to consider the development of regional consultant services. When Charles became CMO in 1950, Godber was promoted to be Deputy CMO, working alongside Weldon Champneys-Dalrymple who had been first Deputy CMO under Jameson. Godber took responsibility for the health service operation within the Ministry. He developed a nationwide network of clinical contacts which he could call upon for advice, a facility he valued highly which enabled him to perform what he saw as the correct role of the CMO – to facilitate rather than to direct.

Godber finally succeeded to the post of CMO in 1960, after Charles' contract was extended for an additional two years (see above). By this time he was proficient at gaining advice and support from his colleagues in the medical profession. One of the best examples of this is his prompting of the Royal College of Physicians in 1958 to form a committee on smoking and lung cancer – thus moving the initiative outside the Ministry of Health where it was stifled by Treasury and tobacco industry self-interest. The 1962 report of Fletcher's Royal College of Physicians committee did more to alert the public of the link between smoking and cancer than any of the government's activities over the previous twelve years.

Godber also benefited from a change of Permanent Secretary at the Ministry. When John Hawton finally retired on health grounds in 1960, he was replaced by Bruce Fraser, a progressive, confident civil servant who worked well with Godber. Together, they steered the reorganisation and modernisation of the hospital services, with Godber reassured that Fraser was competent at managing the financial and administrative side of the business. When Fraser was replaced by Arnold France in 1964, he began a more difficult period of negotiations on the reform of the National Health Service. Godber's philosophy of strong local autonomy and discreet central 'guidance' was at odds with the political ideology of the day.

Godber reverted to Jameson's practice of regular office meetings at the Ministry, a tradition which his predecessor, Charles, had abandoned. He also encouraged the development of the more junior staff in government and facilitated office communication and administration systems. He fostered links outside the Ministry, developing a close friendship with Gordon McLachlan at the Nuffield Provincial Hospitals Trust, which he used to hold 'think-tanks' on current medical issues, and was a Member of Council of the King's Fund. Although a teetotaller, Godber was aware of the importance of the social side of the CMO position and 'endured' his quota of official dinners and functions.

Godber retired in 1973, leaving behind a very different health service from the one he had entered in 1939. His long tenure as CMO spanned the Ministry of Health and the Department of Health and Social Security (from 1968). He worked with six Ministers (Secretaries of State) of Health, including Enoch Powell and

Richard Crossman, who made their mark in the redesign of the National Health Service under guidance from Godber. He consolidated his reputation as a superb CMO, well-grounded in medical and scientific principles and with the widest respect from the medical profession and the government.

Henry Yellowlees

DoB 19.04.1919

CMO 1973–1983 (10 years)
Retired

Henry Yellowlees was born in Edinburgh, son of an eminent psychiatrist. He was educated at Stowe and University College, Oxford, where he graduated in 1950, after his training was interrupted by the Second World War (he served as a pilot in the Royal Air Force from 1941–45). His first medical post was at the Middlesex Hospital, and from there he moved into medical administration at the South West Regional Hospital Board. Following a promotion to Deputy Staff Area Medical Officer at the North West Metropolitan Hospital Board, he met George Godber. Godber recognised Yellowlees' abilities in medical administration and appointed him as a Principal Medical Officer at the Ministry of Health in 1963. He continued his career within the Ministry, promoted to Senior Principal Medical Officer in 1965 and Deputy CMO in 1967.

Godber tutored Yellowlees, intending that he should be his successor as CMO when he retired in 1973. Yellowlees inherited a department which needed to respond to massive National Health Service restructuring and developments in the medical profession. The 1974 reforms included a unification of personal social services and of the previously tripartite (hospital, general practice, public health) health services. Other emerging issues included postgraduate medical education, the role of nurses in management and the transformation of the public health profession into 'community medicine'. Yellowlees was the first CMO not to hold the Diploma in Public Health since the qualification was established in 1889, and to some in the medical profession this signalled a loss of interest in the traditional remit of the CMO's office – to advise on the health of the public as well as managing the National Health Service. Yellowlees suffered in the wake of Godber's successful domination as CMO. It has been suggested that Whitehall deliberately appointed Yellowlees because it could not countenance another powerful CMO.

The state of the National Health Service continued to attract criticism through-out Yellowlees' term as CMO, although the problems were exacerbated by the 1970s oil crisis. He did manage to achieve some policy initiatives, including the translation of the Department of Health and Social Security Working Party on Lead in Petrol advice into legislation. He also accomplished an internal restructur-ing of medical staff at Whitehall to facilitate greater co-operation between departments. In retirement he played a significant role in the 1980s Balkans dispute, when he led a World Health Organization team to successfully negotiate with the Turks and the Bulgarians for the provision of healthcare for refugees.

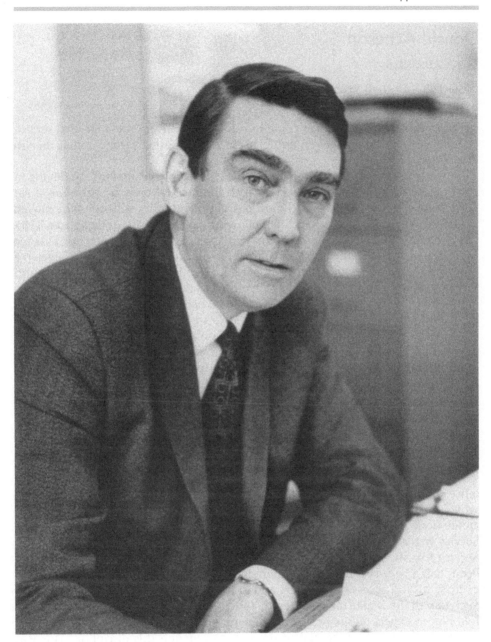

Figure A12 Henry Yellowlees.

Donald Acheson

DoB 17.09.1926

CMO 1984–1991 (8 years)
Retired

Acheson was the first CMO to come into the post with no previous civil service experience. He did, however, bring back to the post a strong public health discipline.

He was educated in Edinburgh and at Brasenose College, Oxford, qualifying in 1951 before doing his national service with the medical branch of the Royal Air Force from 1953 to 1955. After clinical posts at the Middlesex Hospital he moved to Oxford where he held a Radcliffe Fellowship at University College from 1957 till 1959. In 1962 he became the first Director of the Oxford Record Linkage System, which was funded by the Nuffield Provincial Hospitals Trust to develop a powerful tool to use with patient admissions data for epidemiological and health service evaluation purposes. He was appointed as Professor of Clinical Epidemiology at the University of Southampton in 1968 where he also served as Dean of the new Southampton Medical School. From 1979 to 1983 he also served as Director of the Medical Research Council Unit in Environmental Epidemiology, and was a member of the Royal Commission on Environmental Pollution. Prior to his appointment as CMO, he was best known for his 1981 report on primary healthcare in inner London, which urged a fundamental reform of structure and funding.

Acheson's appointment as CMO in 1983 came as a surprise to many in the medical profession, and he himself admits surprise at being 'headhunted'. He came into the Department of Health and Social Security at the end of 1983 for three months to shadow Henry Yellowlees and to learn some of the Whitehall systems and traditions. The CMO post was restructured when Acheson came into office, and he was given a fixed five-year contract rather than permanent tenure which his predecessors had enjoyed. His initial reaction was one of excitement at the scale of the post. The day-to-day management of the National Health Service was a major part of his remit, before the creation of the National Health Service Executive in 1988. Acheson viewed some of his predecessors as having been 'half a pace behind their Permanent Secretaries' and he was determined to exercise his full access to Ministers and to have equal status with the Permanent Secretary in the Department of Health and Social Security. Henry Yellowlees had told him to expect public health to make up only five per cent of his CMO role, yet Acheson saw the potential of the post to redefine this discipline. This was particularly apposite given two major outbreaks in communicable disease early in his time in office. Acheson is best remembered for his proactive and highly professional stance on AIDS. He proved to be the right man in the right place at the right time.

In retirement Acheson has held a number of honorary and visiting positions and completed projects for the World Health Organization, notably in war-torn Bosnia.[1] He also chaired the influential Inquiry into Inequalities in Health, which reported in 1998.

[1] D Acheson, 'Conflict in Bosnia 1992–3', *British Medical Journal*, 1999, 3, 1639–42.

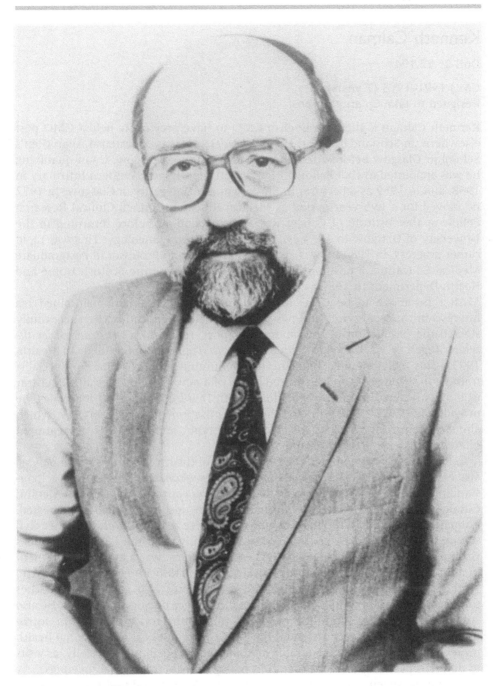

Figure A13 Donald Acheson.

Kenneth Calman

DoB 25.12.1941

CMO 1991–1998 (7 years)
Resigned to take up another post

Kenneth Calman is the only English CMO to have previously held a CMO post elsewhere (in Scotland between 1989 and 1991). He was educated at Allan Glen's School in Glasgow before attending the University of Glasgow. Upon qualifying he was appointed as Hall Fellow in Surgery at the Glasgow Western Infirmary in 1968, and in 1969 as a Lecturer in Surgery at the University of Glasgow. In 1972 he moved for a two-year period as Medical Research Council Clinical Research Fellow at the Institute of Cancer Research in London, before returning to the University of Glasgow in 1974 as Professor of Clinical Oncology. This was rapid career progress. In 1984 he was appointed as Dean and Professor of Postgraduate Medical Education, a position he held until his move to the Scottish Home and Health Department in 1989 as CMO.

After his move to be CMO for England in 1991, Calman maintained his interests in cancer services and postgraduate medical education. He successfully steered the production of the landmark report, *Hospital Doctors: training for the future. Report of the Working Group on Specialist Training* (Department of Health, 1993). This recommended reducing the minimum length of time for specialist training to seven years and the introduction of a new grade of Specialist Registrar in line with new European regulations. With Deirdre Hine, CMO for Wales, he provided in 1995 a blueprint for the reorganisation of cancer services, which aimed at removing the 'postcode' lottery in types and standards of treatment offered to patients across England and Wales.

Calman was instrumental in the Department of Health 1995 report, *Maintaining Medical Excellence: review of guidance on doctors' performance*. This tackled a long-standing issue of poorly performing doctors and encouraged the General Medical Council to begin a fundamental reform of the way doctors' conduct was assessed. Calman also used his Whitehall position to improve relations with the other civil service healthcare professions. His decision to jointly chair the Clinical Outcomes Group with the Chief Nursing Officer, Yvonne Moores, was a major achievement in moving from medical audit into clinical audit, and fully integrating all staff who worked together in clinical settings. He and Moores also gave joint speeches together in a show of unity for National Health Service doctors and nurses. He also strengthened CMO communications with the health service through the introduction of a fax/cascade system and the *CMO Update* publication. Regional health professionals commented favourably on Calman's accessibility, especially his visits to different parts of the country and his policy of regular informal meetings.

During his seven years as CMO for England Calman endured some stringent cuts to civil service medical staffing, almost reminiscent of the struggles which Simon and the first CMOs faced in the late nineteenth century as they sought to secure a team of medical experts within Whitehall. The late twentieth century reforms were not specific to the Department of Health, but part of a much larger Whitehall rationalisation. They left the CMO with a much-depleted staff, no longer directly accountable to him, with which to investigate new health scares such as bovine spongiform encephalopathy (BSE). In spite of these reductions,

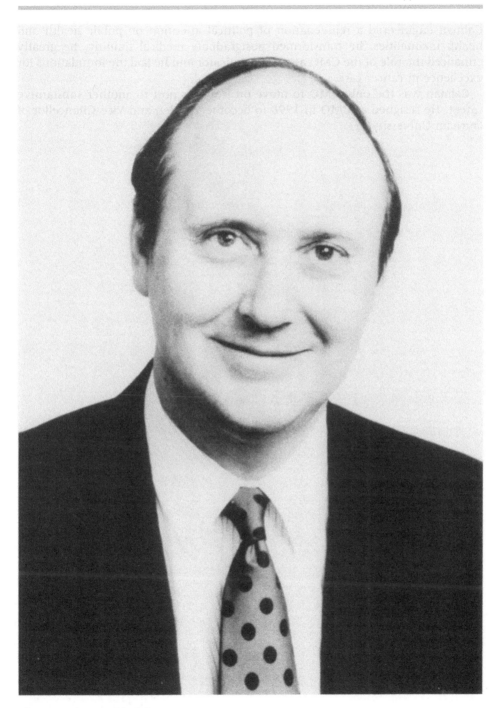

Figure A14 Kenneth Calman.

Calman engineered a rejuvenation of political attention on public health and health inequalities, he transformed postgraduate medical training, he greatly enhanced the role of the CMO as a communicator and he laid the foundations for excellence in cancer care.

Calman was the only CMO to move on from his post to another substantive career. He resigned as CMO in 1998 to become Warden and Vice-Chancellor of Durham University.

Appendix 2

Secretaries of State for Health and Ministers of Health in the Ministry of Health, the Department of Health and Social Security and the Department of Health

Name	Dates in office	Years in office
Christopher Addison (1861–1951) Lib.	1919–1921	2
Alfred Mond (1868–1930) Lib.	1921–1922	1
Arthur Griffith-Boscawen (1865–1923) Cons.	1922–1923	<1
(Arthur) Neville Chamberlain (1869–1940) Cons.	1923–1923	<1
William Joynson-Hicks (1865–1932) Cons.	1923–1923	<1
John Wheatley (1869–1930) Lab.	1924–1924	<1
(Arthur) Neville Chamberlain (1869–1940) Cons.	1924–1929	4
Arthur Greenwood (1880–1954) Lab.	1929–1931	2
(Arthur) Neville Chamberlain (1869–1940) Cons.	1931–1931	<1
Edward Young (1870–1960) Coalition.	1931–1935	4
Howard Wood (1881–1943) Cons.	1935–1938	3
Walter Elliot (1888–1958) Cons.	1938–1940	2
Malcolm MacDonald (1901–1981) Coalition.	1940–1941	<1
Ernest Brown (1881–1962) Coalition.	1941–1943	2
Henry Willink (1894–1973) Coalition.	1943–1945	2
Aneurin Bevan (1897–1960) Lab.	1945–1951	5
Hilary Marquand (1901–1972) Lab.	1951–1951	<1
Harry Crookshank (1893–1961) Cons.	1951–1952	<1
Iain Macleod (1913–1970) Cons.	1952–1955	3
Robin Turton (1903–1994) Cons.	1955–1957	2
Dennis Vosper (1916–1968) Cons.	1957–1957	<1
Derek Walker–Smith (1910–1992) Cons.	1957–1960	3
Enoch Powell (1912–1998) Cons.	1960–1963	3
Anthony Barber (1920–) Cons.	1963–1964	1
Kenneth Robinson (1911–1996) Lab.	1964–1968	4

Name	Dates in office	Years in office
Richard Crossman (1907–1974) Lab.	1968–1970	2
Keith Joseph (1918–1994) Cons.	1970–1974	4
Barbara Castle (1910–2002) Lab.	1974–1976	2
David Ennals (1922–1995) Lab.	1976–1979	3
Patrick Jenkin (1926–) Cons.	1979–1983	4
Norman Fowler (1938–) Cons.	1983–1987	4
John Moore (1937–) Cons.	1987–1988	1
Kenneth Clarke (1940–) Cons.	1988–1991	3
William Waldegrave (1946–) Cons.	1991–1995	4
Stephen Dorrell (1952–) Cons.	1995–1996	1
Virginia Bottomley (1948–) Cons.	1996–1997	1
Frank Dobson (1940–) Lab.	1997–1999	2

Appendix 3

Permanent Secretaries in the Ministry of Health, the Department of Health and Social Security and the Department of Health

Name	Dates in office	Years in office
Robert Morant (1863–1920)	1919–1920	1
William Robinson (1874–1935)	1920–1935	15
George Chrystal (1880–1944)	1935–1940	5
Evelyn John Maude (1883–1963)	1940–1945	5
William Douglas (1890–1953)	1945–1951	6
John Hawton (1904–1981)	1951–1960	9
Bruce Fraser (1901–1993)	1960–1964	4
Arnold France (1911–1998)	1964–1968	4
Clifford Jarrett (1909–1995)	1968–1970	2
Philip Rogers (1914–1990)	1970–1975	5
Patrick Nairne (1921–)	1975–1981	6
Kenneth Stowe (1927–)	1981–1987	6
Christopher France (1934–)	1987–1992	5
Graham Hart (1940–)	1992–1997	5
Christopher Kelly (1946–)	1997–2000	3

CMO chronology and allied historical events

Date	CMOs and their activities	Health and medicine	Social and political
1848		Public Health Act – creates potential for local Medical Officers of Health, Borough Engineers and Inspectors of Nuisances.	
1854		John Snow removes the handle from the Broad Street pump in London, claiming that cholera is transmitted by water. *On Chloroform and other Anaesthetics: their action and administration* by John Snow published.	Crimean War begins (ends 1856).
1855	John Simon appointed Medical Officer to the General Board of Health (the first CMO).	Influenza pandemic. Loius Pasteur publishes his 'germ theory' of fermentation and putrefaction.	Viscount Palmerston becomes Liberal Prime Minister.
1857		*British Medical Journal* first published.	
1858		Medical Reform Act – sets up Medical Register and General Medical Council in Britain. Rudolf Virchow's *Cellularpathologie* demonstrates that every cell is a product of another cell. Public Health Act – ends the General Board of Health and transfers its medical duties to the Privy Council.	'The Great Stink' of London, caused by the sewage pollution of the Thames.
1859	First report of the Medical Officer of the Privy Council.	Charles Darwin's *The Origin of Species* published. *Notes on Hospitals* by Florence Nightingale published. First 'district' nurses appointed in Liverpool.	
1861		Louis Pasteur discovers anaerobic bacteria.	Start of American Civil War. Population of Britain = 28.9 million.
1862	Investigations into industrial diseases.	Manchester and Salford Ladies Health Society appoints the first 'health visitors'.	London to Edinburgh by rail takes 10½ hours. First underground railway, the Metropolitan Railway (Paddington to the City of London), opens. It becomes known as 'The Sewer'.
1863	Investigations into cattle diseases.	Fourth cholera pandemic begins.	

Date	CMOs and their activities	Health and medicine	Social and political
1864	Development of new disease statistical summaries.	Contagious Disease Act – attempts to control venereal diseases by the compulsory medical examination of 'common prostitutes' in garrison towns. *A Manual of Practical Hygiene* by EA Parkes published.	International Red Cross founded.
1865	Simon begins to publish *Pathological Enquiries*.	Joseph Lister introduces phenol as a disinfectant in surgery. Elizabeth Garrett (later Anderson) becomes first woman to qualify in medicine in Britain.	Red Flag Act – introduces a 4mph limit on highways. Start of the main drainage system for London. End of American Civil War and of slavery in USA.
1866		Thomas Allbutt develops the clinical thermometer. Cholera epidemic in Britain. Sanitary Act.	
1867		First international medical congress in Paris. Royal Commission on London Water Supply. New smallpox vaccination regulations.	Russia sells Alaska to USA. Dominion of Canada established.
1868		Sanitary Act. Artisans and Labourers Dwellings Act – first national legislation to tackle slum dwellings. Pharmacy Act – limits the sale of opium to qualified pharmacists.	Trades Union Congress founded.
1869	The Metropolitan Association of Medical Officers of Health founded, with John Simon as President.	Sophia Jex-Blake matriculates in medicine at Edinburgh University (but University reverses decision in 1873). The *Lancet* advocates the creation of a state medical service and a Ministry of Health.	Suez Canal opens. Charity Organisation Society founded, aimed at encouraging self-reliance among the poor.
1870		Over the next three years there are widespread outbreaks of smallpox. About 44 000 people in England, 10 000 of them in London, die from the disease.	Education Act – elementary education for all children. Civil service opened to entry by competitive examination.
1871	Simon appointed CMO to the Local Government Board.	Report of The Royal Sanitary Commission, which had been set up in 1869. The General Medical Council introduces regulations for Diplomas in Public Health.	Darwin's *Descent of Man* published. Census population of Britain = 31.4 million. Local Government Board Act – sets up the Local Government Board.
1872		Public Health Act.	Ballot Act – introduces voting by secret ballot. Licensing Act – introduces licensing of premises selling beer and spirits and limits their opening hours.

Date	CMOs and their activities	Health and medicine	Social and political
1873		The Association of Medical Officers of Health.	
1874		Louis Pasteur suggests placing instruments in boiling water to sterilise them. The first 'home' or 'district' nurse appointed in Liverpool.	Births and Deaths Registration Act – requires medical certification of the cause of death. Foundation of the Cremation Society. First two workmen, both miners, elected to Parliament.
1875		Public Health Act – consolidates and amends previous Acts.	Income tax is 2d in the pound.
1876	Simon, the first CMO, resigns. Edward Cator Seaton appointed as second CMO.	Robert Koch identifies the anthrax bacillus.	The Sanitary Institute (later the Royal Society of Health) founded to promote the health of the people. Alexander Graham Bell patents the telephone.
1879	Seaton, the second CMO, dies.		
1880	George Buchanan appointed as third CMO.	Charles Laveran isolates blood parasite that causes malaria.	
1881		Fifth cholera pandemic begins. Louis Pasteur devises a vaccine for anthrax.	Census population of Britain = 34.8 million.
1882		Robert Koch isolates the tubercle bacillus.	Eruption of Krakatoa in the Sunda Straits.
1883		Robert Koch discovers the cholera vibrio.	
1884			National Society for the Prevention of Cruelty to Children founded. Fabian Society formed.
1885			KF Benz (German engineer) builds the first car using an internal combustion engine.
1886		Contagious Disease Acts repealed.	Gold discovered in the Witwatersrand, South Africa.
1887		British Nurses Association founded.	
1888		Local Government Act – makes the Diploma in Public Health a requirement for Medical Officers of Health.	
1889		Infectious Diseases (Notification) Act.	Brazil ends Portuguese rule.
1890	First edition of *English Sanitary Institutions* by Simon (retired CMO) published.	Emil von Behring and Shibasabura Kitasato develop vaccines against tetanus and diphtheria. William Halsted introduces surgical gloves.	

Date	CMOs and their activities	Health and medicine	Social and political
1891			Volume 1 of *Life and Labour of the People in London* by Charles Booth published. Census population of Britain = 37.7 million.
1892	Buchanan, the third CMO, retires. Replaced by Richard Thorne Thorne, the fourth CMO.		
1893		The Bertillon Classification of the Causes of Death adopted by the International Statistical Institute (previously Congress) at its meeting in Chicago.	Death duties introduced. Manchester Ship Canal opens.
1894			Nicholas II becomes last Tsar of Russia.
1895		Institute of Sanitary (later Public Health) Engineers founded. Wilhelm Röntgén discovers X-rays.	G Marconi makes the first radio transmission over one mile. Manufacture of cars (Wolseley) begins in Birmingham. Cinematography invented.
1896		Antonie Becquerel discovers radiation. Scipione Riva-Rocci invents device for measuring blood pressure.	
1897		Ronald Ross reports that malaria transmitted by anopheles mosquitoes. M Ogata shows that the flea is the principle vector of bubonic plague both between rats and between rats and humans.	National Union of Women's Suffrage Societies formed. The electron discovered by JJ Thomson, Professor of Experimental Physics at Cambridge University.
1898		Pierre and Marie Curie obtain radium from pitchblende. Vaccination Act – introduces a 'conscientious objection' clause. First Infant Welfare Centre opens in St Helens. The Liverpool School of Tropical Medicine established; the first such school in the world.	
1899	Thorne Thorne, the fourth CMO, dies. Replaced by William Power as the fifth CMO.	The London School of Tropical Medicine opens. Aspirin introduced by Bayer. Sixth cholera pandemic.	Boer War begins (ends 1902).
1900		Sigmund Freud's *The Interpretation of Dreams* published. Karl Landsteiner identifies four major human blood groups (A, O, B and AB).	Labour Representation Committee, forerunner of the Labour Party, formed.

Date	CMOs and their activities	Health and medicine	Social and political
1901			Death of Queen Victoria. Census population of Britain = 41.4 million, of whom over 80 per cent live in urban areas. First Nobel Prizes.
1902		William Bayliss and Ernest Starling discover the hormone secretin. Registration of Midwives Act passed.	
1903		Willem Einthoven describes the first electrocardiograph.	Wright brothers fly in petrol-powered aircraft.
1904		Rockefeller Institute for Medical Research founded in New York. Report of the Interdepartmental Committee on Physical Deterioration.	
1905		George Washington Crile performs first direct blood transfusion.	
1906		Frederick Gowland Hopkins starts experiments on 'accessory food factors' (vitamins). Charles Sherrington's *The Integrative Action of the Nervous System* published.	Education (Provision of Meals) Act.
1907	George Newman appointed CMO at the Board of Education.	Creation of first World International Health Organisation in Paris.	
1908	Power retires as the fifth CMO. Replaced by Arthur Newsholme as the sixth CMO.	Sulphanilamide first synthesised. HW Geiger develops a counter to detect radioactivity.	Old Age Pensions Act. Children's (Medical Inspection) Act.
1909		Royal Commission on the Poor Laws reports.	Industrial production of plastics begins after Bakelite developed. Robert Peary and Matthew Henson reach the North Pole. Blériot flies the Channel.
1910		Paul Ehrlich announces his discovery of Salvarsan for treatment of syphilis – the beginning of modern chemotherapy. TH Morgan identifies genes.	Accession of George V.
1911		National Insurance Act – sets up first state medical insurance scheme in Britain. William Hill develops the first gastroscope.	Roald Amundsen reaches the South Pole British census population = 45.2 million.
1912		Harvey Cushing's *The Pituitary Gland and its Disorders* published. Casimir Funk coins the term 'vitamin'. Acute poliomyelitis and tuberculosis become notifiable diseases.	The *Titanic* sinks on maiden voyage.

Date	CMOs and their activities	Health and medicine	Social and political
1913		John Jacob Abel develops first artificial kidney. Establishment of Medical Research Committee (Council from 1920). Blood transfusion becomes possible through the research of A Huston and L Agote.	Rockefeller Foundation creates the International Health Board.
1914		Alexis Carrel performs first successful heart surgery on a dog. Henry Dale discovers the neurotransmitter acetycholine in ergot.	Outbreak of the First World War. Panama Canal opens.
1916		Margaret Sanger founds first American birth-control clinic in Brooklyn, New York.	Albert Einstein's *General Theory of Relativity* published. Conscription of all men of military age introduced.
1917		Carl Jung's *Psychology of the Unconscious* published.	Russian Revolution starts.
1918	George Newman (still CMO at the Board of Education) publishes *Some Notes on Medical Education.*	Start of influenza pandemic.	End of First World War. Women over 30 allowed to vote in Britain if ratepayers or wives of ratepayers.
1919	Newsholme retires as the sixth CMO. Replaced by George Newman, the seventh CMO, and first to serve in a Ministry of Health.	Ministry of Health created. Christopher Addison, Minister of Health.	Ernest Rutherford splits the atom. First crossing of the Atlantic by air.
1920		Report of the Consultative Council on Medical and Allied Services (Dawson Report). General Nursing Council established.	League of Nations established. Alcohol prohibition introduced in USA (abandoned in 1933).
1921		Permanent Secretary Robert Morant dies; Alfred Mond, Minister of Health. Marie Stopes opens first birth-control clinic in London. FG Banting and CH Best isolate insulin.	
1922		Arthur Griffith-Boscawen, Minister of Health.	USSR established.
1923		Neville Chamberlain, Minister of Health. William Joynson-Hicks, Minister of Health. Albert Calmette and Camille Guerin develop the BCG vaccine for tuberculosis.	Turkish republic formed – end of Ottoman Empire.
1924		John Wheatley, Minister of Health. Neville Chamberlain, Minister of Health.	
1925	George Newman publishes *Public Education in Health.*		White lines painted on roads to reduce traffic accidents.
1926		First enzyme (urease) crystallised by American biochemist James B Sumner.	General strike. JL Baird first demonstrates television.

Date	CMOs and their activities	Health and medicine	Social and political
1927		Phillip Drinker and Louis Shaw develop the 'iron lung'. Central Council for Health Education created.	
1928		Alexander Fleming discovers antibacterial effects of penicillin. Albert Szent-Györgyi isolates vitamin C.	Voting age for eligible British women reduced from 30 to 21 years.
1929		Arthur Greenwood, Minister of Health. Henry Dale and HW Dudley demonstrate chemical transmission of nerve impulses. Werner Forssmann develops cardiac catheter. London School of Hygiene and Tropical Medicine opens.	Wall Street crash. World economic crisis.
1930		Mental Treatment Act. Fluoride in water shown to prevent dental caries.	2.5 million unemployed.
1931		Neville Chamberlain, Minister of Health. Edward Young, Minister of Health. The electron microscope invented by M Knolt and E Ruska – enables viruses to be seen.	Census population of Britain = 44.7 million.
1932	Arthur Newsholme (retired CMO) publishes *Medicine and the State*.	Gerhard Domagk discovers the first sulpha drug, prontosil.	Nazis take power in Germany.
1933			30 mph speed limit in built-up areas.
1934			Cheap or free school milk for all school children.
1935	George Newman retires as seventh CMO. Succeeded by Arthur MacNalty, the eighth CMO.	Howard Wood, Minister of Health. Development of prefrontal lobotomy to treat mental illness. First blood bank set up – in the USA at the Mayo Clinic, Rochester. Introduction of sulphonamides.	
1936		Ugo Cerletti describes electroconvulsive therapy. GOM McGonigle and J Kirby publish *Poverty and Public Health*.	George V dies. Edward VIII abdicates.
1937		Development of vaccine against yellow fever by Max Theiler and of first antihistamine by Daniel Bovet. Charles Dodds discovers a synthetic oestrogen (stilboestrol).	Spanish Civil War (1936–39).
1938		Walter Elliot, Minister of Health. New Zealand Social Security Act – provides pioneering state medical service. John Wiles develops the first total artificial hip replacement, using stainless steel.	
1939		Emergency Hospital Service mobilised.	Outbreak of Second World War.

Date	CMOs and their activities	Health and medicine	Social and political
1940	MacNalty retires as eighth CMO. Succeeded by Wilson Jameson, the ninth CMO.	Malcolm MacDonald, Minister of Health. Howard Florey and Ernst Chain develop penicillin as an antibiotic. Karl Landsteiner discovers the rhesus factor in blood.	Invasion of France and Belgium. Air Battle of Britain. Food rationing introduced.
1941	May 5 – CMO radio broadcast on diphtheria.	Ernest Brown, Minister of Health. Ministry of Health hospital surveys begin.	Pearl Harbour.
1942	October – CMO radio broadcast on venereal disease.	*Social Insurance and Allied Services* report by William Beveridge paves way for a National Health Service in Britain. DDT (insecticide) introduced.	Fall of Singapore. Battle of Alamein.
1943		Henry Willinck, Minister of Health. Wilhelm Kolff develops first kidney dialysis machine. Selman Waksman discovers the antibiotic streptomycin.	Russian victory at Stalingrad. Fall of Mussolini.
1944		Goodenough Report on Medical Education.	Allied landings in Normandy.
1945		Aneurin Bevan, Minister of Health. Fluoridation of water observed in the USA to prevent tooth decay.	End of Second World War – 5 May in Europe and 15 August in Japan following atomic bombing. Beginning of Cold War.
1946		Start of first randomised clinical trials of streptomycin for TB treatment. National Health Service Act.	First meeting of United Nations General Assembly in New York.
1947		Alcoholics Anonymous formed.	Independence of India and Pakistan.
1948		World Health Organization (WHO) formed (first assembly in Geneva). National Health Service begins in Britain on 5 July. National Institutes of Health created in the USA.	State of Israel proclaimed. Transistors invented. Railway and electricity industries nationalised.
1949		Cortisone treatment introduced for rheumatoid arthritis.	North Atlantic Treaty Organization (NATO) formed.
1950	Jameson retires as ninth CMO. Succeeded by John Charles who becomes the tenth CMO.		Korean War begins.
1951		Hilary Marquand, Minister of Health. Harry Crookshank, Minister of Health. John Gibbon develops heart–lung machine and successfully operates in 1953.	Election: Attlee's Labour Government replaced by Conservatives under Churchill. Census population of Britain = 53.1 million, including 22 per cent under 15 years and 11 per cent over 65 years. Newcastle United FC win FA Cup (and again 1952 and 1955).

Date	CMOs and their activities	Health and medicine	Social and political
1952		Iain Macleod, Minister of Health. Douglas Bevis develops amniocentesis. College of General Practitioners founded. R Doll and AB Hill publish research on link between smoking and lung cancer in the *British Medical Journal*.	Death of King George VI. Introduction of some charges for NHS services, including a £1 prescription charge. Great Smog of London 5–9 December causes over 4000 deaths.
1953		EA Graham and EL Wynder show that tobacco tars cause cancer in mice. James Watson and Francis Crick determine the double-helical structure of DNA.	Everest climbed. Death of Stalin.
1954		First successful kidney transplant (from identical twin). First government statement on link between smoking and lung cancer. Contraceptive pill, norethynodrel, developed. 250 cases of vaccine-associated poliomyelitis in USA – the Cutter Incident.	Food rationing ends. First business computer (IBM).
1955		Robin Turton, Minister of Health. Ultrasound used in obstetrics.	Winston Churchill succeeded by Anthony Eden as Prime Minister.
1956		Clean Air Act – introduces smokeless zones in urban areas. Medical Act – reforms the General Medical Council. Sanitary Inspectors title changes to Public Health Inspectors. Guillebaud Report on the Cost of the NHS. Society for Social Medicine founded.	Suez Crisis. Hungarian revolt crushed. First British atomic power station opens at Calder Hall, Cumbria.
1957		Dennis Vosper, Minister of Health. Derek Walker-Smith, Minister of Health. Albert Sabin develops a live polio vaccine. Royal Commission on Doctors' Pay. Mass X-ray campaign in Scotland to detect hidden TB cases. *The Uses of Epidemiology* by JN Morris published.	Treaty of Rome, leading to establishment (1958) of the European Economic Community. First satellites, Sputnik I and II, launched by USSR.
1958		Effective treatment of blood pressure. 44-hour week introduced for nurses.	Boeing 707 in service.
1959		Mental Health Act. Immunisation against poliomyelitis general in UK.	Election: Conservative majority 100, 'You've never had it so good'. Morris Mini goes into production. M1 opens. Fidel Castro assumes power in Cuba.
1960	John Charles retires as tenth CMO. George Godber becomes the eleventh CMO.	Enoch Powell, Minister of Health. Royal Commission on Remuneration of NHS Doctors and Dentists.	Berlin Wall built by East Germany.

Date	CMOs and their activities	Health and medicine	Social and political
1961		Oral contraception available in family planning clinics. Human Tissue Act. Thalidomide disaster.	First man in space.
1962		Lasers first used in eye surgery. Royal College of Physicians report *Smoking and Health*. Committee on Safety of Medicines formed. First ten-year plan for hospital building.	Cuban missile crisis.
1963		Anthony Barber, Minister of Health. Measles vaccine licensed for general use in the USA. Thomas Starzl's first human liver transplant.	Kennedy assassinated. The Beatles take America by storm.
1964		Kenneth Robinson, Minister of Health. Home kidney dialysis introduced in the UK and USA. RCN report on reform of nursing education.	Outbreak of Vietnam War between North Vietnam and USA (to 1973). Labour Government; Harold Wilson as Prime Minister.
1965		Charter for family doctors. TV advertising ban on tobacco.	
1966		Measles vaccine in UK. Establishment of cervical cytology service. New GP contract.	Cultural Revolution begins in China. General election: Labour victory. England football team wins World Cup
1967		Christian Barnard performs human heart transplant. Abortion Act. WHO embarks on eradication of smallpox.	Torrey Canyon oil disaster.
1968		Department of Health and Social Security formed. Richard Crossman, Secretary of State for Health. Royal Commission on Medical Education (Todd). Seebohm Report. First Green Paper on NHS reorganisation.	Czechoslovak uprising. Moon orbited. Martin Luther King Jr assassinated. Students revolt in Paris.
1969	First CMO for Wales appointed.	Ely Hospital report published.	Neil Armstrong lands on the moon. Age of majority reduced from 21 years to 18 years.
1970		Keith Joseph, Secretary of State for Health. Second Green Paper on NHS reorganisation.	Conservative Government (Edward Heath)
1971		Coronary artery bypass surgery. Rothschild Report on Government Research and Development. Royal College of Psychiatrists founded. ASH – Action on Smoking and Health formed.	Decimalisation of currency. Census population of Britain = 55.9 million (24 per cent under 15 years and 14 per cent over 65 years).

Date	CMOs and their activities	Health and medicine	Social and political
1972		Computerised axial tomography (CAT) introduced for medical imaging. NHS reorganisation White Paper *Effectiveness and Efficiency: random reflections on health services* by A Cochrane published.	First showing of TV hospital drama, *MASH*, based in Korea. Local Government Act. Watergate burglary. Faculty of Community Medicine formed. School leaving age raised to 16 years.
1973	Godber retires as eleventh CMO. Succeeded by Henry Yellowlees as twelfth CMO.	NHS Reorganisation Act.	Yom Kippur War. OPEC rise in oil prices. UK joins EEC.
1974		Barbara Castle, Secretary of State for Health. NHS and local government reorganised. Post of Medical Officer of Health abolished.	Three-day working week. February election: minority Labour Government; October election: Labour Government with majority of three.
1975		Whole-body CT scanning. Controversy over private medicine.	First North Sea oil extracted. US withdrawal from Vietnam.
1976		David Ennals, Secretary of State for Health. Epidemics of Ebola virus disease in Sudan and Zaire. Royal Commission on NHS established. Royal Colleges' criteria for brain-stem death.	Concorde in service. James Callaghan as Prime Minister.
1977		'Health for All by 2000' declaration. Communicable Disease Surveillance Centre formed.	Elvis Presley dies.
1978		First 'test-tube' baby born in England. Alma-Ata declaration: 'Health for All'.	Winter of discontent.
1979		Patrick Jenkin, Secretary of State for Health. World declared free of smallpox. Royal Commission on the NHS reported *Patients First*.	Conservative election victory (first term). Margaret Thatcher as Prime Minister.
1980		Black Report on Inequalities in Health. Magnetic resonance imaging (MRI).	SAS storm Iranian embassy. John Lennon shot dead in New York.
1981		AIDS first recognised by US Centers for Disease Control. Primary Health Care in Inner London (Acheson Report).	Prince Charles and Lady Diana marry. Population of Britain = 59.2 million.
1982		NHS restructuring; abolition of areas. Warnock Inquiry.	Falklands War.

Date	CMOs and their activities	Health and medicine	Social and political
1983	Yellowlees retires as twelfth CMO. Succeeded by Donald Acheson as thirteenth CMO.	Norman Fowler, Secretary of State for Health. NHS management inquiry (Griffiths). Mental Health Act.	Conservative election victory (second term). More than 3 million unemployed. Seat-belts in cars compulsory. Compact discs developed.
1984		Warnock Report. Implementation of General Management Function. Limited List introduced.	Miners' strike. Band Aid concert for Ethiopia famine.
1985		WHO (Europe), *Targets for Health for All*. Stanley Royd salmonellosis outbreak.	Mikhail Gorbachev takes power in USSR.
1986		BSE identified in cattle. *Primary Health Care* (Green Paper). AIDS campaign starts.	Chernobyl nuclear disaster. Stock market 'big bang'.
1987		John Moore, Secretary of State for Health. *Promoting Better Health* (White Paper).	Conservative election victory (third term).
1988		Kenneth Clarke, Secretary of State for Health. Measles/mumps/rubella (MMR) vaccine introduced. Mrs Thatcher announces NHS review on *Panorama*.	Cows with BSE slaughtered. Pan Am Lockerbie bomb. 'Poll Tax' protests.
1989		*Working for Patients* (NHS reforms). Hepatitis C virus discovered.	Fall of the Berlin Wall. Tiananmen Square massacre.
1990		Calman Report on Hospital Staffing.	Rapid expansion of World Wide Web. John Major becomes Conservative Prime Minister.
1991	Acheson retires as thirteenth CMO. Succeeded by Kenneth Calman as fourteenth CMO.	William Waldegrave, Secretary of State for Health. *The Health of the Nation* consultation document published.	Collapse of USSR. Gulf War.
1992			Fourth consecutive Conservative election victory.
1993			Council Tax replaces the Poll Tax.
1994		Fourteen NHS regions reduced to eight.	Mandela made President of South Africa. Channel Tunnel opens.
1995		Stephen Dorrell, Secretary of State for Health. Debate on rationing of healthcare. GP 'out-of-hours' dispute.	

Date	CMOs and their activities	Health and medicine	Social and political
1996		Virginia Bottomley, Secretary of State for Health. Dolly the sheep – first mammalian clone. NHS (Primary Care) Act. nvCJD identified.	Hong Kong reverts to China. Creation of the Food Standards Agency. Death of Princess Diana. Scots vote for devolution.
1997		Frank Dobson, Secretary of State for Health. First Minister of Public Health (Tessa Jowell) appointed.	General election – first Labour Government in 18 years. Tony Blair as Prime Minister.
1998	Calman retires as fourteenth CMO. Succeeded by Liam Donaldson as fifteenth CMO.		Human Rights Act National Minimum Wage Act.

Index

Page numbers in *italics* refer to figures.

Abrams, Michael 83, 90, 128, 133
accountability in Whitehall 62–3
Acheson, Donald 206, *207*
  honours *18*
  length in office *xii*
  media involvement 161–3
  on 1995 restructuring 85, 87
  on access to Ministers 65–6
  on AIDS crisis 36, 124–34, *130*
  on BSE crisis 135–45, 162–3
  on CHO authority 87
  on drug 'limited lists' 113
  on public health 171
  on Whitehall reviews 78
  relationship with medical establishment
    103, 113
  reputation 36
  selection 35–6
  workload 127, 135–7
Acton Society Trust surveys 74
Addison, Christopher 25–7, 42–3
administrative staff
  'cogwheel' reports 174
  pay and status 72–4, 82–3, 84–5
  structural hierarchy 74–5, 84–5
advisory committees
  influence of CHOs 118–20
  SEAC (Spongiform Encephalopathy
    Advisory Committee) 139–44
AIDS crisis 123–34
  Acheson's involvement 36, 124–34
  as metaphor for society 133
  screening and testing 131–2
Alderslade scrutiny of Department of
    Health Medical Division (1990) 78–9,
    85
Alexander Fleming House (Elephant and
    Castle) 88–9, *88*
Allbut, Clifford 95
Andrews, Sir Derek 135
Annual Reports 147, 149–53, 163
  suppression 151
  treasury threats 152–3
  see also On the State of the Public Health
    reports
appraisal and revalidation schemes 113–14

archives, state medicine xviii
armed forces, Hygiene Laboratory
    (Sandhurst) 30
Association of Metropolitan Medical
    Officers of Health 4–5, 20

Bampfylde, Saxton 36–7
Banks Review (1994) 83–6, 144
Banks, Terri 83
Barber, Anthony 58
Barberis, Peter 39–40, 61–3
Barlow, Thomas 95
Benner–Godfrey Review (1988) 78, 81–2,
    135
Benner, Patrick 81–2, 135
Benn, Tony, on Permanent Secretaries 63
Berridge, Virginia 125–7, 129
Bevan, Aneurin 61, 63–5, 96, 101–3
  on consultants 103
Beveridge, William 96, 100
biographies and histories xi, 165
  autobiographies xvii
Black Report on Inequalities in Health (1980)
    170–1
Black, Douglas 120
Board of Education 24–5
Boer War recruits 41
Bottomley, Virginia 133
botulism warnings 162
Brackenbury, Sir Henry 94
Bradford Hill, Austin 45–7, 50
Bridges, Edward 61
Bristowe, John 8–9
British Medical Association (BMA)
  on AIDS testing 130–1
  formation 93
  functions post NHS formation 105
  membership 93
  and National Health Service 96–103
  support for John Simon 6–7
British Medical Journal
  on Aneurin Bevan 103
  on Enoch Powell 58
  on George Buchanan 21
  on George Godber 56
  on George Newman 27

British Medical Journal cont.
  on John Simon 6
  on smoking 154–5
  timing of press releases 159–60
Brotherston, John 171
Brown, Ernest 100
Bruce, HA 148
BSE crisis 134–45, 168–9
  Acheson's involvement 135–45
  precedents 69
  Southwood working party 136–9
Buchanan, George 20–1, 181–3, *182*
  association with John Simon 8–9, 10, 14
  early career 8–9, 10, 20
  honours *18*
  lifespan *xii*
  published reports 153
  retirement 21
  selection 20
  time in office *xii*
  workload issues 20–1, 68–70, 153
Buchanan, Sir John *173*
The Building of a Nation's Health (Newman)
  xvii
BUPA, pay beds 108
Burdon Sanderson 15
Burns, John 22
Butler, Sir Robin 36
Buzzard, Sir Farquhar 30, 100

Calman, Kenneth *143*, 208–10, *209*
  honours *18*
  length in office *xii*
  nomination to GMC 92
  on AIDS crisis 133–4
  on BSE crisis 141–5
  on cancer services 170
  on poor performance 113–14
  on postgraduate medical education 113
  on risk management 169
  post-retirement 37–8, 175–6
  retirement 115
  selection 36–7
cancer services, Cochrane efficiencies 170
Cartwright, Ann 75
Castle, Barbara 61, 108–11, *110, 112*
Cave Committee (1921) 99
Central Health Services Council 104
Chadwick, Edwin xi, 1, 12, 40, 148–50
Chamberlain, Austin 42
Chamberlain, Neville 31, 64, 73
Charles, John 199–201, *200*
  honours *18*

legacy 49
length in office *xii*
lifespan *xii*
reputation 32, 49–50
retirement 55
post-retirement 49, 175
selection 32
on smoking risk 44–9
Chernobyl radiation incident 90
Chief Medical Officers
  key qualities 165–6
  key roles 40–1, 176
  Annual Reports 147, 149–53, 163
  'as gatekeeper' xii, 96, 129, 145
  as communicator 104–7, 147–63, 166
  direct management responsibilities 86–7
  engaging external experts 117–45
  freedom of speech 148–9
  future options 174–5, 176
  lifespan and length in office xii
  overview of roles 40–1, 104–5, 176
  pay 19, 37, 42–3, 68–74
  policy 'making' 167, 176
  post-1870s career progression 18
  relationships with Permanent Secretaries
    39, 43–4, 55–7
  representation on NHS Executive 81–3,
    86, 175–6
  risk management 140, 144–5, 163
  selection and succession issues 17–38
  status and recognition 6, 17–18, *18*, 33,
    37, 42–3, 71–2
  statutory powers 136
  Whitehall reviews (post 1980–) 80–3
  see also Deputy CMO posts
Chief Scientist appointment 77, 120
child and infant clinics, introduction 23
chiropody services 75
cholera epidemics 1–2, *2–3*
  threat of 69, 70
Circular Letter 24
The Civil Service: continuity and change
  (1994) 60, 65
civil service
  post-Fulton reforms 59–61, 65
  reviews of senior personnel (1980–)
    80–3, 135
  see also administrative staff
Clarke, Kenneth 79–80, 113, 147
  AIDS crisis 128, 133
  BSE crisis 140, 162
Cochrane, Archie 120, 170
'cogwheel' reports 174

Cohen, Dick 120
Cohen, Henry 32
Collier, James 35
communication issues
  key role of CHO 104–7, 147–63, 166
  Annual Reports 147, 149–53, 163
  circulars and letters 155–6
  email and websites 156
  government–doctor initiatives 104
  radio 156–60, 167
  and risk 168–9
  television 160
  see also 'networking' by CMOs
consultant advisers 121
consultants
  contracts 109
  pay beds dispute 107–11, 110
  position on NHS formation 102–3
Cook, Dr Clarence 50
coterminosity 76
Cousins, Frank 61
Cowan, Kenneth 53, 173
Cox, Dr Alfred 94
Creutzfeldt–Jakob disease see BSE crisis
crisis management 173–5
  see also AIDS crisis; BSE crisis
Crossman, Richard 58–9, 76, 88–9
  on external expertise 117
  relationship with Godber 58–9, 106–7
  reputation 59
Cruickshank, Alistair 136
Cumberledge, Baroness 142
Currie, Edwina 162, 168

Daily Mail 154
Daily Telegraph, on Imperial Tobacco 53
Daley, Allen 99
Dalrymple-Champneys, Sir Weldon 29–30, 32
Davies, Joan 136
Dawson, B 30, 94–5
Dawson, Dr John 130
Dawson's report (1920) 94–5
Day, Patricia 83
'Dear Doctor' letters 155–6
Delane, JT 150
dental representation, Godber's influence 59
Department of Health 79–80
  budgets 80
  creation 79–80
  recruitment issues 82, 90
  reviews (1981–93) 78–9

reviews of 1994 (Banks) 83–6
restructuring (1995) 84–6
scope of responsibilities 80
separation of NHS Management
  Executive 82–3, 86
Department of Health and Social Security
  75–8
  location issues 87–9
  reviews (1981–93) 78–9
  role 77
Deputy CMO posts 28
  and additional CMO posts 33
  representation on NHS Executive Board
    81–3, 86
  reviews and cutbacks 78, 80–3
Dilke, Sir Charles 21, 68–9
diphtheria immunisation 21, 27
disease surveillance, early history 15
disputes
  government–medical profession 112
  see also pay beds dispute; pay and
    conditions
Disraeli, Benjamin 13, 152
Doll, Richard 45–7, 50, 131
Dorrell, Stephen 142–4
Douglas, Sir William 61, 65, 101
Drummond, Sir Jack 122
Duncan, Sir William xi

Eden, Sir Anthony 50
Efficiency Unit report (1988) 60
The Elite of the Elite (Barberis) 39–40
Elliot, Walter 121
email 156
Emergency Beds Service 123
Emergency Medical Services, MacNalty's
  contribution 29
Emergency Public Health Laboratory
  Service 119–20
English Sanitary Institutions (Simon) xvii
Ennals, David 111, 112, 170–1
  on Crossman 59
Epidemiological Society of London 5
Epstein, (Michael) Anthony 137–8
European Law, and postgraduate medical
  education 113
Evans, Dr John 35, 84, 144
Expert Advisory Group on AIDS 127–8,
  132–3
experts see external expertise; technical
  experts in government
external expertise 117–45
  advisory committees 118–20, 127–8

external expertise *cont.*
consultant advisers 121
Evans review 144
Royal Commissions 118
Standing Committees 120–1
working groups 117
Eyler, John 26

family planning services
influence of Charles 118
influence of Godber 118
Farr, William 148
Fifty Years in Public Health (Newsholme) xvii
Fisher, Sir Warren 28
Fleming, Henry 12
Fletcher, Charles 52, 160
Fletcher, Walter 119
food hygiene
Jameson's contribution 31
Simon's contribution 150
food scares 90, 162
see also BSE crisis
Foot, Michael 61
Ford, Dr Gillian 34–5
Forrest, Sir Patrick *130*
Fowler, Norman *112*, 113, 171
on AIDS crisis 124–5, 129, *130*, 161
Fox, D xi
*A Framework for Government Research and
Development* (1972) 120
France, Arnold 73
France, Sir Christopher 36, 79, 138
Fraser, Sir Bruce 56, 58, 61
freedom of speech 148–9
Fulton Committee report (1966) xv, 60
Functions and Manpower Review (1993)
79
funding issues 68–72

Galbraith, Spence 136
Gamgee, John 150
Gardner, Sylvia 136
'Gas Bag' Committee 99
gatekeeping role xii
General Board of Health
Benjamin Hall's presidency 2–3
Edwin Chadwick's involvement 1–2
medical representation (Simon) 3–4
political threats of 1850s 4
see also Local Government Board
General Medical Council 91–2
Simons opposition 151
Thorne Thorne's legacy 22

General Medical Services Committee 105
general practice 105
contracts 58
Godber's influence 107, 121–2
standards 121
Girdlestone, Gaythorne 96
Gladstone, William 10, 12, 151
Godber, George *173*, 201–4, *202*
early experience 57, 100
honours *18*, 38
length in office *xii*
on Charles 49–50
on general practice 107
on MacNalty 29
on medical specialities 105
on NHS capital investment 57–8, 170
on NHS restructuring 76
on past Ministers 64
on pay 106
on smoking and lung cancer 52–5
on Turton 57–8
published reports 154–5
relationship with Bevan 63
relationship with Crossman 58–9, 106–7
relationship with doctors 155–6
relationship with King's Fund 122–3
relationship with media 159–60
relationship with MRC 120
relationship with Royal Colleges 95
reputation 32–3, 56
retirement 34
post retirement 175
salary 73
selection 32–3
working practices 33, 37, 56
Godfrey, Malcolm 35, 81–2, 135
Goldfinger, Ernö 89
Goodman, Arnold 109–11
Goodman, Neville 48, 55
government of healthcare *see* state
medicine
Gowans, Sir James *130*, 140–1
Graham, Edwin 46
Green, Dr FHK 47
Greenfield and Hale Report (1991) 79
Greenhow, Dr Edward Headlam 7, 8–9,
10, 148
Griffith, JAG 74–5
Griffiths Report 171
Griffiths, Roy 35, 86, 114
The Guardian 154
guidance for doctors 155–6
Guillebaud Report (1955) 74

Gummer, John 140, 168
Gwynn, Heather 78, 83

Haddow, Douglas 53
Hailsham, Lord 54
Haldane Report (1918) 103–4
Haldane, Lord 25
Hall, Sir Benjamin 2–3
Hall, Sir Douglas 73
A Handbook of Vaccination (Seaton) 19
Harris, Dr Ed 35, 90, 136, 138
Hart, Sir Graham 36, 84, 115
Hawton, John 44, 48–9, 50–1, 55–6
Hayhoe, Barney 128
Healey, Denis 40
health circulars 155–6
health inequalities, CHO's role 170–1
Health Inquiry Office 161
The Health of the Nation white paper 171
health promotion
    anti-smoking campaigns 54
    see also preventative medicine
health services *see* National Health Service;
    state medicine
Health Trends, on role of Department of
    Health and Social Security 77
health visiting 94
Helps, Arthur 8, 39
Henderson, Arthur 63
Hennessy, Peter 44, 80
Herbecq Review (1990) 78
Higgins, Peter 107
Hill, Charles 101, 160
Himsworth, Sir Harold 48, 99
Hine, Deirdre 142, 170
The History of State Medicine (MacNalty) xvii
Hogg, Douglas 142, 144
Honigsbaum, Frank xi, 26, 29
Hospital Building Programme (1962) 57–8,
    170
hospital dramas and documentaries 160
hospital surveys (1941–44) 100
housing issues 75
Hygiene Laboratory (Sandhurst) 30

Imperial Tobacco Company 47, 49–50
*Improving Management in Government: the
    next steps* (Efficiency Unit 1988) 60
infant welfare programmes 94
    Newman vs. Newsholme 24–5
information withholding 167–8
    see also risk management
international collaborations 22, 23, 172–3

international sanitary agreements 22, 23
Internet use 156

Jameson, Wilson *157*, 196–9, *197*
    education 30–1
    honours *18*
    interests 31
    legacy and achievements 31, 103, 166,
        167
    length in office *xii*
    lifespan *xii*
    networking 99–100
    NHS development role 98–103
    on mass immunisation 120
    relationship with King's Fund 122
    relationship with Newman 28–9
    reputation 32
    retirement 103, 122
    post-retirement 175
    selection 28–31
    use of media 31, 156–9, *157*, 167
Jarrett, Clifford 59, 107
Jenkin, Patrick 62, *112*, 171
JESP (Job Evaluation for Senior Posts)
    84
Joint Consultants Committee 104–5, 114
Jones, Robert 96
Joseph, Keith 64, 76, *112*
Joules, Horace 47

Kearns, Gerry 26
Kendell, Robert 145
Keppel Club 99
Kerr, James 24
King's Fund 29, 121–3
King's Fund Institute 123
Kitson Clark, G 73–4
Klein, Rudolph xi, 78, 83, 113

Lambert, John 12–14, 19, 151–2
    retirement 21
Laming, Sir Herbert 115
Lancet, on John Simon 6, 13, 151
Langlands, Sir Alan 115
Lawrence, Lord 99
leaded petrol 34
Lectureship in Public Health 7
Lewin, Walpole 109
Liberal Government
    background to health policy reforms
        (1866–70) 10–11
    welfare legislation (1905–14) xvii, 23–4
The Listener 158–9

Lloyd George 23, 25–7, 71–2, 91
  national health insurance 72
Local Government Act (1929) 99
Local Government Board
  formation 11–14
  funding shortfalls 20, 21, 68–72
  staffing 21, 68–72
  suspension 42
Local Government Board Act (1871)
  11–12
local government health services
  early history xiv–xv, 11–14
  public health officer appointments 14
  relationship with central policy making
    15, 74–5
  see also Local Government Board
London Epidemiological Association 7
London School of Hygiene and Tropical
  Medicine 28–9, 31
Low, Bruce 23
Lowe, Robert 5, 10, 150–1
lung cancer see smoking and lung cancer

McColl, Prof Ian 123
MacDonald, Malcolm 30, 98
MacDonald, Ramsay 29
McGonigle, GCM 170
MacGregor, John 135
MacLachlan, Gordon 121
MacLeod, Ian 47, 57
MacNalty, Arthur 193–6, *194*
  honours *18*
  legacy 28
  length in office *xii*
  lifespan *xii*
  on health service development 98
  published works xvii
  reputation 29, 98
  retirement 29
  selection 28–9
Major, John 143
Marlborough, Duke of 9–10
Martin, William 137–8
Maude, Sir John 101
Mawhinney, Brian 133
Maxwell, Robert 63
media 147–8, 156–60, 167–8, 174
  AIDS crisis 125, 129–30
  BSE crisis 161–3
  salmonella scares 162, 168
  use by Jameson 31, 156–9, *157*, 167
  use by Simon 149–52
Medical Act (1983) 92

medical experts see external expertise;
  technical experts in government
medical inspectors, background history
  8–9, 11–12
Medical Officers of Health xv, 4–6
  qualification reforms (Simon) 4
  see also Chief Medical Officers
Medical Register 91–2
Medical Research Council 77
  relationship with Ministry of Health
    118–20
  on smoking 45–8, *48*, 50–1
Medical Staff Association, on pay parity
  72–3
medical training see training of doctors
Medicine and the State (Newsholme) 165
Medicines Control Agency 83
Meldrum, Keith 141–2
Mellanby, Sir Edward 30, 99, 119
Metters, Jeremy 83, 133
Milroy lecture (1887) 69
Ministers for Health *211–12*
  relationship with CMOs 56–9, 63–6
  'success' characteristics (Maxwell) 63–4
Ministry of Agriculture, Fisheries and
  Food (MAFF), BSE crisis 134–45, 162
Ministry of Health
  location issues 87–9, *87–8*
  origins 25, 93
  relationship with local government 74–5
  relationship with Medical Research
    Council 118–20
  see also Department of Health;
    Department of Health and Social
    Security; Local Government Board
Ministry of Health Bill 25
Ministry of Health Establishment File 42
Ministry of Housing and Local
  Government 75
Moore, John 79, 136
Moores, Yvonne 115
Morant, Robert 26–7, 42–3, 72–3
Morning Post 151
Morrison, Herbert 62
Moseley Report (1986) 78, 80–3, 135
Moseley, Sir George 80

Nairne, Sir Patrick 61, 62–3, 110
National Archives at Kew xviii
national health insurance 72
National Health Service 86–7, 169–71
  development 96–103
  management 74–5

relationship with BMA 96–103
reorganisation plans (1964–73) 76
reviews (1981–93) 78–9
reorganisation (1990s) 84–6
role of Jameson 74, 98–103, 166, 167
National Health Service Act (1946) xvii,
    120
National Health Service Management
    Board, CMO representation 81–3,
    175–6
National Health Service (Management)
    Executive 86
    formation 82, 86
National Health Service (Reorganisation)
    Act (1973) 76
National Insurance Act (1911) 96, *98*
National Vaccine Establishment 19
Netten Radcliffe, John 10, 20
'networking' by CMOs xvi, 114, 166, 176
    Charles 52
    Godber 52, 95
    Jameson 99–100
    Newman 25, 41–2, 96
New Labour, role of special advisers
    114–15
Newman, George 41–3, 191–3, *192*
    diaries 25, 41
    honours *18*, 26–7
    legacy 27–8
    length in office *xii*
    lifespan *xii*
    media 'control' 156
    networking skills 25, 41–2, 95
    on malnutrition 170
    on 'Preventive Medicine' 41–3, 75,
        93–5, 147–8
    on status and pay of CMOs 42–3, 72–3
    published works xvii
    relationship with Addison and Morant
        42–3
    relationship with Newsholme 24–6
    selection 24–7
Newsholme, Arthur 188–90, *189*
    honours *18*, 26–7
    legacy 72
    length in office *xii*
    lifespan *xii*
    memoirs 23
    on technical expertise 67
    post-retirement 172
    published works xvii, 23, 165
    relationship with BMA 94
    relationship with Newman 24–6

reputation 26
retirement 26
selection 22–3
workload issues 23
Next Steps agencies 60–1, 83
Nightingale, Florence 12, 148–9, 150
Northcote–Trevelyan Report (1854) 60
Nuffield Provincial Hospitals Trust 29, 100,
    121–2
nursing representation, Godber's influence
    59
Nutrition Committee 118–19

O'Brien, Dr Michael 36
On the State of the Public Health reports
    154–5
    see also Annual Reports
*On the Study of Epidemic Disease, as
    Illustrated by the Pestilences of London*
    (Greenhow) 7
orthopaedic services 96
Owen, David 64, 108–10
    on Yellowlees 110
Owen, Hugh 21

Packer, Richard 142–4
Pall Mall Gazette 151
Panel Doctors Scheme 23
Parliamentry Report on Physical
    Deterioration (1904) 41
Parran, Thomas 158
Parsons, Franklin 23
Partridge, (Ernest) John 50
Partridge, Michael 79
Pater, John 32, 100
Pattison, Prof John 142
pay beds dispute 107–11, *110*
pay and conditions 19, 37, 68–74
    Buchanan's efforts 69–70
    Newman's influence 42–3, 72–4
    pension rights 69–70, 122
    reviews 82–3
Permanent Secretaries 39, *213*
    relationship with CMOs 39, 43–4, 55–7
    relationship with Ministers 39, 44, 61–2,
        62–3
    responsibilities 44, 62–3
    selection 61–2
    tenures 44, 65
pharmaceutical industry, restricted list
    proposals 113
pharmacy representation, Godber's
    influence 59

Phillips Inquiry Report 135–6, 140, 144–5
Phillips, Sir Nicholas 135–6
Pickering, George 99
Pickles, Hilary 132, 138–9
Platt, Robert 52, 114
Policy Strategy Unit 78
Political and Economic Planning (PEP)
    think-tank 99
Poor Law Board 8, 11–12
Poor Law reforms 40, 94, 99
Port Sanitary Authorities 12
Porter, Dr Charles 31
postgraduate medical education 113, 121
Powell, Enoch 64
    and Godber 53–4, 58
Power, William Henry 186–8, *187*
    early career 22
    honours *18*
    length in office *xii*
    lifespan *xii*
    on appointment of non-professional
        staff 71
    retirement 22
    selection 22
Practitioner 152
Press Officers 157
Preston-Thomas, Herbert 151
preventative medicine, Newman's vision
    41–3, 75, 93–5
Preventive Committee (MRC 1939) 120
Privy Council 5–6, 7, 8–9, 12–13
'professionalisation of government' *see*
    technical experts in government
Public Health Act (1848) 1
Public Health Act (1858) 5
Public Health Act (1859) 5–7
Public Health Act (1872) 12
Public Health Act (1875) 13–14
Public Health Function inquiry (1987) 171
Public Health Group Board (1995) 85
Public Health journal 24
Public Health Link System 156
public health officers 14

radio, use by Jameson 31, 156–9, *157*, 167
Rayner, Bryan 113
Raynerism xvi, 60–1, 62
Rayner, Sir Derek xvi, 60
recruitment issues, Department of Health
    82, 90
Regional Health Authorities 76, 86
Reid, John 33–4

*Reports of the Medical Officer of Health for the
    City of London* (Simon) 4
research programmes (LGB/MoH/DHSS/
    DH)
    background history 10, 15, 150
    funding 69, 77, 120
    relationship with MRC 120
Resource Allocation Working Party 64
Richardson, John 114
risk management, BSE crisis 140, 144–5,
    163, 168–9
Rivett, G xi
Robinson, Arthur 43
Robinson, Kenneth 58, 64, 76
Rock Carling, Ernest 99
Roffey, Norman *173*
Rogers, Sir Phillip 34, 108–9
Royal College of Physicians (RCP) 95–6
    smoking and lung cancer 52–4
Royal College of Surgeons 95–6
Royal Commissions, influence of CHOs
    118
Royal Sanitary Commission (1868) 8, 9,
    10
Royal Sanitary Commission (1869) 11
Russell Smith, Dame Enid 51

St Thomas's Hospital, Lectureship in Public
    Health 7
salaries *see* pay and conditions
salmonella warnings 162, 168
Sanderson, John Burdon 8–9
Sanitary Act (1866) 9, 10
Sanitary Engineers, qualification reforms 4
Sanitary Papers (Simon) 5, 148–9
scarlet fever surveys 68
school medical inspections, introduction
    23
Sclater Booth, George 13–14, 70, 152
Scotland, lung cancer and smoking 53
Scott-Douglas, Sir William 44
Scott, Dr JA 53
SEAC (Spongiform Encephalopathy
    Advisory Committee) 139–44
Seaton, Edward Cator 19–20, 179–81, *180*
    association with John Simon 14, 19
    honours *18*
    length in office *xii*
    lifespan *xii*
    published works 19
    remuneration 19
    resignation 19–20
    post-resignation 172

selection 19
work on smallpox vaccine 7, 9, 19
workload issues 19–20, 68
Secretaries of State for Health *211–12*
senior civil servants, reviews 80–3, 135
Serota, Bea 118
sexually transmitted disease programmes
23
radio education broadcasts 157–9
Shore, Dr Elizabeth 34–5
Shore, Peter 35
Simon, John 1–15, 177–9, *178*
background and education 1
early career 1–3
honours *18*
key appointments 3–7
lecturing positions 1, 3, 6
legacy 13–14, 15, 166
length in office *xii*
lifespan *xii*
links with medical profession 1, 3, 6–7,
150–1
main aims 4–5
Privy Council involvement 5–6, 7, 8–9,
12–13
published works and reports xvii, 4, 7,
148–52
relationship with Chadwick and
Nightingale 1, 12, 40, 148–50
relationship with GMC 151
remuneration 19
resignation 14, 68
threats and challenges 9–11, 13–14, 68,
148–9
use of media 149–52
working methods 4, 15, 150–1
workload 9–11, 13–14, 68
smallpox eradication 34
smallpox vaccination programmes 148–9
Buchanan 21, 68
Seaton 5, 7, 9, 19
Simon 148–9
Yellowlees 34
smoking cessation clinics 54
smoking and lung cancer 32, 44–56
early research 45–6
influence of Godber 52–5
influence of Hawton 44, 48–9, 50–1
mortality rates 50–1
RCP report 52–4
Snow, Sir John xi
Social Insurance and Allied Services
(Beveridge 1942) 100

Social Science Association 5
Southwood (BSE) working party 137–9
Southwood, Richard 137
special advisers (New Labour) 114–15
Standing Committees 104, 120–1
Cancer and Radiotherapy 46–50
Stansfield, James 12–13, 151–2
state medicine, historical overview xiv–xv,
92–5
Stevenson, Derek 108
Stocks, Percy 47
Stowe, Sir Kenneth 35, 62, 79, 80, 136
AIDS crisis 129
Straw, Jack 110
Sunley, Bernard 107

Taylor, Tom 4
technical experts in government 67–8
background history xvi, 6, 15
status and pay 68–74
television 160
Terrence Higgins Trust 127–8
Thatcher, Margaret 60, 62, 124
Thompson, Landsborough 99
Thorne Thorne, Richard 184–6, *185*
association with John Simon 14
honours *18*
legacy 22
length in office *xii*
lifespan *xii*
on status of CHOs 70
published reports 152–3
selection 21
unexpected death 22
workload 21–2, 70–1
Thudichum, JLW 15, 150
The Times
on Simon 14, 149–52
on Thorne Thorne 22
Timmins, N 108
tobacco advertising ban 54
tobacco industry 32, 47, 49–50, 55
Tomlin Commissioners 73
Topley, WWC 99
training of doctors
contribution of Thorne Thorne 22
postgraduate medical education 113, 121
Treasury
on CHO status and funding 20, 21,
68–73
on funding annual reports 152–3
role of Permanent Secretaries 63
tobacco industry influence 32, 49, 55

Treasury Review (1982) 80, 82
Trefoil Report (1990) 78, 83
tuberculosis programmes 23, 26
Turton, Robin 50–1, 57
typhus fever 1
Tyrrell Committee 139
Tyrrell, David 139

underfunding *see* funding issues
UNESCO 172

Vaccination Act (1853) 19
Vaccination Committee 119
vaccination programmes *see* smallpox
    vaccination programmes
Vaughan-Morgan, JK 51–2
venereal disease, public education 157–9
von Liebig, Justus 6
von Pettenkofer, Max 6
Vosper, Dennis 51–2, 57

Waldegrave, William 141–2
Walford, Dr Diana 37, 83, 86
Walker-Smith, Sir Derek 52
Walton, Sir John 137–8
Wardale Review (1982) 78, 80
Warner, Norman 110
Washington Post 167–8
Watson, Bill 136
Webb, Beatrice 23
Webb, Sidney 93
websites for CHOs 156
Webster, C xi, 74
Whitehall
    accountability structures 62–3
    health department reviews 78–9
Whitelaw, William 124, 161
Whitley Council 73
'Wider Department' 82

see also Department of Health
Wilson, Harold 76, 109
Winyard, Graham 86, 115
Wolfson, Sir Isaac 107
Wood, Sir Kingsley *64*
working groups
    difficulties setting up 117–18
    Southwood Working Party (BSE) 137–9
    see also external expertise; technical
        experts in government
workload issues 68–72
    Acheson 127, 135–7
    Buchanan 20–1, 68–70, 153
    Newsholme 23
    Power 71
    Seaton 19–20, 68
    Simon 9–11, 13–14, 68
    Thorne Thorne 21–2, 70–1
World Health Assembly 172–3, *173*
World Health Organization 172
    John Charles 49, 175
    John Reid 34
Wynder, Ernst 46

Yellowlees, Henry 204, *205*
    honours *18*
    legacy 34
    length in office *xii*
    on health inequalities 171
    on interdepartmental links 77
    on medical manpower planning 77
    on pay beds dispute 108–11, *112*
    published reports 155
    relationship with doctors 155–6
    reputation 34, 110–11
    selection 33–4
Yeo, Tim 133
Yes, Minister 39, 60
Your Life in Their Hands 160